The
WHOLE
BODY
CURE

The
WHOLE
BODY
CURE

The Simple Plan to Prevent and Reverse Disease, Eliminate Pain, and Lose Weight for Good

DR. COREY W. KIRSHNER

with the editors of Prevention® and Catherine Knepper

RODALE.

Printed in the United States of America

Rodale Inc. makes every effort to use acid-free ∞, recycled paper ♺.

Exercise photos by Mitch Mandel/Rodale Images

Participant photos on pages 25, 75, 76, 95, 357, and 359 by Ryan Olszewski

Author photo on page xi and other participant photos by Matt Rainey/Rodale Images

Book design by Carol Angstadt

Library of Congress Cataloging-in-Publication Data is on file with the publisher.

ISBN 978-1-62336-849-4

4 6 8 10 9 7 5 3   hardcover

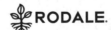

We inspire health, healing, happiness, and love in the world.
Starting with you.

Acknowledgments

Kirshner Health Solutions would not be possible without the involvement of my wife Lisa who has been integral in developing and refining the methods used in our office. Thanks also to the staff at KHS, who greet our patients with a smile every day.

Thanks to Anne Egan for conceptualizing my program as a book to bring health and healing to a much larger audience and to Catherine Knepper for her brilliant writing. Kudos to the entire team at Rodale who created this terrific book, especially designer Carol Angstadt, assistant editors Sabrina Mastronardo and Kristina Gonzalez, project editor Marilyn Hauptly, and photographers Mitch Mandel, Matt Rainey, and Ryan Olszewski. I appreciate Hilary Smith's expertise with qigong.

Finally, I would like to thank my hundreds of patients who had the faith in this program and are now living healthier, happier lives. And a special thanks to the test panelists who followed the plan—your great success confirms and inspires my work.

Contents

Introduction

Anti-Inflammatory Living, For Life

Of the 10 leading causes of death in the United States, 8 of them—heart disease, cancer, chronic lower respiratory diseases, stroke, Alzheimer's disease, diabetes, pneumonia/influenza, and kidney disease—are directly linked to the same root cause, inflammation.[1] In fact, we now know that the long-term, low-grade inflammation can persist in all of our cells and tissues, also playing a key role in everything from acne to arthritis, from celiac disease to psoriasis, from chronic pain to depression, from insomnia to lupus, from multiple sclerosis to osteoporosis—and the list hardly stops there. These incredibly diverse health conditions all share a common denominator—chronic inflammation.

Health Conditions Linked to Chronic Inflammation

- Accelerated aging
- Acne
- Age-related macular degeneration
- Allergies
- Alzheimer's disease
- Anxiety
- Asthma
- Attention-deficit/hyperactivity disorder
- Bipolar disorder
- Bronchitis
- Cancer
- Carpal tunnel syndrome
- Celiac disease
- Chronic fatigue
- Chronic obstructive pulmonary disease
- Chronic pain
- Chronic stress
- Conjunctivitis
- Crohn's disease
- Depression
- Diabetes
- Eczema
- Fibromyalgia
- Gallbladder disease
- Gastritis
- Hair loss
- Heart disease
- Hepatitis
- Insomnia
- Irritable bowel syndrome
- Lupus
- Metabolic syndrome
- Multiple sclerosis
- Muscle loss
- Osteoporosis
- Overweight/obesity
- Periodontal disease
- Pneumonia
- Psoriasis
- Rheumatoid arthritis
- Schizophrenia
- Scleroderma
- Sinusitis
- Tendonitis
- Ulcerative colitis

The number and scope of illnesses with an inflammatory component is certainly alarming—especially considering that inflammation can simmer away for years without producing overt symptoms, silently causing damage without our knowing it. But there's a bright side to consider, and it's a powerful one: *Knowing the common culprit in so many of our health problems illuminates the way to a common cure.*

Can we stem the rising tide of heart disease, cancer, Alzheimer's, type 2 diabetes, and other major killers by quenching the fires of inflammation? Or better yet, prevent that spark before it erupts into the flame of full-blown illness?

The short answer is yes. The longer answer involves living a lifestyle that helps keep inflammation—and thus, a host of debilitating symptoms and deadly health conditions—at bay for the long term. And that's just what *The Whole Body Cure* is all about.

We're going to tell you everything you need to know about inflammation—from exactly what it is and how it contributes to such a diversity of health conditions to what you can do to prevent or reverse inflammatory illnesses. Within these pages you'll learn:

- The different types of inflammation and how they affect your health
- How to detect elevated inflammation before disease creates further problems
- The causes of inflammation and how you can avoid and reverse them
- The role that inflammation plays in perpetuating pain, fatigue, weight gain, memory problems, mood disorders, and allergies
- The surprising connections between inflammation and stress
- How inflammatory illnesses increase the risk of certain types of cancer—and what you can do to reduce your risk
- Which foods and beverages cause inflammation—and which prevent and reverse it
- Which forms of exercise can reduce and reverse inflammation—and which worsen it

We'll also give you the very latest exciting clinical research on inflammation and health, and we'll give you delicious, easy-to-prepare recipes based on foods that can eradicate smoldering inflammation and keep it from reigniting.

But most important of all, we're going to give you a simple yet powerful plan for turning down the heat on inflammation and regaining whole-body health. For more than 30 years, Corey W. Kirshner, DC, has been helping patients make total health transformations and stay healthy for the long term. A licensed, board certified chiropractic neurologist and wellness consultant with advanced training in nutrition, Dr. Kirshner responded to the steep rise in chronic, degenerative diseases by formulating a comprehensive plan that guides people in reducing inflammation safely and quickly. The plan also helps identify hidden food sensitivities that may be causing symptoms and stoking the fires of inflammation. Hundreds of Dr. Kirshner's patients are living healthy, vibrant lives by following the same plan you'll find here, and throughout the book you'll hear firsthand accounts from our special group of test panelists who followed the Whole Body Cure wellness plan and experienced remarkable health turnarounds. We're talking greater energy; weight loss of up to 25 pounds; a complete cessation of joint pain, heartburn, and acid reflux; improved gastrointestinal health; the elimination of allergy symptoms; lower blood pressure, total cholesterol, and triglycerides; and a marked reduction in biomarkers of inflammation—all in just 12 weeks.

How are such extraordinary

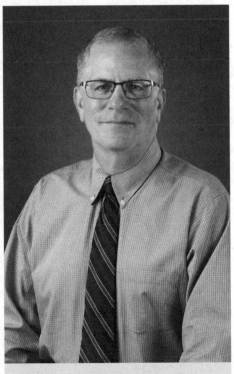

DR. COREY W. KIRSHNER

results possible? Because of that powerful bright side of inflammation: Knowing the common culprit behind so many health conditions illuminates a common cure. It means we can help you address the root cause of illness rather than temporarily relieve symptoms. You can turn down the heat on inflammation at any point, whether you're healthy and want to stay that way or already suffering from a chronic illness and want to improve. And ultimately, this is what *The Whole Body Cure* is all about. It's about enjoying life to your fullest capacity for many years to come.

PART I

Inflammation, Inside and Out

CHAPTER 1

Smoldering Cells

Some Inflammation Basics

In the past several years—certainly since *Time* magazine featured "the secret killer" as its February 23, 2004, cover story—inflammation has become an important topic; it seems we're greeted every week with breaking news about another piece of the inflammation puzzle. If there once was a clandestine killer on the loose, the secret is long since out!

While popular coverage on inflammation runs the gamut from the silly to the sound, the buzz is well deserved, and we can assure you that inflammation isn't just the next fad in health and wellness. In fact, based on the emerging science, it may become the next frontier in medicine. Understanding how inflammation affects your body; how chronic, low-grade inflammation *will* eventually make you sick; and most importantly, what you can do to reduce or avoid chronic inflammation are among the most important health lessons you can learn.

So let's begin our journey into anti-inflammatory living by learning exactly what inflammation means. If you're just glancing at the headlines, it would be very easy to assume that inflammation is all bad, all the time. But the truth is, without inflammation none of us would be around to celebrate our first birthdays.

Good versus Bad Inflammation? Not So Fast!

One of the most common ways to talk about inflammation is to pit "good" inflammation against "bad" inflammation. That distinction can be useful to a certain extent, but the real picture is more complex—and far more helpful—than that.

What the medical community is referring to when they talk about "good" inflammation is *acute inflammation*. And considering you could hardly live a day without good (acute) inflammation, it's very good indeed.

Above all, your body wants to maintain a state of *homeostasis*. This is a fancy way of saying that your body wants to remain in a state of balance and stability. In other words, it wants to maintain conditions for optimal health and wellness. If things are going well, no problem! But if something affects homeostasis—say you come down with a cold or you cut your finger—then your body reacts swiftly to restore it. Your body's first line of defense is none other than acute inflammation, which is short term, and it's your body's built-in way of handling anything it perceives as a threat—whether that's an infection, an injury, or an irritation.

Infection results from pathogens—any disease-causing microbe, such as bacteria, viruses, parasites, or fungi—that enter the bloodstream and multiply. Injury is self-explanatory, but it's worth remembering, for reasons we'll explain below, that acute inflammation will occur whether that injury is as minor as a scraped knee or as catastrophic as a head injury. Whatever the degree of injury, the immune system launches into action to prevent infection and to start mending wounded tissue. As for irritation, here's where things can start to get complicated because what the body perceives as an irritation can range from a food sensitivity or allergy (such as to peanuts or the ever-present gluten protein found in most grains), to a seasonal allergen (such as pollen), to an environmental toxin (such as radon), to a foreign substance (such as a drug or a splinter). And sometimes the body can mistakenly perceive its own tissues as a threat and launch an attack, which is what happens with autoimmune disorders, such as celiac disease, lupus, or rheumatoid arthritis. (We'll be covering autoimmune disorders at length in Chapter 7.)

No matter the cause, *all* of these instances of inflammation reveal how the body tries to eliminate a threat and restore homeostasis, and it does so in predictable ways. To understand how this process works, let's set up a fall (just bear with us) and look at what happens to the body, inside and out, when it encounters a threat that calls for an acute inflammatory response.

Let's say you're out for an evening stroll and you're so enthralled by the sunset you don't notice the broken sidewalk four paces ahead. You fall down, scraping your knee and twisting your ankle in the process. Thankfully the injuries are minor, but even before you get back on your feet (perhaps indulging in a bit of inflammatory rhetoric as you brush yourself off), your immune system is kicking into high gear. The *immune response* is how your body deals with anything it perceives as a threat. And when a threat is detected, the first course of action is for your body to launch an extraordinary cascade of events known collectively as the *inflammatory response*. The inflammatory response is another way of describing acute inflammation.

The external hallmarks of acute inflammation are unmistakable: pain, swelling, heat, and redness. These terms were known to ancient physicians as *dolor, tumor, calor,* and *rubor,* respectively, and they happen to be the four classical signs of *inflammo* ("I ignite") as described as far back as the first century CE. While none of these signs of acute inflammation is pleasant to experience, they indicate your body is doing exactly what it's supposed to do. Even before you brush yourself off, your body is hard at work healing itself and trying to restore homeostasis. Let's look at each of these signals a little closer.

Dolor, or pain, is immediate. This is your body's way of signaling to you, loud and clear, that something is amiss and needs attention. As we all know, pain can take many forms and range in severity, from scrapes and bruises to pinched nerves to migraines to the agony associated with serious injury and illness. And while we're at it, let's not forget that mental or emotional pain is no less potent—in later chapters we'll explain how stress, depression, and anxiety all cause inflammation, too. No matter its source, type, or severity, pain is the body's unmistakable call for attention: *Help me!*

Tumor, Latin for swelling or the condition of being swollen, is the source of the word we use to describe a cancerous "swelling," or tumor. In the case of acute inflammation, swelling is the body's built-in way of immobilizing the injured area. That twisted ankle obviously shouldn't be used again until it's healed, and both pain and swelling make sure you keep injured body parts out of commission. Swelling happens in part because fluid rushes to the injured area, transporting white blood cells, the foot soldiers of the immune system, to fight any incoming pathogens that could gain access through that scraped knee. Fluid also transports histamine, a compound that triggers small blood vessels to become more permeable; hormones called prostaglandins that trigger blood clots to stop any bleeding; and any extra nutrients required to begin repairing damaged tissue.

Calor and *rubor*, heat and redness respectively, both occur when those small blood vessels become permeable, essentially opening the gates for the rest of the players in your immune system to move more easily between cells and go where their work is required. Sometimes, increased heat is body-wide in the form of a fever. This is Mother Nature's way of making your insides inhospitable to pathogens.

Acute inflammation is your body's brilliant, all-natural way of fending off invaders, repairing damage, and healing itself. We absolutely want this kind of immune response to occur as often as necessary. We quite literally couldn't live without it.

But we also want these inflammatory and protective events to switch off when the threat subsides. Most of the time that's just what happens as soon as homeostasis is restored. Sometimes, however, the alarm bells keep ringing long after they're necessary because of a breakdown in communication. The body simply doesn't receive the usual cue to turn off its acute inflammatory response. In these days of increased pollution, too much stress, not enough sleep, reliance on prepackaged foods, and hidden food sensitivities, the common triggers that threaten homeostasis are part of a daily lifestyle for many of us. Whatever the reason, when inflammation persists past its point of usefulness, trouble inevitably follows.

Too Much of a Good Thing

There are basically two ways that the kind of inflammation you want—acute inflammation, your body's short-term inflammatory response—can slip over to the dark side and become the type of inflammation that can make you sick rather than well.

We'll just briefly mention the first because Chapter 7 will focus on the complex world of autoimmune disorders and allergies. Those conditions arise when the body launches the inflammatory response in the face of something that normally isn't a threat, such as shellfish, eggs, or the body's own tissues, allergies and autoimmune disorders result.

The type of harmful inflammation we want to focus on here is the one you've heard so much about and the reason you're reading this book. This is *chronic*, or *long-term, inflammation*—inflammation that sticks around past the acute stage. Think for a moment back to those four classic symptoms of acute inflammation: pain, swelling, heat, and redness. We saw why they were good for the short term, but no one wants to *remain* in this state, right? It's a bit like having your cells and tissues stuck indefinitely on a low simmer, which leads us to consider why chronic inflammation is also sometimes referred to as *persistent, low-grade inflammation*. Further, acute inflammation is well and good for a scraped knee or twisted ankle, but now picture your *whole body* overheated, irritated, and inflamed. When chronic inflammation affects the entire body, it's referred to as *systemic inflammation*. Often, people will use these four terms—chronic inflammation, persistent inflammation, low-grade inflammation, and systemic inflammation— interchangeably. They all boil down to body-wide inflammation that sticks around for the long term, causing damage that may not yet be apparent.

By any name, chronic inflammation is what happens when, for a variety of reasons we'll explore throughout this book, the acute inflammatory response doesn't shut down. What should have been temporary inflammation smolders on, keeping the body in a state of red alert and keeping the inflammatory response revved high. If you stop and think about this scenario at its most basic level, the problem is immediately evident: Too much of *anything* causes problems, even if it's too much of a good thing. A short course of antibiotics is just what the doctor ordered to zap a bacterial infection, but overuse can lead to antibiotic-resistant bacteria along with a slew of other problems. A sweet treat for a special occasion is pure delight, but a slice of cake every day will inevitably lead to weight gain. There are a million examples of how too much of a good thing becomes a bad thing, and such is the case with inflammation.

There are two aspects of chronic inflammation that make it especially insidious. First off, inflammation often assumes a long, quiet phase, thus earning nicknames like "the silent killer," "the hidden epidemic," or "the underlying cause of illness." For months or even years, chronic inflammation produces no perceived symptoms. While acute inflammation is immediate and hard to ignore, chronic inflammation can simmer away in our cells, blood vessels, nerves, tissues, and organs for quite some time before symptoms become apparent. And by then, a disease process is already well under way.

The other reason chronic inflammation leads to so many problems? It essentially exists in lockstep with illness, a vicious, unending cycle that's hard to break. Essentially, chronic inflammation is both a cause *and* an effect of many diseases. As chronic inflammation begets disease, that same disease begets further inflammation, which begets worsening disease, which begets further inflammation, and so on and so forth, with no good outcome unless something breaks the cycle. To look at just one brief example, consider one of the most common health challenges facing people today: being overweight. It may surprise you to learn that carrying too much weight causes chronic inflammation, but that's because fat cells release a variety of compounds that cause inflammation, affect your ability to use insulin effectively, and throw other hormones off balance. These changes can promote more weight gain, effectively producing more body fat to create even more chronic inflammation—and you see where all this is headed. In the end, we have chronic inflammation, excess weight, and insulin problems reinforcing one another and making us fatter *and* sicker, eventually resulting in type 2 diabetes. Not to mention that type 2 diabetes *itself* promotes inflammation—and off we go again.[1]

Think of chronic inflammation as the accelerant that can make a fire burn out of control. Your body can handle a struck match and even put it to good use, such as when your body temperature rises in the case of infection. This is acute inflammation. However, it cannot handle the ongoing blaze of chronic inflammation, which destroys cells and tissues, renders the body unable to function properly, and ultimately can cause disease.

How Do I Know If I Have Chronic Inflammation?

It's a sobering fact that more than half of Americans likely live in a state of chronic inflammation without even knowing it.

How can we make such a bold assumption? Because of the staggering rates of overweight/obesity, type 2 diabetes, heart disease, cancer, chronic lung disease, Alzheimer's, arthritis, allergies, chronic gastrointestinal disorders, and many more illnesses whose primary driver is inflammation. Further, we know that the standard American diet—or SAD, an appropriate acronym if there ever were one—is by its very nature proinflammatory. The typical American (or Western) diet—consisting of fast food, processed food, industrially produced meats, sugar and high-fructose corn syrup, and a disproportionate ratio of unhealthy to beneficial fats—is a fast track to chronic inflammation and thus to illness. So, if you're a person who eats "SADly" on a regular basis, and/or if you're already suffering from a chronic condition, it's very likely that chronic inflammation is present.

Fortunately, it's possible to reduce chronic inflammation on your own, no doctor's visit or prescription needed, with simple lifestyle practices that we'll teach you in this book. And through research about chronic inflammation and various illnesses, we'll show you how to identify some very early signs and symptoms of rising systemic inflammation. Many are easy to miss, either because they're subtle or because you may not have known to associate them with chronic inflammation. You can find these signs and symptoms listed in the next section. Treat them as *possible* indicators. Exactly how and when chronic inflammation manifests will vary from person to person and depends on a host of additional factors, such as genetics, environmental factors, body mass index (BMI), and lifestyle habits such as exercise, nutrition, and smoking. These signs and symptoms do not *guarantee* that you'll come down with a serious illness. But they *do* indicate that your body is trying to get your attention.

Remember, your body is always talking to you. Heed these cues and you can intervene well before serious illness sets in.

Possible Early Warning Signs
of Chronic Inflammation

Chronic inflammation will inevitably make itself known through illness. But if you know what symptoms to look for, it's entirely possible to detect systemic inflammation in its earliest stages, before health problems emerge. Here are some possible signs of hidden inflammation at work. Treat these as red alerts, your body's way of asking for help, and you may be able to prevent many major illnesses and maintain optimal wellness.

- **DIGESTIVE COMPLAINTS, ESPECIALLY IF THEY'RE NEW.** Though diarrhea, constipation, nausea, excessive gas, and abdominal pain can be caused by a variety of factors, gastrointestinal symptoms are also classic signs of chronic inflammation. Irritable bowel syndrome, inflammatory bowel disease, leaky gut syndrome, gluten sensitivity or intolerance, or individual GI symptoms (especially if they seem to have developed "out of nowhere") are all indications that inflammation is at work.

- **INTERMITTENT JOINT PAIN.** Joint pain is a classic symptom of arthritis, in which case an inflammatory process is already well under way. But if you're just starting to experience joint pain not due to injury, especially when you first get up in the morning, it's a sign that inflammation is increasing.

- **A NEW FOOD SENSITIVITY.** Food sensitivities will usually make themselves known through GI symptoms (see above). Determining which food is causing the symptoms may take some detective work, though, and that's just what the whole-body eating plan (in Chapter 11) is designed to do. A new food sensitivity is a reliable sign that inflammation is occurring on a cellular level.

- **A "SPARE TIRE."** If you have central adiposity—otherwise known as belly fat or a spare tire—you can safely assume inflammation is present. Abdominal fat cells are known to be a potent source of the proinflammatory chemicals your body produces.

(continued on page 12)

DIAGNOSTIC TESTS FOR ELEVATED INFLAMMATION

There are several diagnostic tools your doctor can use to assess the level of inflammation in your body, as well as determine your risk for certain inflammation-related illnesses. They're all performed by a simple blood test, which will look for *biomarkers* of inflammation. A biomarker (short for biological marker) simply refers to something that can be measured to help determine a medical state. Pulse rate, blood pressure, cholesterol values, and body temperature are all biomarkers. In the case of inflammation, biomarkers come in many forms, but the primary ones used to diagnose inflammation are special molecules that circulate in your blood called *cytokines*.

Cytokines are proteins that function as cell-signaling molecules. When the cells of your immune system need to communicate with each other, they use cytokines to deliver the message. Because cytokines are produced any time the inflammatory response is under way, doctors can test for their presence as an indicator of inflammation. The level of cytokines can also tell us something about the *severity* of the inflammation. The higher the level of proinflammatory cytokines in the blood, the higher the level of systemic inflammation. As it happens, there are different types of cytokines, and some are better than others at revealing particular types of inflammation and predicting certain diseases; we'll show you what each test is used for below.

C-reactive protein (CRP) and high-sensitivity C-reactive protein (hs-CRP): The CRP test is by far the most commonly used tool to detect levels of inflammation in the body, and this is the test we used to measure before-and-after inflammation levels in our test panel. This test measures the amount of a substance called C-reactive protein, which the liver produces in response to inflammation. When CRP levels are high, we know that inflammation is occurring in the body. Another, more recent test, the hs-CRP test, is able to detect even smaller amounts of inflammation than the basic CRP test. Both are among the standard means doctors use to monitor heart disease risk. Optimally, CRP levels should be below 3 mg/l.

Fibrinogen (also known as factor I): Fibrinogen is a protein the liver produces to help form blood clots. Like CRP, fibrinogen is elevated in the presence of systemic inflammation, and high levels of fibrinogen are strongly associated with heart disease. Normal fibrinogen levels are between 1.5 and 3 g/l. Too much fibrinogen can make the blood "sticky," resulting in a higher risk of blood clots, heart attack, and stroke. Fibrinogen is also a particularly good indicator of heart disease and chronic obstructive pulmonary disease (COPD), which can involve chronic inflammation of bronchioles, lung tissue, and pulmonary blood vessels.

Erythrocyte sedimentation rate (also known as sed rate or ESR): The sed rate test indirectly measures the level of inflammation in the body by measuring the rate at which red blood cells (erythrocytes) settle (or sediment) in a test tube in 1 hour. Because inflammation causes red blood cells to clump together (mostly due to fibrinogen), these dense clumps of cells settle more quickly. The higher the sed rate, the higher the amount of systemic inflammation in the body. Because the sed rate alone can't be used to diagnose a specific illness, it's often conducted alongside other tests, like the CRP test. The normal sedimentation rates are listed below; rates above these indicate inflammation.

- Women up to the age of 50: 0–20 millimeters per hour (mm/hr)
- Women 50 and above: 0–30 mm/hr
- Men up to the age of 50: 0–15 mm/hr
- Men 50 and above: 0–20 mm/hr

Homocysteine: Homocysteine is an amino acid produced when we eat protein. As with the other biomarkers, elevated homocysteine indicates systemic inflammation. Normal levels are anywhere between 4.4 and 10.8 micromoles per liter (µmol/l) of blood. Homocysteine levels are typically higher in men than in women, and they increase with age, smoking, the use of certain drugs, and a vitamin B_{12} or folate deficiency.

A high level of homocysteine is strongly associated with coronary heart disease, especially blood clots, strokes, and heart attacks. In fact, elevated homocysteine is now considered an independent risk factor for heart disease.[2] High homocysteine is also considered an independent risk factor for a variety of inflammatory diseases, including kidney failure and cancer,[3] and high levels are also strongly associated with neurological illnesses in which inflammation plays a role, such as Alzheimer's and schizophrenia.

- **WORSENING OF SEASONAL ALLERGIES OR ASTHMA.** When hay fever or asthma worsens with no apparent trigger (such as pollen or smog), inflammation is a likely culprit.

- **BRAIN FOG.** If you notice that you're feeling "spaced out," becoming more forgetful, or experiencing a general lack of mental clarity or difficulty in concentrating, these could be early indicators of rising inflammation. Fluctuating hormones, insomnia, stress, and poor nutrition can also cause brain fog, and each of these factors is individually associated with inflammation.

- **UNEXPLAINED FATIGUE.** Many things can cause fatigue beyond the usual suspects of overexertion, insomnia, or illness. If you're run-down for no apparent reason, however, it can be an early sign of systemic inflammation.

- **MOOD DISTURBANCES.** Research shows that people who are depressed have more inflammation than those who aren't, and those who are in a state of medically induced inflammation, such as for skin cancer treatments or some vaccinations, report higher levels of depression and fatigue. We also know that stress causes the release of proinflammatory compounds into the bloodstream, and if stress and the resulting inflammation become chronic, anxiety results.

- **SLEEPING DIFFICULTIES.** Sleep deprivation and sleeping for short periods, as well as sleeping for more than 9 hours a night, can promote inflammation. And there is a vicious cycle at work: Chronic inflammation contributes to sleeping difficulties.

- **A RASH, ACNE BREAKOUT, AND/OR RED, BLOTCHY SKIN.** Not every blemish or rash is an indication of disease. But especially if breakouts or other skin complaints are unusual for you, or a rash or hives arrive suddenly, it's a signal that the inflammatory response is under way. Remember, too, that skin complaints can be the result of an allergic response and are seen in some autoimmune disorders; in either case, inflammation is at work.

- **PERSISTENT BLOODSHOT AND/OR PUFFY EYES.** Eyes that are often red, irritated, and bloodshot (not due to infection) may be an outward sign of increasing inflammation. Puffy eyes can indicate fluid accumulation. And of course, all of these symptoms are associated with chronic insomnia, so you can safely assume that inflammation is elevated.

If you do notice some early warning signs, consider making immediate lifestyle changes to decrease inflammation, even before you call your doctor. Altering what you eat; getting some low-impact exercise, or at least adding more movement to your daily routine; and taking care to avoid or remedy chronic stress will make a difference. You'll be surprised by how quickly you may notice results, too. Part III of this book will guide you in our full anti-inflammatory wellness plan.

Single-Source Health and Wellness

While the body's acute inflammatory response is designed to work quickly to restore homeostasis, and thus return us to health, inflammation that becomes chronic will eventually make us sick. However, knowing the simple fact that chronic inflammation lies at the root of so many illnesses also provides us with a single-source means of preserving health by keeping inflammation levels low. If you are already living with a chronic illness, taking steps to "turn down the heat" and reduce chronic inflammation will bring symptom relief and perhaps even a full recovery.

But to avoid or reduce chronic inflammation, we need to know exactly what causes it in the first place. So it's to the many causes of chronic inflammation—most of them so ingrained in our culture that we'd hardly think twice about them—that we now turn our attention.

CHAPTER 2

Sparks That Start the Flame

Causes of Chronic Inflammation

We know that the body launches an immune response in the face of anything it perceives as a threat. Most often, threats arrive in the form of an infection, injury, or irritant. When the body encounters harmful bacteria, for instance, the "inflammation army" goes on the attack. White blood cells rush to engulf and kill off the invaders, and the body's temperature rises to create an environment in which the bacteria can't survive. We'll encounter countless pathogens over the course of a lifetime, and in most cases our bodies will successfully fight them off through the process of acute inflammation.

But what if the threat isn't a straightforward case of an invading bacteria? And what if the threat is something we encounter again and again on a daily basis? In our day and age, our bodies are called on to do battle against a legion of foes, and many of them aren't nearly as clear-cut as a bacterial infection. To understand the many causes of chronic inflammation and how beneficial acute inflammation can progress to the damaging form of chronic inflammation, we need to expand our idea of what the body considers a threat.

It turns out many things can undermine optimal conditions for health and wellness, including quite a few of our routine activities. If we're engaging in these activities daily—if they're *chronic*, in other words—the resulting inflammation will be chronic. The immune system will remain revved up, on high alert, until the threat is removed and balance is restored.

Below you'll find a list of the top primary causes of chronic inflammation. These root causes can lead to secondary causes of inflammation. For example, poor sleep habits are strongly associated with depression and anxiety, which in turn trigger the inflammatory response all on their own. Along the same lines, overconsuming unhealthy saturated and trans fats and sugar leads to excess weight, which in turn generates its own inflammation. There is a vicious cycle at work, wherein chronic inflammation is both the cause and effect of so many illnesses.

If we can stop inflammation at its root by avoiding these primary causes, we may be able to avoid many deadly diseases and enjoy many more years of health and wellness.

The Top Primary Causes of Chronic Inflammation

Ultimately, a variety of factors will determine your body's individual inflammatory response, including genetics, lifestyle factors, and your health history. However, from case to case, the same external factors are often at play. Take a moment to compare your lifestyle habits and health history to the top 14 causes listed below. How many factors might affect you?

1. Processed foods, including processed meats, prepackaged foods, and fast foods
2. Unhealthy fats—saturated fats and trans fats
3. Sugar
4. Overconsumption of alcohol
5. Underconsumption of fresh fruits and vegetables
6. Grains
7. Food sensitivities
8. Intestinal permeability (leaky gut syndrome)
9. Exposure to environmental toxins and pollutants
10. Smoking
11. Extremes in exercise, either too much or too little, but especially a sedentary lifestyle

12. Poor sleep habits, either too much or too little

13. Chronic stress

14. Advancing age

There are a couple of things worth pointing out about this list. First, most of these causes of chronic inflammation are very much under our control. We choose what we eat and drink. We choose to smoke or not. We choose our level of exercise—or how often we sit around. We can practice excellent sleep hygiene, and we can work to reduce the sources of chronic stress in our lives and to learn coping strategies that help us deal with stress when it occurs. We can learn which foods trigger inflammation and eliminate those—and replace them with delicious anti-inflammatory foods that turn down the heat. And while many of us live in polluted areas or are routinely exposed to toxins in the everyday products we use, we can protect ourselves and minimize the damage. The bottom line here is that many of the causes of chronic inflammation are lifestyle-related, and that means the power to maintain optimal health and prevent many diseases lies in our hands.

Second, most of the primary causes of chronic inflammation are about nutrition—what we're eating and drinking, and in some cases what we're *not* eating and drinking. Food plays a powerful role in causing chronic inflammation—and in putting an end to it. In Chapter 11, you'll find specific guidance on our anti-inflammatory approach to eating, which includes a wide range of delicious foods that extinguish the fires of inflammation. For now, let's take a brief look at each of the primary causes of chronic inflammation, and we'll start with the biggest area where you may be unwittingly inviting inflammation into your life, your diet.

You Truly Are What You Eat: Dietary Sources of Chronic Inflammation

Processed foods is a term that refers to any foods that have been altered from their natural state. Foods are processed to preserve their shelf life, to alter their taste, and/or to make their preparation and consumption more "convenient." Are some foods more processed—and therefore more harmful—than others? Most definitely. At the "low harm" end of the spectrum are minimally processed foods, such as frozen vegetables, seeds or nuts that have been pressed to make oil, or dairy products that have been pasteurized to neutralize harmful pathogens.

On the other end of the spectrum are processed foods that have been chemically altered in some way—by smoking or curing or by adding preservatives, food coloring, or other artificial ingredients. Also on the harmful end of the spectrum are foods that have been "enhanced" with additives such as salt, sugar, and/or unhealthy saturated or trans fats.

Processed meat—which is any meat that has undergone salting, curing, or smoking or that has been treated with some other form of preservative or flavor enhancer—is particularly harmful. Common examples include bacon, salami, sausage, hot dogs, corned beef, ham, and some deli or lunchmeats. Essentially, these meats constitute a five-alarm fire when it comes to inflammation. And then there's the smoking or curing process, which exposes the meat to an array of inflammatory or even cancer-causing chemicals and leaves it with staggeringly high amounts of sodium. A single ounce of pan-fried bacon, for example, contains 647 milligrams of sodium, or 27 percent of the Recommended Dietary Allowance.[1] Compare that to the 62 milligrams of sodium found in *4 ounces* of cooked grass-fed beef.[2]

Further, there's now substantial evidence that processed meats raise the risk of cancer, an illness that's driven by inflammation from start to finish. In 2015, the World Health Organization's International Agency for Research on Cancer added processed meats to its list of Group 1 (carcinogenic to humans) agents. This means that processed meats join the list of familiar human carcinogens, such as tobacco products, formaldehyde, and mustard gas. Research has shown that eating even small amounts of processed meat every day, such as one small hot dog, increases the chance of colorectal cancer by 18 percent compared to eating none. Scientists have also observed a link between processed meat and an increased risk of stomach cancer.[3] Want to hazard a guess as to how these types of cancer often begin? With inflammation of the colon and stomach lining. We'll explore the link between an inflammatory diet and cancer in detail in Chapter 10. But the bottom line for now is that for anti-inflammatory eating, it's best to avoid processed meat entirely. If you're a fan of red meat, the American Institute for Cancer Research recommends that you eat no more than 18 ounces per week.[4] The Whole Body Cure Plan encourages you to enjoy grass-fed, organic meat, as these animals aren't raised with food that's been treated with pesticides, fertilizers, and other chemicals, and they tend not to have been treated with antibiotics and other drugs that can be passed on to consumers. Meat from grass-fed animals also tends to have lower saturated fat and cholesterol contents than conventionally raised meat.

As for prepackaged foods, many contain ingredients that trigger an inflammatory response. Among them are artificial sweeteners, chemical preservatives, artificial dyes, refined carbohydrates, emulsifying agents (thickeners), omega-6 fatty acids, trans fats, and saturated fats. Take a look at some of the evidence.

- In the past 50 years, the use of artificial food dyes has increased by 500 percent. When the body encounters these synthetic chemicals and recognizes them as foreign agents, it launches an inflammatory response, which can lead to new allergies, autoimmune conditions, a disruption of the microbiota that colonize the gut, and even neurobehavioral disorders such as ADHD (attention-deficit/hyperactivity disorder) and increased aggression.[5]

- One of the staple ingredients in prepackaged foods, refined carbohydrates (including white rice, instant mashed potatoes, and the white flour that's nearly ubiquitous in processed crackers, breads, cake and muffin mixes, packaged desserts, and even some granola bars and energy bars), refers to ingredients that are stripped of nutrients and fiber through a chemical process. Refined carbs are particularly problematic because they are high in sugar and contain high amounts of advanced glycation end products, known by the wonderfully apropos acronym AGEs. AGEs are compounds that are created by a chemical reaction between sugars and proteins. They provoke an inflammatory response, and elevated levels have been linked with cardiovascular disease, diabetes, kidney disease, and excessive skin wrinkling.[6]

- A recent preclinical study showed that common food emulsifiers (thickeners) such as polysorbate 80—which can be found in ice cream, margarine, and mayonnaise—alter the gut microbiota, induce low-grade systemic inflammation, and can contribute to diseases such as colitis and metabolic syndrome—not to mention that the study animals became obese when these chemicals were added to their water.[7]

- Omega-6 fatty acids trigger an inflammatory response; they're found in corn oil, safflower oil, soybean oil, sunflower oil, and vegetable oil, which are mainstay ingredients in many processed foods. The disproportionately high ratio of proinflammatory omega-6s to anti-inflammatory omega-3s that's so typical of the Western diet plays a role in many chronic inflammatory conditions, including heart disease, rheumatoid arthritis, autoimmune diseases, certain types of cancer, and asthma.[8] (Anti-inflammatory omega-3s can be found in cold-water fish, walnuts, and flaxseeds.)

- Artificial sweeteners such as saccharine and sucralose have been linked with the rise in Crohn's disease and ulcerative colitis, the two main forms of inflammatory bowel disease.[9]

- In animal studies, sodium benzoate, a common preservative in soft drinks, fruit juices, jams, salad dressings, pickles, and sauces, was found to impair motor function and increase anxiety.[10] A laboratory study found that sodium benzoate and potassium benzoate caused DNA damage and were toxic to human lymphocytes, a type of white blood cell involved in the immune response.[11]

Saturated and trans fats provide a hotbed for inflammation. Saturated fats are typically solid at room temperature, and they come mostly from animal sources. (A couple of exceptions are palm oil and coconut oil, which are high in saturated fat but don't contain cholesterol.) Examples include butter, lard, cheese, and cream. Red meat (beef, lamb, pork) and poultry with skin are also high in saturated fat. Eating saturated fats triggers the release of several proinflammatory cytokines and raises the risk of metabolic diseases, such as type 2 diabetes. Saturated fats also stimulate fat cells to become inflamed, which promotes insulin resistance.[12]

However, for all the problems saturated fats can cause, trans fats are even worse. They're made by adding hydrogen to liquid vegetable oils to render them more solid, such as with margarine or shortening. Most often, trans fats are identified on packaging as "partially hydrogenated vegetable oils." As health concerns about trans fats have mounted, manufacturers have relied on them less, but they are typically used in processed foods such as packaged desserts, chips, crackers, fried food, creamers, and popcorn to extend shelf life and enhance flavor. Trans fats wreak havoc with your vascular system by boosting harmful LDL cholesterol and decreasing beneficial HDL cholesterol, as well as increasing CRP (C-reactive protein) levels and other biomarkers of inflammation that lead to atherosclerosis. Not surprisingly, trans fat consumption is associated with an increased risk of heart disease as well as type 2 diabetes.[13] A study conducted by the Harvard T.H. Chan School of Public Health's Department of Nutrition concluded that the elimination of trans fats from the American diet could prevent up to one in five heart attacks and related deaths. This translates to a quarter-million lives saved per year.[14]

Sugar and foods high in added sugar can raise blood sugar levels, which is also referred to as blood glucose levels. Even small increases in blood glucose levels trigger a spike in inflammation—and the effect is more pronounced in people who have any form of impaired glucose tolerance, including diabetes and metabolic syndrome.[15] Nutrition experts commonly use the glycemic index to compare the sugar content in various foods. Foods that are high on the glycemic index—such as sugar-sweetened drinks, white rice, and anything made with white flour—prompt a quick release of glucose into the blood. These foods have been associated with greater waist circumference, more belly fat, greater risk of metabolic syndrome, high BMI, and higher inflammation. On the other hand, low-glycemic (low-sugar) diets have been shown to improve insulin resistance, promote weight loss and smaller waist circumference, and reduce CRP levels.[16]

Frequent overconsumption of alcohol affects the entire body and promotes system-wide inflammation as well as inflammation in specific areas. It's known to inflame the oral cavity, esophagus, larynx, throat, and liver, which raises the risk of cancer in each of these areas. Excessive drinking can disrupt the healthy composition of bacteria in the gut; cause changes in brain structure and function; raise blood pressure; and increase the risk of stroke, heart disease, type 2 diabetes, pancreatitis, metabolic syndrome, and chronic liver disease, all inflammation-related conditions.[17] Anything above the current definition of "moderate alcohol consumption," which is no more than two drinks per day for men and one drink per day for women, is considered excessive. A drink is defined as one 5-ounce glass of wine, one 12-ounce glass of beer, or one 1.5-ounce serving of 80-proof spirits.

Underconsumption of fresh fruits and vegetables gets less attention than the frequent recommendations we hear to eat an abundance of fresh fruits and veggies, but it's equally important to remember that *not* eating enough fresh produce contributes to inflammation. How? First, there is evidence that a diet lacking in fruits and vegetables triggers the immune system. With poor nutrition, the body is in a state of ill health, so it responds in the way it always does when homeostasis is threatened: It ramps up the inflammatory response.[18]

Second, without these foods in your daily diet, you're missing out on the anti-inflammatory and healing benefits of phytochemicals, which are found only in plant sources. Scientists have identified more than a thousand phytochemicals, and the list continues to grow. Some of the well-known classes of phytochemicals you may already be aware of include antioxidants, flavonoids, carotenoids, and isoflavones. Many individual phytochemicals boast a wide range of health-promoting and disease-protecting effects, from the anticancer effect of sulforaphane, found in cruciferous veggies (broccoli, cabbage, kale, cauliflower, Brussels sprouts, etc.), to the antibacterial effect of allicin, found in garlic. And certainly, many phytochemicals have an anti-inflammatory effect. The antioxidant flavonoid quercetin, for example, is a powerful anti-inflammatory found in onions, capers, dark cherries, blueberries, blackberries, apples, peppers, and citrus fruits. Ginger and turmeric are also powerful all-natural inflammation fighters—ginger because of polyphenolic compounds called gingerols and turmeric because of the polyphenol curcumin.

Some people wonder if they can get all their fruits and veggies in a pill form. There are supplements and vitamins made from fruits and veggies, but they're best used as an add-on rather than a replacement for whole foods. While these pills may offer some micronutrients, you also miss out on the fiber, the full complement of nutrients, and certainly the feeling of satiety that eating whole foods brings. Further, eating whole foods is far better for your digestion. The digestive process begins as you chew your food. Swallowing a pill does not allow the enzymes in your mouth to begin digestion, nor does it trigger the process of peristalsis, or gut motility, which is how the body moves food through the digestive system. Optimal gut motility means that food is moving neither too quickly nor too slowly and that nutrients are being adequately absorbed along the way.

Grains are a staple of most people's diets, and many healthy eating plans advocate eating whole grains because of their high fiber content and their association with a reduced risk of diseases like type 2 diabetes and heart disease. Whole grains unquestionably contain health-promoting vitamins and minerals, but accumulating evidence suggests that wheat and other grains can also contribute to chronic inflammation and autoimmune diseases by increasing intestinal permeability (we'll talk more about that later in this chapter) and keeping the inflammatory response stuck in the "on" position. Scientists have identified certain "antinutrients" in cereal grains, such as the proteins gluten, lectin, and gliadin, which are responsible for intestinal irritation and keeping the immune system in overdrive. This situation applies to everyone, too—not just those with a wheat allergy or gluten intolerance.[19]

Food sensitivities can be a hidden source of inflammation for many people according to a body of quickly accumulating research. A food sensitivity, also known as a food intolerance, is different from a true food allergy, though it can cause some of the same symptoms (such as a runny nose or hives). Usually, however, symptoms of a food sensitivity are gastrointestinal in nature, and they take longer to show up than an allergic reaction to a food, which can happen within minutes Further, a food allergy can provoke a life-threatening whole-body response in some people called anaphylaxis, and this does not happen with a food intolerance. For more on this topic, please see Chapter 7.

When it comes to inflammation, however, both food sensitivities and allergies provoke the inflammatory response, and experts are finding that food sensitivities are more prevalent and harmful than we once thought. Food sensitivities can result from increased intestinal permeability or leaky gut syndrome (see the next section), and left unaddressed, they may lead to a worsening of leaky gut syndrome and a worsening of inflammation generally. Many people find, however, that once they identify their food sensitivities and eliminate that problematic food or food category from their diets, their symptoms quickly resolve. Our Whole Body Cure Eating Plan is designed to simultaneously provide two important benefits: You'll learn how to identify your unique food sensitivities and turn down the heat on inflammation.

Increased Intestinal Permeability: The Cause and Consequence of Chronic Inflammation

Increased intestinal permeability, which is often used interchangeably with the term **_leaky gut syndrome,_** or just _leaky gut_, works hand in hand with inflammation on several levels. It's been associated with many chronic inflammatory conditions, including autoimmune diseases such as type 1 diabetes, rheumatoid arthritis, celiac disease, and multiple sclerosis; allergies; chronic fatigue syndrome; inflammatory bowel disease; irritable bowel syndrome; overweight and obesity; type 2 diabetes; fatty liver disease; and even depression.[20, 21]

Leaky gut syndrome appears often in health-related news, but what exactly is it, and how does a gut that's become more permeable lead to so many different health problems? First of all, in a healthy intestine, you want _just enough_ permeability—enough for fluids and nutrients to be able to pass

(continued on page 27)

Tammy Pfeiffer

AGE: 55

- Constant joint and neck pain, muscle soreness, and a sense of puffiness relieved
- Regular blurred vision gone
- Fatigue and mental fatigue relieved
- Daily cough rarely occurs
- Persistent bloating after meals eliminated
- Balance problems relieved
- WEIGHT LOST: 20 pounds
- INCHES LOST: 13¼

I had reached a point where I didn't feel good and knew I had to do something. My blood pressure had been borderline high for 5 years, I'd gained 20 pounds, I had arthritis in my hands, and I just felt tired. I also had a problem with allergies and postnasal drip. I was constantly coughing and clearing my throat—to the point that it had become embarrassing. I tried a juice cleanse, and then I did some research and found out that dairy can cause those allergy symptoms, so I started eliminating dairy. This was hard to do on my own—I was a person who'd drive through a snowstorm for ice cream!—and it was right about that time that I heard about the Whole Body Cure study. It was perfect timing

because I was devoted to doing something for my health, but I needed help.

For those first 2 weeks, my husband and I ate really high-quality fruits and vegetables, and I got so much more creative with my cooking. I'm a gardener and had the advantage of a wide variety of plentiful vegetables. I loved the freedom this program offered of being able to pick your own foods and make your own meals—you don't have to pick certain foods or eat at certain times, and the choices of vegetables and fruits is nearly endless. It was during those first 2 weeks that I started to notice how much better I was feeling. But it was when I had a friend over for dinner about 2½ weeks in that I had my wow moment. I happened to look down at my hands

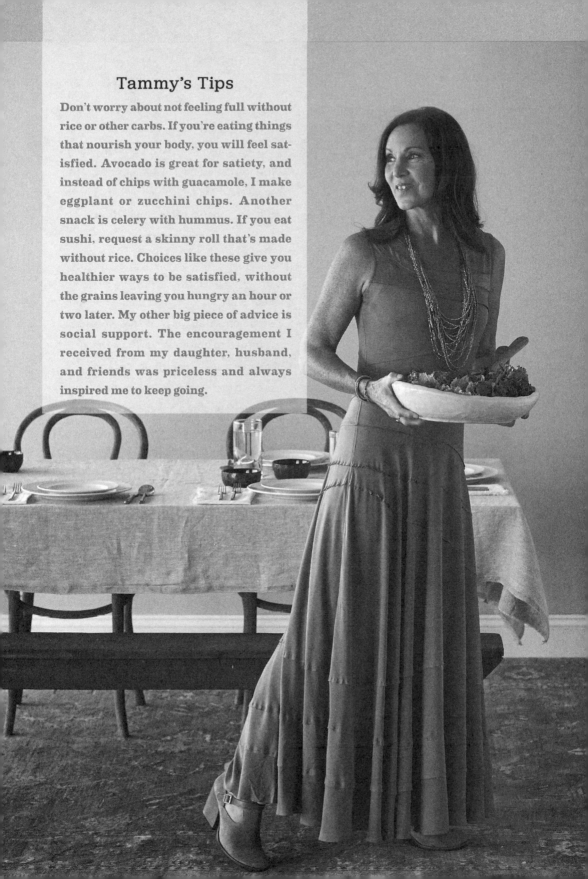

Tammy's Tips

Don't worry about not feeling full without rice or other carbs. If you're eating things that nourish your body, you will feel satisfied. Avocado is great for satiety, and instead of chips with guacamole, I make eggplant or zucchini chips. Another snack is celery with hummus. If you eat sushi, request a skinny roll that's made without rice. Choices like these give you healthier ways to be satisfied, without the grains leaving you hungry an hour or two later. My other big piece of advice is social support. The encouragement I received from my daughter, husband, and friends was priceless and always inspired me to keep going.

and realized they were no longer swollen. The arthritis had got to the point that my hands constantly ached, and sometimes I'd have to come home from work and put cold compresses on my hands. But in less than 3 weeks, my hands didn't hurt and they were visibly smaller.

Another aha moment came when we added eggs back into our diets. I had missed eggs and was so excited to reincorporate them. But that very first day I felt very tired. On Day 2, I was even more tired. By Day 3 I felt downright fatigued—just horrible. That was enough for me. I've now permanently omitted eggs from my diet, and I don't miss them at all.

I had a similar moment with sugar. When we could have dark chocolate, I ate a bit, 4 days in a row. The next day my arthritis pain was back, so bad that I had to use the cold compresses again. It was unbelievable. I had almost forgotten what pain was like because I hadn't had it for over a month. I suspected the culprit might be sugar, and

sure enough, when I looked at the ingredients on the chocolate, the kind I'd purchased had quite a bit of organic sugar. I'm sure the sugar brought my inflammation back. I don't ever want to have that feeling in my hands again, so it hasn't been hard to eliminate sugar because of how good I feel.

I ended up losing 20 pounds during the first 2 months of the plan, and I've kept it off. I'm no longer bloated, and my stomach is flat. My blood pressure has returned to normal, and I think the qigong practice contributed to that. I also do restorative yoga, which continues to be a huge part of my wellness plan. I have more energy, and I feel so much better about myself. I even dumped all my vitamins—I just don't need them anymore because I'm eating the right things instead of relying on breads and sweets. My allergies are gone, and to keep them gone, I have hot lemon water with a teaspoon of local honey every morning. I'm convinced that food can heal us. I look and feel like my old self again. ■

from the small intestine into the bloodstream, but not enough that harmful substances such as toxins, disease-causing microbes, or antigens can get through. (An *antigen* is anything that can provoke an immune response.) When any of these harmful substances finds its way into the rest of the body, it automatically provokes an inflammatory response.

Factors that can increase intestinal permeability probably won't surprise you, as they're many of the very same factors that spark chronic inflammation. For example, any of the dietary issues just mentioned can inflame your gut and make it more permeable ("leaky"), as can stress, infections, changes in the gut bacteria (see Chapter 4 for more on this), and, over time, any chronic inflammatory disease. Here's another occasion of the vicious cycle of chronic inflammation at work: Once the gut becomes inflamed and leaky, it contributes to more inflammation, which contributes to disease, which contributes to more inflammation. You'll see leaky gut come up several times throughout the book. In fact, the state of your gut is so influential in regaining and maintaining whole-body health that we've devoted an entire chapter to it.

Environment: The Inflammation Triggers All Around Us

Pollutants and toxins are an obvious inflammation trigger, but for many of us, avoiding exposure is no easy task. Toxins abound in the air we breathe, the food we eat, the water we drink, and in some cases, the ground we walk on. Smog, radon, lead, mercury, pesticides, and herbicides are just a few of the common pollutants we potentially encounter every day, but there are also plenty of hidden toxins lurking in the health and beauty products and household cleaners that we use daily. (Our wellness plan recommends organic, non-GMO fruits and vegetables whenever possible to avoid exposure to toxins.)

As we've already covered, when your body is exposed to pollutants or toxins, it responds by trying to protect itself from the offending agents. This is a classic case of the acute inflammatory response sparked by an irritant. When small particulate matter in polluted air is drawn into the lungs, for example, the inflammation army goes on the attack to neutralize the threat, and the airways become inflamed. When exposure occurs every day, the inflammation becomes chronic, and eventually, there will be a price to pay in terms of a chronic inflammatory condition. Asthma, allergies, bronchitis, chronic obstructive pulmonary disease (COPD), pulmonary hypertension (high blood pressure that affects the arteries in the lungs and heart), and eventually lung cancer are all potential consequences, and they're all inflammation-mediated conditions.

There's also the role that our environment plays in triggering chronic inflammatory conditions, such as with some autoimmune conditions. Chronic exposure to heavy metals such as mercury, cadmium, lead, nickel, and gold can spark autoimmunity in some people. These metals all occur naturally in our environment, but they're also commonly used in many industrialized products such as batteries, paints, pesticides, and plastics. Radiation is another common trigger of autoimmune conditions. Ultraviolet (UV) radiation from sunlight triggers the production of proinflammatory cytokines, and in skin cells it triggers an inflammatory response that causes DNA damage, cell death, and the release of autoantigens, which are any immune response triggers that arise from the body's own tissues.[22] Systemic lupus erythematosus, an autoimmune disorder that affects some 5 million people worldwide, is thought to be caused by a complex interplay of genetic and environmental factors. Among the environmental toxins and factors that can induce lupus or trigger a flare are tobacco smoke, UV light, silica dust (released when construction materials such as bricks, tile, concrete, and mortar are cut, ground, or drilled), mercury, liquid solvents, pesticides, and phthalates (found in many cosmetics).[23] There is even some evidence that in susceptible individuals, exposure to certain environmental toxins and chemicals—such as air pollution; tobacco smoke; bisphenol A (BPA), found on the interior lining of metal food cans; and polybrominated diphenyl ethers (PBDEs), flame-retarding chemicals used in building materials and furniture—may trigger and/or accelerate type 1 diabetes.[24]

Though we can't avoid toxins and pollutants entirely without living in a sterile bubble, there are things we can do to reduce our exposure and to minimize the damage. Eating organic foods will eliminate many toxins automatically as these foods are grown without them. So will using "green" household products that don't contain harsh chemicals. (Read labels carefully, however, as even products labeled "all-natural" can sometimes contain toxins. For a guide to household products that are good for the health of your body and the environment, check out the Environmental Working Group's (ewg.org) comprehensive guide.) A water filtration system will help purify water drawn from a chemical treatment facility (use one if there's any doubt about your well water, too). You can have your house and lawn tested for certain heavy metals and chemicals, such as lead, mercury, and radon, and take abatement measures if necessary. There are also many ways to detox the body through diet, periodic fasting, supplements, and in rare cases, chelation therapy, a medical procedure in which a synthetic binding agent is injected into the bloodstream in order to remove heavy metals. We'll cover the methods that involve detoxing, fasting, and supplements in the chapter on anti-inflammatory eating. Chelation therapy should be done under a doctor's supervision.

Smoking is a bad habit you'll hear us talk about all throughout the book. It's truly one of the deadliest habits around, and it is so harmful—for the primary smoker as well as anyone exposed to secondhand smoke—that it deserves a place in the spotlight as a top cause of chronic inflammation. Smoking inevitably inflames the mucous membranes of the oral cavity and the lungs, resulting in a markedly increased risk of bronchitis, asthma, allergies, chronic respiratory illnesses, lung cancer, and oral cancer. It also irritates the endothelium, the highly sensitive inner lining of the blood vessels, resulting in inflammation, hypertension, and arterial stiffness, which in turn creates the conditions for atherosclerosis, heart attack, and stroke.

A recent study on 1,819 people, comprised of smokers, former smokers, and nonsmokers, examined the effect of smoking on the immune system. Current smokers exhibited a reduced level of seven different immune markers, indicating a suppressed immune system, and a higher level of CRP, an indication of systemic inflammation specifically linked with lung cancer and heart disease. But there was good news from this study, too. The folks who kicked the habit eventually reached an immune and inflammatory profile similar to those who'd never smoked. The longer the time without smoking, the more normal the immune and inflammatory markers.[25]

The Goldilocks Effect: How Extremes in Exercise, Sleep, and Stress Lead to Chronic Inflammation

Extremes in exercise—overdoing it at the gym or working out infrequently—can both lead to chronic inflammation. You want to aim for that Goldilocks effect of "not too much, not too little" when it comes to exercise to avoid chronic inflammation. We'll discuss this further in Chapter 12, but in brief, it's important to know that both overexertion and a sedentary lifestyle spark inflammation and worsen any existing inflammation. On one extreme, over-exertion causes site-specific inflammation in joints and wherever injuries occur. Elite athletes face a greater chance of developing osteoarthritis than the general population,[26] and there is some evidence that during times of intense training or athletic performance, athletes are more susceptible to infection.[27]

But let's face it: The far greater risk for most of us lies on the other end of the spectrum—leading a sedentary lifestyle. And the inflammation risks associated with this extreme are far more harmful than those associated with overexertion. Both body and mind suffer from a lack of regular exercise, leaving us at higher risk for every chronic illness wreaking havoc on a global scale—cardiovascular disease, cancer, stroke, diabetes, overweight/obesity, Alzheimer's, depression, and anxiety chief among them. Notice that chronic inflammation is a key player in the development of *all* of these conditions, and we know that regular physical activity provides protection against every one of them. That pattern is hardly a coincidence. Studies show that while exercise produces a temporary inflammatory response, regular physical activity reduces CRP levels over time.[28]

Regular, weight-bearing exercise also helps preserve bone density and muscle mass, the loss of which causes two of the hallmark signs of aging, and it's been shown to improve brain function and reduce the risk of dementia. It's even been shown to increase the size of the hippocampus, the part of the brain associated with learning and memory.[29] The hippocampus can shrink in the face of aging, stress, depression, and inflammation—but regular exercise and healthy eating can prevent that from happening.[30]

What's the takeaway for us? Aim for the happy medium: Get regular physical activity with adequate rest periods in between. Most health experts recommend that adults get at least 150 minutes of moderate-intensity aerobic exercise per week, or roughly half an hour 5 days per week. Given the overwhelming health benefits of exercise and the overwhelming cost of inactivity, however, it's best to get in some form of physical activity daily. Even if you can't get to a dedicated workout on all or most days, make sure you're up and moving and not sitting for prolonged periods of time. Any form of movement—a brief walk, gardening, cleaning, taking the stairs when you can—is better than none.

Sleep can be harder to come by as we age, and research shows that sleep disturbance and chronic insomnia won't just leave you groggy the next day. Over time, poor sleep can accelerate aging, boost chronic inflammation, and increase the risk of heart disease, depression, hypertension, obesity, type 2 diabetes, cancer, stroke, and even death.[31]

As with exercise, you should avoid the extremes when it comes to sleep, as both too much and too little sleep contribute to chronic inflammation, and research has determined that "long sleepers" face some of the same dangers as "short sleepers." A study of more than 2,550 adults found that those who slept more than 10 hours a night—not those with insomnia—had the highest levels of proinflammatory cytokines CRP and interleukin-6 (IL-6).[32] Similarly, a study of nearly 25,000 people ages 15 to 85 found that those who slept 10 or more hours a night were more likely to suffer from depression and elevated BMI than those who slept a desirable 7 to 8 hours a night. However, this same study found that sleeping too little—fewer than 5 hours a night—was far more harmful than oversleeping. Short sleep duration was significantly associated with cancer; respiratory diseases; pain and rheumatologic diseases; digestive, hormonal, and metabolic diseases; and psychological diseases.[33]

As with exercise, health outcomes seem to be worse for those who are getting too little sleep rather than too much. Even short-term insomnia—such as sleeping 4 to 5 hours a night for a week or two—may activate the inflammatory response and induce insulin resistance.[34] Similarly, some studies have shown that even a modest reduction in sleep, from 8 hours a night to 6, may increase proinflammatory cytokine levels as well as stress hormones. There is also a documented association between insomnia, inflammation, and depression. People living with depression have higher levels of inflammatory biomarkers, and people with immune diseases report greater rates of depression.[35] Insomnia has also long been known as a risk factor for heart disease, and in addition to the inflammation it causes, research now suggests that insomnia also indirectly lowers beneficial HDL cholesterol.[36]

So in an ideal world, how much sleep should we get? The National Sleep Foundation recommends 7 to 9 hours of sleep per night for adults ages 26 to 64 and 7 to 8 hours for adults 65 and over.[37] Talk with your doctor if you seem to consistently get more or less than this amount.

Stress, believe it or not, also displays a correlation to that Goldilocks effect of "not too much, not too little." There are several interesting parallels between the acute inflammatory response and what we can call the acute stress response, or the way the body handles an isolated stressful event. Keep in mind that the acute inflammation response and the acute stress response are *good* for us—this is the "not too little" end of the spectrum. Acute inflammation and the acute stress response help us handle immediate threats, whether that's an invading pathogen or the proverbial tiger lurking in the bushes, a threat our ancestors once routinely faced that has left our brains hardwired to react quickly. When we encounter a stressful situation, the hypothalamus, an area of the brain that produces many of the body's hormones, activates the stress response. The sympathetic nervous system kicks into high gear and triggers the adrenal glands to release epinephrine (adrenaline) into the bloodstream. Epinephrine then triggers a cascade of effects. Heart rate increases, blood pressure rises, breathing rate quickens, and extra oxygen is delivered to the muscles and the brain. Sugar and fats are also released into the bloodstream. These changes happen in less than a second, and they prepare the body for quick action. This is the classic fight-or-flight response.

Now, let's say you catch a lucky break and the tiger melts back into the underbrush. With the threat eliminated, there's no longer any need to remain charged up, ready to fight or flee. This is when the parasympathetic nervous system kicks in, signaling the body to calm down. While the sympathetic nervous system cues fight-or-flight, the parasympathetic nervous system cues rest-and-digest. It's a beautiful system that serves us well, as long as the "on" and "off" switches function properly. We're built to handle these short bursts of stress followed by rest and recuperation. Without the acute stress response and the acute inflammatory response, humans would've died off long ago.

But what if the threat persists, or the switch gets stuck in the on position? Few of us will ever encounter a lurking tiger, but all too often, we face long-term stressors such as work-related anxiety, financial worries, concerns about a loved one, or relationship difficulties. For some, heightened anxiety can make a relatively minor stressor *feel* as dangerous as a tiger. In both cases, the stress response is the same. Remember that anything that threatens the body's ability to maintain optimal conditions for health and wellness (homeostasis) can trigger the inflammatory response. The same is true of the stress response. So when a stressor remains, so does the ensuing stress response—and the system-wide inflammation that comes with it.

And as we know, any time inflammation sticks around, we get into trouble. Your body can't maintain that initial burst of adrenaline, so the HPA axis—which consists of the hypothalamus, pituitary gland, and adrenal glands—takes over. The HPA axis is involved in many body processes, including the stress response and the immune system. The adrenal glands flood the system with cortisol, also known as the stress hormone. If the stress response system remains revved up, the body is constantly flooded with cortisol, and inflammation remains elevated. Stress and inflammation absolutely work hand in hand. Chronic stress interferes with the body's ability to regulate the inflammatory response, which can easily rage out of control. Accumulating research shows that a revved-up HPA axis and rampant cortisol secretion play a role in heart disease.[38] Further, chronic stress can turn on genes that prepare immune cells to fight even though infection isn't present. In studies on animals and humans under stress, immune cells show an increased expression of genes that activate inflammation and a decreased expression of genes that suppress inflammation.[39] The effects of chronic stress are numerous. It can cause or contribute to an enormous range of illnesses, including depression, anxiety, insomnia, hypertension, heart attacks, skin conditions, gastrointestinal conditions, and stroke, and it can make us more vulnerable to infections and even to autoimmune disorders, such as rheumatoid arthritis and multiple sclerosis.[40]

Like chronic inflammation, chronic stress leads to physical changes that occur so gradually that you may not be aware of them until you're sick. But you can take steps to counteract the negative effects of stress; eventually, with practice, you can alter your body's reaction to the stress response. Chapter 13 gives a full list of noninvasive means to tamp down inflammation. It's no coincidence that they're ways to reduce stress, as well.

Age: Advancing Years and Escalating Inflammation

While there are many different aspects of our lives where we can at least partially control the level of inflammation we experience, there remains one area where we inevitably lose ground every day. It's a fact of life that chronic, low-grade inflammation increases as we age. There's even a term for it: *inflammaging*. **Increasing age** is associated with higher concentrations of several biomarkers of inflammation, but the star of the show is IL-6, which is so closely associated with age-related inflammation that it's been referred to as "the cytokine of gerontologists." We'll cover IL-6 and inflammaging in detail in the chapters that follow, as well as in our discussion of the age-associated conditions we know so well: cognitive decline, Alzheimer's disease, cancer, osteoporosis, macular degeneration, type 2 diabetes, atherosclerosis, and osteoarthritis. Inflammaging is considered a highly significant risk factor for incidence of illness as well as overall mortality.[41]

Fortunately, while inflammaging is inevitable, the rate at which it occurs is within our control. And, not surprisingly, the same lifestyle strategies that reduce inflammation can also lower age-related inflammation: following a healthy diet, keeping stress levels in check, engaging in regular moderate exercise, maintaining a healthy BMI, and getting adequate sleep.

Anti-Inflammatory Living: The Key for Long-Term Health

Abundant scientific evidence assures us that we can make positive, effective interventions at any point in the inflammatory process. Obviously it's far better, and far easier, to stamp out the initial sparks of inflammation than it is to try and put out a five-alarm fire in the form of an inflammatory illness. To maintain optimal conditions for health and wellness, adopt an anti-inflammatory way of living. Here's a cheat sheet of the chapter summarized for quick reference.

Quick Reference Guide for Avoiding Chronic Inflammation

- Stay away from all processed foods, including processed meats, prepackaged foods, and fast foods.
- Steer clear of trans fats entirely, and keep saturated fats to a minimum.
- Don't eat too much sugar.
- If you drink alcohol, stick to a moderate consumption: no more than one drink per day for women and no more than two for men. Red wine is the healthiest option.
- Eat fresh fruits and vegetables in abundance.
- Eliminate or cut back on grains.
- Take some time to identify any food sensitivities or allergies, and eliminate those foods.
- As much as possible, avoid exposure to toxins and pollutants.

- Don't smoke, and avoid secondhand smoke.

- Get regular, moderate exercise, and make sure to be up and moving every day.

- If you're an adult up to the age of 64, get 7 to 9 hours of sleep a night. If you're over 64, aim for 7 to 8 hours per night.

- Reduce the stress in your life, and use coping techniques such as meditation, yoga, deep breathing, journaling, talking and laughing with friends, or counseling to deal with life stressors.

CHAPTER 3

Fuel to the Fire

How Chronic Inflammation Accelerates Aging and Reduces Life Span

Thanks to medical advances and better living standards, statistics reveal a dramatic increase in human life span. Japan is the current world leader, with an average life expectancy from birth of nearly 84 years. In the United States, people can expect to live an average of 79 years. As of 2015, worldwide average life expectancy from birth was 71.4 years, and it's expected to climb as more people gain access to better health care, clean drinking water, better nutrition, and medicines that prevent or treat infectious diseases.[1] What's more, it seems that if you can make it to a certain age, the likelihood of your longevity increases. In fact, the fastest growing demographic in many countries is people ages 85 and above. Globally, the 85 and over population is expected to increase 351 percent between 2010 and 2050, compared to just a 22 percent increase for the population under 65.[2]

Believe it or not, this phenomenon could be connected to inflammation. It seems that once you reach the age of about 85, inflammation doesn't have the same effects on the body. In this demographic researchers call "the oldest old," rising inflammation is no longer predictive of age-related conditions such as dementia, frailty, and even death.[3] Some researchers have even suggested that in the oldest age groups, high levels of inflammation may be protective and actually an indicator of a well-functioning immune system.[4] We'll look at this intriguing phenomenon more closely a little later, when we take a look at what centenarians and supercentenarians can teach us about successful aging.

The dramatic increase in human life span, heralded by many as one of the greatest achievements of the 20th century, is certainly impressive.

WHO LIVES THE LONGEST?

As of 2015, here are the top 28 countries with the highest life expectancies and their average life spans from birth.

COUNTRY	YEARS
Japan	83.7
Switzerland	83.4
Singapore	83.1
Australia	82.8
Spain	82.8
Iceland	82.7
Italy	82.7
Israel	82.5
France	82.4
Sweden	82.4
Republic of Korea	82.3
Canada	82.2
Luxembourg	82
Netherlands	81.9
Norway	81.8
Malta	81.7
New Zealand	81.6
Austria	81.5
Ireland	81.4
United Kingdom	81.2
Belgium	81.1
Finland	81.1
Portugal	81.1
Germany	81
Slovenia	80.8
Denmark	80.6
Chile	80.5
Cyprus	80.5

Source: Data from the World Health Organization.[5]

However, not surprisingly, the prevalence of age-related diseases has climbed alongside this remarkable rise in life span. But a look at the top causes of death in people ages 65 and over reveals something very interesting. As of 2015, the top killers in this demographic were *all* inflammation-mediated illnesses: heart disease, cancer, and chronic lower respiratory illnesses (such as asthma, chronic bronchitis, emphysema, and chronic obstructive pulmonary disease).[6] With what we now know about chronic inflammation and how to prevent and reverse it, there is ample evidence that we may be able to slow the aging process and delay many age-related conditions by adopting an anti-inflammatory lifestyle.

With so many of us living longer lives, doctors and researchers are now focusing a great deal of energy into defining the concept of "successful aging," which in broad terms has four components: (1) retaining independence, (2) retaining physical capability, (3) retaining cognitive function, and, rather obviously, (4) postponing mortality. In real-world terms, we can think of successful aging as living in a state of physical and mental wellness as long as possible. It means living independently and disease-free, with our mental faculties intact; enjoying more time with the people we love; and pursuing activities we enjoy. This kind of life isn't a pipe dream, and it isn't just for those who've hit the genetic jackpot and ended up with so-called longevity genes. Successful aging is very much a result of keeping chronic inflammation in check.

Aging + Inflammation = Inflammaging

Inflammaging refers specifically to the chronic, low-grade inflammation that rises with age *independently of illness*. It seems that simply growing older causes a surge in all of the proinflammatory biomarkers discussed in previous chapters, especially IL-6. Elevated levels of this biomarker are so common in older people that some experts refer to IL-6 as "the cytokine of gerontologists." Unfortunately, the fact that these biomarker levels naturally increase with age also means that the problems associated with inflammation rise, as well. Consider the following studies.

In Canada researchers followed over 3,000 middle-aged people for 10 years and found that having a high IL-6 level cut the odds of successful aging nearly by half. High IL-6 also increased the risk of both future heart disease and death due to noncardiovascular causes. What's more, those who had higher inflammation at the outset of the study had worse outcomes with respiratory functioning, musculoskeletal functioning, and mental well-being, as well as lower odds of avoiding diabetes and disability. Researchers concluded that maintaining a low IL-6 level over the years—which comes from keeping inflammation suppressed—directly supports successful aging.[7]

Another large study, this one based on nearly 5,000 people ages 65 to 90-plus produced similar results. As expected, IL-6 and CRP levels rose as age increased, and higher IL-6 and CRP levels were associated with poorer physical and cognitive performance. This association remained even after the researchers took into account participants' age, gender, BMI, cholesterol levels, smoking status, and kidney function. On the other hand, the researchers found that lower IL-6 and CRP levels were associated with longer survival rates—regardless of whether participants were healthy and aging successfully *or* living with an age-related disease or disability.[8] Levels of inflammation were *that* influential.

In many ways, inflammaging is associated with some of the general features of the aging process, as well as age-related diseases, such as Alzheimer's, osteoporosis, cancer, type 2 diabetes, and heart disease. And it doesn't stop with disease. Many of the typical manifestations of aging, including cognitive decline, anemia, and even accelerated skin wrinkling, involve an inflammation component, too.[9] Inflammaging is the key underlying factor in muscle loss, frailty, and the impaired ability to build muscle in older people.[10] In a study that focused on healthy men ages 65 to 78, researchers found that even a slight rise in CRP levels resulted in a decline in physical fitness and increased insulin resistance.[11] Inflammaging has even been identified as a significant risk factor for death![12] In a recent study, IL-6 and another well-known proinflammatory cytokine, tumor necrosis factor-α receptor-1 (TNF-α R1), were shown to be the best predictors of death from any cause after 10 years—and this was after adjusting for age, sex, education, race, smoking, and BMI.[13]

Given this body of research, why is inflammaging so deadly? One reason is that chronic inflammation increases our susceptibility to infection. Although inflammaging results in an increase in circulating white blood cells, the constant exposure to proinflammatory cytokines results in immune cells that just don't work as well as they did when we were younger. This understanding of inflammation also helps explain why older people are so much more susceptible to infection than younger people.

In a study conducted on mice, researchers examined how a young versus an aging immune system responded to pneumonia, one of the leading causes of death among the elderly. First of all they found that older mice had higher numbers of monocytes—immune cells that help rid the body of pathogens and cellular debris—in their bone marrow and circulating in their blood. And as is characteristic in inflammaging, they observed higher levels of IL-6 and tumor necrosis factor (TNF) in the blood of older mice, as well as in blood samples from older human donors.[14]

The researchers then infected mice with pneumonia. They found that although older mice had higher inflammatory biomarkers and higher monocytes, they couldn't fight off the infection as efficiently. But when researchers reduced the number of monocytes or removed TNF—in effect, when they reversed inflammaging—the mice's immune systems functioned like those of younger mice and they were able to fight off the pneumonia effectively. The researchers also observed that the chronic, age-related exposure to TNF caused the monocytes to leave the bone marrow prematurely. In turn, these immature monocytes released even *more* proinflammatory cytokines. These results echo other studies that have shown that adults who have higher levels of circulating TNF and IL-6 are at far higher risk for pneumonia than those with lower levels of these proinflammatory cytokines. Higher levels of TNF and IL-6 are also associated with more severe pneumonia and higher death rates.[15]

But it isn't just in the realm of infectious diseases and immunity that inflammaging causes trouble. It's also directly implicated in noncommunicable age-related diseases—cancer, type 2 diabetes, Alzheimer's, arthritis, osteoporosis, and atherosclerosis, just to name a few. How can chronic inflammation wreak such havoc? What's the common thread?

Cellular Aging

At the most basic level, the aging process is the result of the slow degradation of cells and tissues over time, ultimately ending in death. Let's stop right there and talk for a moment about what the phrase "degradation of cells" means because it provides a key clue to age-related disease driven by inflammation. Damaged, dysfunctional cells are a threat to homeostasis—to optimal health and wellness. The body can't allow these damaged cells to stick around because the damage will spread to neighboring healthy cells, and eventually to tissues, setting the stage for disease and dysfunction.

Damaged or abnormal cells are therefore threats that must be eliminated, and this will happen in one of two ways, both of which involve the immune response and inflammation. The first way the body will try to rid itself of damaged cells is through the ordinary functions of the immune system. Sensing the presence of suspicious cells, the inflammation army goes on the attack to eliminate the threat. It's out there fighting the daily routine battles, scavenging damaged cells, with us none the wiser. The second way your body will deal with the threat is through cell death. This kind of programmed cellular death is called *apoptosis*. It's a built-in way the body rids itself of abnormal or damaged cells. But there's one wrinkle: Any time cells die, whether from disease, damage, or simply old age, they trigger the release of proinflammatory cytokines. In this case, the cytokines alert the inflammation army to go out and clear away the "debris" of dead cells.

And there, in miniature, is a snapshot of how aging and inflammation are two inextricably related processes that operate in tandem. Aging cells spark inflammation, and rising inflammation accelerates aging. Understanding this cycle helps explain why there are so many age-related diseases. Because at the body's most basic level of operation, the single cell, damage and dysfunction naturally occur as we age; eventually cell and tissue function become compromised, setting the stage for disease. Consider this: What's the most profound risk factor for all noninfectious diseases, such as heart disease, diabetes, and neurological diseases? Age.[16] What's the single most significant risk factor for developing a malignant tumor? Age.[17]

Let's go another level deeper. While we're worrying over deepening wrinkles or more fatigue or how it's getting harder and harder to recall family birthdays, even more cellular changes are under way. Those aging cells give rise to the outward signs of aging we know so well. The technical term for the process cells undergo as they age is called *cellular senescence*, and it refers to the stage when normal cells cease to divide and replicate. Like cats with their nine lives, there is a limited number of times cells can replicate, and once they reach that threshold, they die.

But while cells are getting older and nearing the end of their life cycles, they remain active, and they go through significant alterations. They secrete some 40 to 80 bioactive compounds—among them proinflammatory cytokines and interleukins—that send messages to other cells. This specific mix of chemical messengers is known collectively in the scientific world as the *senescence-associated secretory phenotype*, or SASP. When the SASP kicks into gear, it generates chronic, low-grade inflammation. Aging cells become veritable factories of proinflammatory cytokines, especially IL-6. The SASP may also directly impair tissue structure and function and indirectly overtax the immune system. And as aging cells accumulate, they trigger even *more* inflammation from an already overstimulated immune system.[18] As we see so often, chronic inflammation is both the cause and effect of deterioration and illness.

Beyond the normal life cycle of a cell, what triggers cellular senescence—and thus inflammation and eventually disease? Many things can activate a cell into reaching its senescent phase. DNA damage, oxidative stress (an imbalance between the production of harmful free radicals and our antioxidant defenses), and exterior stressors such as smoking, poor nutrition, high BMI, and chronic stress are just a few of the things that can trigger the senescence process that leads to cell death.

Another factor you may not have heard about is called telomere erosion, and it plays a significant role in DNA damage. An important part of the chromosomes in each cell, telomeres are repeating DNA sequences that "cap" the ends of chromosomes. They help make the chromosome stable and protect DNA from damage when cells replicate. Over time, the length of telomeres naturally shortens each time a cell divides and copies its DNA. Thus telomeres shorten as we age, and the rate at which they shorten can be used as an indicator of the pace of aging. (We all know people who seem to age more quickly than others!) Telomere length also seems to be a reliable predictor of life expectancy, similar to the way elevated proinflammatory biomarkers are. Once our telomeres fall below a critical length, the cell is no longer able to divide and can begin to malfunction. And when *that* happens, the process of cellular senescence occurs, sparking inflammation.

So what can affect the rate at which our telomeres shorten? Many of the very things that cause chronic inflammation! We're talking about increasing age, high cholesterol or triglyceride levels, smoking, a proinflammatory diet, high BMI, lack of exercise and chronic stress, as well as inflammation itself. The presence of disease also accelerates the rate of telomere shortening. Age-related diseases such as heart disease, diabetes, lung disease, some cancers, and osteoporosis are all associated with shorter telomeres. Elderly people who have shorter telomeres are at significantly higher risk of death than those with longer telomeres.[19] To keep telomeres long and help keep the effects of aging at bay, treat yourself to an anti-inflammatory lifestyle.

The Ins and Outs of Aging

Thus far we've focused on the *ins* of aging—that is, aging that takes place on a cellular level and that eventually gives rise to age-related decline and disease. But what about the *outs* of aging, the most visible sign of getting older? We can't have a chapter on aging without talking about our skin. And while we'll leave an antiwrinkle regimen to the skin care experts, we can tell you that science has uncovered some very interesting connections between chronic inflammation and the wrinkles you see when you look in the mirror.

Did you know that your skin can provide a reliable indicator of the state of your physical health and even your emotional well-being—and in ways you wouldn't necessarily expect? For example, people with diabetes are at higher risk for accelerated aging because chronic high blood sugar leads to an increase in advanced glycation end products (AGEs for short). As we saw in the previous chapter, AGEs provoke an inflammatory response and increase oxidative stress. Their effects on the skin can be seen in dryness and decreased elasticity.[20] And as for mental and emotional well-being, skin can certainly be a barometer of what's going on within. Stress or emotional upset can trigger hives, rashes, redness, and acne breakouts. Chronic stress is also known to trigger or aggravate inflammatory skin conditions, such as acne, psoriasis, dermatitis, alopecia (a type of hair loss), and skin that tends to be itchy, red, or flushed.[21]

Skin can also be a better indicator of your biological age than your chronological age. We all know people who look far younger, as well as people who look much older, than their years. Genetics certainly plays a role, but inflammation is just as much of a driving factor. What causes excessive and/or early skin aging? As always, there are "ins and outs" to that answer, meaning there are intrinsic and extrinsic causes of aging. For the "ins," we're talking about factors such as the decline in hormone levels and the natural rise in age-related inflammation, a poor diet, chronic stress, and sleep deprivation. For the "outs," the number-one extrinsic driver of aging is damage from the sun, or UV light exposure. The number-two spot goes to smoking, and a third cause of extrinsic aging is exposure to pollutants and toxins. Let's look at some of these factors in more detail, and we'll begin with those aptly named AGEs, one of the key drivers of skin aging.

Some AGEs form naturally within the body when sugar and proteins react, and these are referred to as endogenous AGEs. But we also get AGEs through the foods we eat, and these are known as exogenous AGEs. Heat-processed foods and foods that are high in animal protein, fat, and/or sugar are high in AGEs. AGEs are believed to be a culprit in all sorts of problems with aging skin, including wrinkling, decreased resistance to stress, slower wound healing, impaired collagen function, and changes to the delicate blood vessels just beneath the skin. On the cellular level, lab experiments have observed that human skin cells age and die prematurely in the presence of AGEs.[22]

What can we do to combat AGEs—and thus, aging from the inside out?

We must first consider the old adage "you are what you eat." Diets that are high in sugar, which is already brimming with exogenous AGEs, also prompt the body to produce endogenous AGEs on its own. Similarly, cooking methods that involve high heat or high fat, such as frying and grilling, boost the amount of AGEs your body must handle. Other cooking methods, such as boiling or steaming, produce far fewer AGEs, and raw foods contain negligible amounts of AGEs. (This may help explain why elderly Asian populations, which rely on water-based cooking methods, have such a relatively youthful appearance.)[23]

Still, the most powerful factor that accelerates skin aging is exposure to sunlight, a phenomenon referred to as photoaging. The sad reality is that there's no such thing as a "healthy" tan. A tan is a sign that UV rays have penetrated the inner layer of skin, damaging the collagen fibers that keep your skin taut. Repeated UV exposure will ultimately result in slack, sagging skin, wrinkles, freckling, and age spots.

The danger of UV exposure shouldn't be underestimated. According to the Skin Cancer Foundation, even one blistering sunburn during childhood more than *doubles* a person's chances of later developing melanoma.[24] And remember that the lighter your skin, the higher your risk of UV radiation damage.

The American Academy of Dermatology recommends that *everyone* use sunscreen with an SPF of 30 or higher when outdoors. Not only will you protect yourself from premature skin aging and the inevitable inflammatory response that UV radiation triggers, you'll also protect yourself from skin cancer, which affects roughly one out of every five Americans.[25]

After the sun, the second most powerful exogenous factor associated with accelerated aging is smoking. Because tobacco use exposes us to an array of harmful chemicals that compromise cellular function and irritate mucous membranes, this bad habit sends the inflammatory response into overdrive. The effect of smoking on the skin is plain to see. Know any long-term smokers? Chances are their skin is much more wrinkled than the skin of nonsmoking friends the same age.

Research has even shown this to be true. By comparing sets of identical twins, either with only one twin who smoked or one twin who smoked at least 5 years more than his or her sibling, researchers consistently found that the smokers had far more signs of extrinsic aging than their nonsmoking twins: more wrinkles, more age spots, more eye bags, more skin sagging, and the presence of jowls.[26] Plus, laboratory tests confirm that smoking boosts levels of IL-6, which is indisputably associated with accelerated aging and a higher risk of age-related illness.

And if you stop to consider that tobacco smoke, at its most basic level, is essentially a form of air pollution, then it's easy to extend that logic and understand how exposure to other forms of pollution and toxins can also accelerate extrinsic aging. Dust, traffic emissions, smoke, and soot have all been linked with pigment spots, collagen damage, and wrinkles. Researchers suspect that air pollution triggers oxidative stress and boosts levels of proinflammatory cytokines.[27]

So given the potential damage we face every time we step outside and take a stroll, what can we do to protect ourselves? Here's a list of suggestions; number one is nonnegotiable.

First, use sunscreen any time you go outdoors, especially if you'll be in direct sunlight or if you'll be in a polluted environment. Pollution *doubles* the damage to skin from UV radiation, so sunscreen protection is a must.[28] Second, use a topical antioxidant product (many antiaging or acne prevention creams and serums rely on antioxidants as their active ingredients), which can help counteract some of the free radical damage created by pollution and UV exposure. Look for products that list vitamins A (retinol), C, or E.

Pay attention to what you put inside your body, too. (A diet that is rich in antioxidants—think fresh fruits and vegetables and green tea—will also help counteract free radical damage.) Third, use a lotion to preserve and restore the skin's protective barrier function and to retain moisture. Fourth, make sure to wash your skin at the end of each day with a gentle, nontoxic cleanser that rinses off easily. This will ensure you've removed any pollutants that have accumulated on your skin. At the same time, don't overdo it. Vigorous, frequent washing is likely to remove the protective oils your skin needs as a natural barrier.[29]

What Can We Learn from Centenarians and Supercentenarians?

Given the extensive health consequences of chronic inflammation, combined with the normal aging process that all of us experience, what can we learn from the folks who live into their hundreds and even beyond? (At the time of this writing, Italian supercentenarian Emma Morano was entering her 117th year.) What can they teach us about successful aging, anti-inflammatory living, and even delaying the aging process? As it turns out, plenty.

In one study, researchers observed 1,554 people who ranged in age from 50 to 115. The group included 684 centenarians (ages 100 to 104) and supercentenarians (ages 105 and above); 536 "very old" individuals (ages 85 to 99); and finally, the children of the centenarians. Participants were assessed to determine their cognitive status, independence, presence of disease, and longevity. The follow-up time on this study was 4 years, during which 123 participants died. Here's what researchers learned.

As expected, chronic inflammation was associated with accelerated aging and increased risk of death. But once a person reached 100, a fascinating paradox came into play: Though centenarians *do* show elevated levels of inflammation, chronic inflammation appears to lose its power by then. Put another way, up until the age of roughly 100, all the old rules apply: Chronic inflammation accelerates aging, drives the development of disease, and contributes to disability. But in centenarians and supercentenarians, chronic inflammation seems to pose no increased risk. Researchers also noticed that the centenarians' children displayed low levels of chronic inflammation, leading to the theory that those who are fortunate enough to become exceptionally old probably don't develop elevated levels of inflammation until very late in life. And right there is the key for the rest of us: Keeping chronic inflammation at bay for as long as possible is an extremely powerful way to slow aging, delay or avoid age-related diseases, and attain longevity. The researchers concluded that "suppression of inflammation" is "the most important driver of successful longevity."[30]

As we mentioned at the beginning of the chapter, other studies have found the inflammaging tipping point to be age 85 and above. Whatever the age at which inflammation becomes protective rather than harmful, or at least doesn't exert the same debilitating effects, it seems that those who attain the longest life spans were successful at keeping inflammation low *earlier* in their lives. This means that you don't have to be a winner in the genetic jackpot to attain a long life and to stay healthy all the way through your ripe old age. The far more influential factor in successful aging is a healthy lifestyle that keeps inflammation low throughout your life. Let's look at how we can do just that.

How to Slow Aging, Anti-Inflammatory-Style

There are plenty of noninvasive, all-natural strategies that can reduce chronic inflammation and delay the pace of aging, from dietary choices to lifestyle considerations. As we've already discussed the importance of getting enough sleep, getting enough exercise, and avoiding smoking, we won't repeat them here, but don't forget that these three healthy habits are among the most powerful for staying healthy and vibrant well into your golden years. Here are some other strategies you can add to your health and wellness routine.

Try Going Without

Before we get into specific dietary advice about what you should eat (and not eat), let's first examine some of the substantial evidence that indicates eating less can decrease inflammation and slow aging. In lab studies, calorie restriction without malnutrition has been shown to delay the onset of age-related illnesses, decrease the production of AGEs, and increase life span.[31] Similar research has shown that intermittent fasting (you'll learn more about this later) may prevent or delay the progression of heart attack, stroke, diabetes, cancer, Parkinson's disease, and Alzheimer's disease—all inflammation-mediated illnesses. It also slowed bone mineral density loss and improved cognitive ability.[32]

Long-term studies on fasting in real-world scenarios aren't nearly as plentiful for obvious reasons, but a just-released study found that cutting calories by 25 percent for 2 years significantly lowered chronic inflammation over time. The study was conducted with 220 nonobese volunteers; one group maintained their normal diets, while the second group restricted calories and took multivitamin and mineral supplements to prevent malnutrition. Inflammation levels were assessed at the outset of the study, at 12 months, and at 24 months. Interestingly, while weight, fat mass, and leptin (the "satiety hormone") levels were all down at 12 months for the calorie-restriction group, inflammatory biomarkers CRP and TNF-a didn't decrease until 24 months, which may suggest that long-term calorie restriction triggers the body to lower inflammation through other ways beyond initial weight loss.[33]

Other studies on people willing to live below their normal calorie ranges reveal that intermittent fasting may reduce markers of oxidative stress and inflammation, reduce weight and body fat, lower blood pressure, and improve memory. Studies have observed a decrease in glucose, insulin, and a hormone called insulin-like growth factor 1 (IGF-1). (IGF-1 along with insulin is associated with accelerated aging and cancer.) One of the most dramatic benefits associated with fasting, however, affects people living with the inflammatory condition rheumatoid arthritis. Many studies indicate that during periods of fasting, rheumatoid arthritis patients experience less inflammation and pain. Their symptoms return, though, once the fast is over—unless the fasting period is followed by a vegetarian diet.[34] Which leads us to the next strategy.

Fight Aging with Phytochemicals

Diets rich in fruits, vegetables, teas, herbs, and spices can help decrease inflammation and promote health at a cellular level through a variety of biologically active compounds called phytochemicals that are only found in plants. Anthocyanins—the antioxidant flavonoids that give red, purple, or blue fruits their color—protect brain cells from free radical damage and reduce the secretion of proinflammatory cytokines. Studies indicate that consuming flavonoid-rich fruits (think blueberries, blackberries, raspberries, and strawberries) may delay the onset of age-related dementia and improve memory.[35] Data from a long-term study suggests that blueberries and straw-berries may delay cognitive aging by as much as 2.5 years—and the greater the intake, the slower the cognitive decline.[36]

Another study based on nearly 2,000 women found that higher anthocy-anin and flavone (a pigment found in white and yellow plants) intake was associated with significantly lower insulin resistance and markers of chronic inflammation, along with higher levels of adiponectin, a protein that helps regulate glucose levels. The anthocyanins and flavones cited in this study came from berries, grapes, oranges, pears, peppers, and wine.[37]

Flavonols, another type of flavonoid found in a wide variety of fruits and vegetables, may protect the nervous system and provide antioxidant, anti-inflammatory, and neuroprotective benefits, as well.[38] To get more flavonols, concentrate on adding more yellow onions, scallions, kale, broccoli, apples, berries, tea, and guava to your diet.[39]

The polyphenols known as resveratrol, curcumin, vanillic acid, and iso-rhamnetin all have the power to reduce the release of proinflammatory cyto-kines. Researchers have highlighted onions, turmeric, red grapes, green tea, and acai berries as sources of these anti-inflammatory polyphenols. They also found that combinations of these polyphenols were even more effective, supporting the oft-repeated advice to enjoy a varied diet.[40] Other sources of these polyphenols include almonds, chives, fennel, and dark leafy greens. Green tea polyphenols get bonus points for slowing aging: They protect against UV-accelerated skin aging and confer antiwrinkle, anti-inflamma-tion, and antioxidant effects.[41]

Spice It Up

Curcumin, the active compound found in the aromatic spice turmeric, is com-mon in South Asian cuisine, but given its health benefits, it would be wise to feature this spice in many types of dishes. Part of the ginger family, this bright yellow seasoning boasts powerful anti-inflammatory effects. A recently pub-lished analysis of nine randomized controlled trials on the effect of curcumin supplements demonstrated a significant reduction in IL-6 levels. And the

IL-6-lowering effect was found to be greatest in the patients who needed it most—the ones with the highest levels of inflammation.[42] To supercharge the effect of curcumin, whether you're getting it through turmeric or a supplement, combine it with black pepper. Black pepper has anti-inflammatory and antioxidant properties all on its own,[43] and combining it with turmeric increases the amount of curcumin the body can absorb and use by as much as 2,000 percent.[44] As turmeric is fat-soluble (meaning it dissolves in fat), another way to increase absorption is to combine it with a healthy fat like olive oil or coconut oil. Essentially, this allows curcumin to avoid being broken down by stomach acids or the liver and to make it into the bloodstream, where it can be absorbed.[45]

Other herbs and spices with demonstrated anti-inflammatory effects include capers, garlic, ginseng, ginger, parsley, rosemary, and sage. Some studies show that certain seasonings, including cinnamon, cloves, oregano, allspice, ginger, and garlic, slow down the body's production of those troublesome AGEs discussed earlier.[46]

Enjoy Olive Oil—Daily

Another all-natural anti-inflammatory powerhouse that may help slow the aging process is olive oil, one of the main staples in the heart-healthy, anti-inflammatory Mediterranean diet. Mediterranean populations have the lowest rates of chronic inflammatory disease in the world, while their life expectancy is among the highest. Virgin and extra-virgin olive oil contain higher polyphenols than refined olive oil, including a phenolic compound called oleocanthal, with anti-inflammatory properties comparable to ibuprofen. Oleocanthal decreases inflammatory biomarkers in arthritis, helps protect the nervous system, and provides anticancer effects.[47]

Another study conducted with overweight and obese people found that replacing their regular cooking oils with extra-virgin olive oil for 3 months resulted in lower systolic blood pressure, higher beneficial HDL cholesterol levels, and improved immune function. The researchers specifically measured how well a type of cell in the immune system known as T-cells reproduced. A decline in T-cell function is associated with obesity and may be the central defect in immunosenescence, the gradual age-related weakening of the immune system that we discussed earlier.[48]

Boost Your Omega-3s

You've read the health headlines. Many studies indicate that there's a strong benefit to getting a type of fatty acid known as omega-3 into your diet. A high intake is related to lower levels of CRP and IL-6, and thus lower inflammation. Other studies have found a low intake of omega-3s is associated with poorer cognitive function and higher CRP levels. You can boost your omega-3s and lower inflammation by adding cold-water fish such as salmon, mackerel, herring, and sardines to your diet. Vegetarian sources of omega-3s can be found in flaxseeds and walnuts and their oils and in extra-virgin olive oil.[49]

Cut Back on Sugar and Animal Protein

Eating less sugar and animal protein is a great idea all around, as both spark inflammation and increase the risk of many other negative health conditions, including heart disease, type 2 diabetes and other metabolic disorders, and high BMI. But a high consumption of sugar (especially refined sugar) and animal protein has also been found to stimulate cell-signaling pathways that can accelerate the aging process. Sugar, animal protein, and saturated fat have all been linked with DNA damage, specifically the telomere shortening discussed earlier.[50]

In a study of more than 5,300 people ages 25 to 60, all with no prior history of heart disease or diabetes, researchers found that drinking sugar-sweetened soda was associated with shorter telomeres. Given that the normal aging process results in telomere shortening of about 13.6 base pairs per year, researchers estimated that drinking a 20-ounce soda on a daily basis was equivalent to 4.6 additional years of aging per year of soda consumption. They concluded that drinking soda regularly could influence metabolic disorders associated with cellular aging.[51] Consuming high amounts of sugar has also been shown to accelerate sagging skin by damaging the delicate collagen fibers that help support your skin and render it more elastic.[52]

Where animal protein is concerned, we've already discussed how processed meats (and to a lesser degree, red meat) are carcinogenic and promote systemic inflammation. However, animal protein is also known to boost levels of the proinflammatory molecule homocysteine, which plays a major role in the development of cardiovascular disease. Guess what else homocysteine has been linked with? Dementia. A recently released study found that centenarians with dementia had significantly higher homocysteine levels than those with normal cognition. A look at other inflammatory biomarkers revealed that those with dementia also had higher levels of CRP, IL-6, and ESR, unequivocally linking dementia with chronic inflammation.[53]

Cultivate Your Social Network

A large body of research has established that social relationships and connections are vital to both physical and mental wellness. Now a recent study that followed a group of people over a period of 24 years has revealed some important insights on the effect of social relationships on inflammation. Based on a study pool of 647 adults, researchers found that support from family, friends, and one's spouse provided some protection against inflammation but that social *strain* from family and friend relationships substantially increased the risks of inflammation. In other words, social strain exerted a more powerful negative effect on inflammation than the positive effect of good social relationships. All of this is fascinating in and of itself, but a look at the details of the study is even more revealing. Check out these highlights.

- The overall inflammation burden was 27 percent lower for those with strong spousal support.

- Even after adjusting for age and sex, strain experienced in family relationships was associated with "vastly elevated odds" of inflammation.

- Strain experienced between friends was associated with a 97 percent higher risk of one inflammatory biomarker and a 50 percent higher inflammation burden overall.[54]

Reduce Stress

It's well established that chronic stress is an independent risk factor for chronic inflammation, heart disease, and mood disorders such as anxiety and depression. We also know that chronic stress contributes to sleep problems and that chronic inflammation is associated with not getting enough rest. Now studies have shown that stressful life events (such as divorce, employment problems, illness, and bereavement) also contribute to the aging process, specifically because stress is associated with telomere shortening.[55]

Fortunately, some stress-reducing techniques may help you slow down the aging process. A recently published study sought out stressed-out people to study the effect of stress-reducing techniques and IL-6 levels. They found them in the form of 35 unemployed adults who were job-hunting. Volunteers were taught either a mindfulness meditation technique or a relaxation technique and were assessed at the outset of the study and again 4 months later. The relaxation training made no difference, but those who decreased their stress through mindfulness meditation exhibited lower IL-6 levels by the end of the study period.[56]

Mindfulness meditation techniques are simple to learn and appear to be very effective in reducing stress and enhancing sleep. A new comprehensive review of randomized controlled trials based on over 1,600 participants has found that mindfulness meditation lowered CRP levels, increased telomerase activity (which can protect against premature aging), and improved immunity. Researchers theorize that exposing a dysfunctional or hypersensitive immune system to mindfulness meditation could improve health by enhancing immune defenses that protect against infection as well as various age-related conditions, including heart disease, osteoporosis, arthritis, type 2 diabetes, frailty, and some cancers.[57] In Chapter 12 you'll find a full qigong exercise routine, which is an incredible way to reduce stress and inflammation through gentle exercise, and in Chapter 13 we'll cover a full range of all-natural, noninvasive means to lower stress and inflammation simultaneously.

The Fountain of Youth Revealed

Is there a fountain of youth? If we're talking about lifestyle practices that can douse the fires of chronic inflammation, the answer is yes!

An increase in inflammation, just like an increase in candles on a cake as the birthdays keep coming, can't be avoided entirely. But we do have plenty of evidence that lifestyle choices can reduce the effects of inflammaging and slow down the process. Keeping inflammation levels in check throughout your life can't extend your life forever—not yet, anyway—but it *can* help delay age-related diseases and age-related decline. So drink liberally from this anti-inflammation fountain of youth to keep feeling *and* looking more youthful for the rest of your life.

PART II

Inflammatory Conditions

CHAPTER 4

Fire in the Belly

Gut Health and Chronic Inflammation

Some of the most game-changing medical breakthroughs of the past decade have converged upon the gut—by which we mean the gastrointestinal (GI) system, but especially the intestines. And we're not just talking about GI problems. Allergies, type 2 diabetes, overweight/obesity, autoimmune diseases, and mood disorders such as anxiety and depression have all been linked to a gut that's gone out of whack.

The knowledge that an unhealthy gut is involved in so many illnesses has given us a very powerful insight for how to heal ourselves, and there's an analogy with the brain to help us understand. When inflammation occurs in the brain, it can wreak havoc because the brain is the body's central command center, in charge of everything from heart rate and lung function to regulating mood, sleep cycles, and memory. Now recent research has confirmed that we have a *second* command center, and it's located in none other than the digestive system. This "second brain" is just as complex as the "first brain" and the central nervous system, and it controls far more in the body than how food gets from point A to point B. However, before we launch into the details of gastrointestinal inflammatory disorders and how we can keep our guts—and thus, the rest of our bodies—in tip-top shape, let us bring you up to speed on what's happening down below with our second brain.

The Gut-Brain Axis

Have you ever acted on a "gut feeling"? "Gone with your gut" when assessing a situation, or decided something based on "gut instinct"? Science tells us these aren't just figures of speech.

The "second brain" in the literal gut boasts some 500 million neurons (nerve cells), operates independently of the central nervous system, and can even influence behavior. It has its own protective barrier much like the blood-brain barrier, and it has glial cells (special cells that support neurons) that function very much like the astroglial cells of the brain. The gut produces 40 different neurotransmitters—including half of the body's supply of dopamine, which regulates movement and motivation and is involved in feelings of reward and pleasure, and 95 percent of the body's serotonin, the "feel-good" neurotransmitter that's key to mood regulation, sleep, GI function, and pain perception.[1] The technical name for the second, gut-based command center is the *enteric nervous system* (ENS).

The enteric nervous system is embedded in the walls of the entire gastro-intestinal tract, from the esophagus all the way down to the anus, but most of the activity takes place in the intestines. (The word *enteric* refers to anything relating to the intestines.) The ENS has long been known to regulate gastro-intestinal function, but we now know that it influences mood and well-being, motor function, the coordination of reflexes, immune function (including the inflammatory response), and endocrine function, and it plays a major role in many neurological disorders.

With so much under its control, imagine the consequences if something goes wrong with the enteric nervous system. A second brain that's on the fritz can potentially result in gastrointestinal problems like diarrhea, constipation, nausea, bloating, bowel incontinence, intestinal permeability (leaky gut syndrome), gut inflammation, and abdominal pain. But a faulty ENS has also been linked to many of the inflammatory conditions we'll explore in this book, including mood disorders, an increased sensitivity to pain, and Alzheimer's disease.

One of the most vivid examples of this connection between the first and second brains—between the central nervous system up top and the enteric nervous system down below, that is—occurs in Parkinson's disease (PD), an incurable degenerative condition. While the most visible symptoms are tremors and movement dysfunction, PD also produces a bevy of gastrointestinal problems. These problems span the entire GI tract, from abnormal salivation to loss of appetite to diarrhea and constipation. For years experts thought that the loss of dopamine was the primary driving factor of Parkinson's (and it certainly causes the movement problems), but newer research has shown that neuron loss in the enteric nervous system, the second brain, could be a prominent factor, as well.[2] Further, the protein clumps that do so much damage in PD, called Lewy bodies, show up in both the brains and the gut neurons of people living with PD. Some researchers are even investigating the possibility that Parkinson's disease begins from an infection in the gut that passes from the enteric nervous system to the central nervous system by way of the vagus nerve, a major cranial nerve that extends from the brain to the abdomen. This theory was first put forward in the early 2000s based on brainstem studies of patients with PD, but a more recent animal study confirmed that the key protein component of Lewy bodies can indeed travel from gut to brain.[3]

The mechanism connecting our two brains, and by which they communicate through biochemical signals, is called the *gut-brain axis*. We used to think it was only the brain that sent out messages, while the rest of the body received them and acted accordingly. But now we know that the communication is a two-way street. It's the gut-brain axis that links the cognitive and emotional centers of the brain to the gut and vice versa. Want to see an easy example of the gut-brain axis at work? Think about how closely the experience of fear is felt in your gut. "Butterflies" in the stomach, nausea, vomiting, diarrhea, loss of appetite, heartburn, indigestion—these are all physical GI symptoms triggered by the cognitive-emotional experience of fear. Along the same lines, stress, anxiety, and depression often coincide with GI disorders such as irritable bowel syndrome and inflammatory bowel disorder, which further demonstrates just how closely the central nervous system and the enteric nervous system are connected.

The Gut Microbiome

So, just as you're getting your first brain wrapped around the fact that you've got a second brain in your guts, let's add the truly mind-blowing notion that there are roughly 100 trillion microbes living in your gut, and these microscopic critters exert untold influence on health and behavior.

Most of these microbes are bacteria—anywhere between 300 and 1,000 different species of bacteria inhabit your gut at any given time—but there are viruses, fungi, and single-celled organisms, as well. Most of these microbes reside in the large intestine. In what may seem like science fiction, the bacteria living in your gut are directly involved in many gut-brain interactions, including gut-brain axis communication, mood regulation, cognitive function, immune system function, the way you gain or maintain weight, and your risk of developing certain diseases. Most of us think of bacteria and other microbes as harmful "germs," but the reality is that most "germs" do not make us sick and we literally could not live without them.

The gut microbiome is so important to our overall health and wellness—in fact, to our very survival—that some researchers now describe it as our "forgotten organ." (And by the way, that organ weighs anywhere between 2 and 6 pounds, or up to twice the weight of the human brain.) The gut microbiome helps to *protect* us from disease; it influences behavior; it influences how efficiently (or not) we convert calories into energy or store them as fat; and, as you'll see later when we discuss allergies, it plays a crucial role in teaching the immune system which substances constitute a true threat and which can be safely ignored. A living, dynamic organ unto itself, the gut microbiome is constantly evolving in response to diet, stress levels, environmental factors, aging, the introduction of antibiotics and probiotics, and certainly the presence of inflammation. Disturb the delicate balance of the gut microbiome, and there's no telling what sort of health consequence you'll face.

All of which begs the question: What constitutes a healthy gut microbiome? First of all, there is no *single* answer because every person's gut microbiome is unique, much like a fingerprint, and even among family members in perfect health (family members show similarities in gut microbiota), there are substantial differences. And in fact, research indicates that the more diverse the gut microbiota, the better. So a healthy gut microbiome boils down to two characteristics above all else: We want our gut microbiota to be *diverse*, and we want them to be *balanced*. When the microbiome is off in some way—when one strain of bacteria grows unchecked and/or if another strain is deficient—it's referred to as *dysbiosis*, a term that means a state of imbalance in the gut microbiome.

What can happen when dysbiosis occurs? Believe it or not it's a factor in every condition we'll cover in this chapter, from irritable bowel syndrome to overweight to certain neurological and mental health problems. Let's start with a simple and all too familiar example, the antibiotic-induced yeast infection. Antibiotics are of course necessary to treat some types of bacterial infections, but they can't distinguish between the bacteria that are making us sick, the bacteria that keep the GI system functioning well, and the bacteria that keep the growth of yeast in check. Therefore, while an antibiotic will effectively obliterate harmful bacteria, the fungi-eating bacteria are wiped out, as well, resulting in the overgrowth of yeast and the unforgettable symptoms of a yeast infection. Gut microbiome dysbiosis is also part of the reason many people experience GI-related side effects such as diarrhea, nausea, flatulence, and indigestion while on antibiotics.

But dysbiosis can also result in serious illness. It's closely associated with chronic illnesses of the intestinal tract, including Crohn's disease, ulcerative colitis, celiac disease, food allergies and sensitivities, and irritable bowel syndrome. It's been linked to impaired immunity, both type 1 and type 2 diabetes, and obesity.[4] Dysbiosis can also lead to malnutrition by impairing the way our bodies extract calories from the food we eat.[5] And alterations in the gut microbiome have been linked to autism spectrum disorders, Parkinson's disease, anxiety, and depression. In the elderly, those who were frail or who showed signs of mental decline exhibited the lowest gut microbial diversity. There is even some indication that our gut microbial composition affects the way we interact (or don't) with others and how we handle stress.[6]

Before we look at some of the research, it's important to note that altering the gut microbiome works both ways. Some of our actions induce dysbiosis and set the stage for ill health. But there are also actions we can take to restore balance in the gut microbiome and increase its diversity, setting the stage for optimal health and wellness. Here are some of the top factors that can change the gut microbiome, for good and for ill.

1. Drugs, especially antibiotics

2. Probiotics

3. Diet

4. Alcohol

5. Illness

6. Inflammation

7. Stress

8. Environmental factors (such as toxins)

9. Degree of hygiene (excessive washing can compromise gut microbiota)

10. Fecal transplants and fecal transplant pills

Though the details mentioned in Item 10 may be the most attention-grabbing (see the sidebar on page 64 if you're dying of curiosity), the thing you should pay the most attention to is Item 3, diet. Why so? Because we all eat and drink multiple times a day, and everything we consume affects our gut microbiota. Those 100 trillion gut microbiota are highly sensitive to what we feed them.

To evaluate just how rapidly food can affect the gut microbiome, researchers designed an experiment to compare two diets on opposite ends of the human-eating-habits spectrum—one plant-based that was rich in grains, legumes, fruits, and vegetables, and the second, an animal-based diet composed of meats, eggs, and cheeses. Changes to gut microbiota occurred as early as 24 hours after eating, and foodborne microbes from both diets were seen to rapidly, if temporarily, colonize the gut. Fecal samples from volunteers revealed that the animal-based diet had a greater impact on gut microbiota, and it increased bile-tolerant microorganisms, including *Bacteroides*, and decreased levels of Firmicutes. (Take note of these two bacterial strains, as they'll come up again.) The animal-based diet also sparked several gut microbiome changes that are known to contribute to inflammatory bowel disease.

THE SCOOP ON POOP: FECAL TRANSPLANTS

Transplanting poop from one person to the other may sound (a) disgusting and (b) like some crazy newfangled procedure, but the practice has been around at least since the 4th century. Modern medical practices have cut down on the gross factor by administering the fecal transplant in a clinical setting, and now recipients can receive their dose of healthy gut microbiota through freeze-dried "poop pills."

Why is this bizarre-sounding treatment effective? It's quite simple. Fecal matter from a healthy person is transferred to the gut of a person with dysbiosis (an imbalanced gut microbiome). When the healthy microbiota land on the scene, they recolonize the gut, restoring microbial diversity and balance. Transplants can take place through an enema, through a colonoscope, through a tube passed through the nose, or, in the most recent form, through capsules containing freeze-dried fecal matter from healthy donors.

Fecal transplants have shown incredible success in combating intractable *Clostridium difficile* infections, which cause inflammation of the colon and can cause life-threatening diarrhea. They're also used to treat a range of GI illnesses, such as ulcerative colitis, irritable bowel syndrome, severe constipation, and neurodegenerative conditions like multiple sclerosis and Parkinson's disease. Researchers at MIT are currently testing fecal transplants on humans as a treatment for obesity. And while results of this trial aren't final at this printing, there's good reason to be optimistic about the results. Preclinical trials on mice have shown that transferring gut microbiota from lean and obese humans resulted in, respectively, lean and obese mice (see the "Weight Management May Begin in the Gut" on page 73 for more), and transplanting the fecal microbiota of lean humans into men with metabolic syndrome resulted in significant improvement in insulin sensitivity and increased gut microbiota diversity.[7]

Taken together, these results demonstrate that diet does indeed cause rapid changes in the gut microbiome.[8]

It's also just one study of many that demonstrates that the typical Western diet reduces gut microbiome diversity. Diets that are high in fat and sugar are known to cause gut dysbiosis and negatively impact the immune system. When mice on a low-fat, plant-rich diet were switched to a high-fat, high-sugar Western diet, they experienced an overgrowth in Firmicutes and a reduction in *Bacteroides*, a ratio that is associated with obesity in animals and in humans. By comparison, the gut microbiome composition of people who eat a diet rich in complex carbohydrates tends to be lower in harmful bacterial strains and higher in beneficial bifidobacteria, while diets high in sugar create gut conditions that are more favorable for the overgrowth of harmful pathogens.[9]

Melancholic Microbes and Stress-Busting Bacterial Strains

Recent research has connected the dots between gut microbiota and psychological conditions like anxiety, depression, and elevated stress. Most of this research comes from preclinical trials conducted with animal models; studies with human volunteers are ongoing and still in the early stages. Here are a few highlights of what we know so far.

First, changes in animal behavior that indicated anxiety or depression were always associated with an altered gut microbiome. In just one example, when researchers transferred fecal microbiota from depressed people to experimental rats, the rats began to display behaviors typical of depression, including anxiety and a loss of pleasure in activities.[10] Second, as expected, antibiotics and diet have a profound effect on the gut microbiota. In particular, a high-fat diet is associated with both anxiety and depression. When microbiota from mice fed a high-fat diet were transferred to mice raised on a regular diet, the latter group developed anxiety-like behaviors. Further, the mice that ate the high-fat diet displayed increased signs of developing leaky gut and higher levels of inflammation.[11] These results echo the results from human studies on the neurological impact of a high-fat diet. A long-term high-fat diet has been shown to reduce the size of the hippocampus, which may impair cognitive function, including causing memory and attention deficits, and increase vulnerability to both depression and anxiety.[12]

But research about altering the gut microbiome has also revealed some exciting possibilities for prevention and treatment. We're still in the early days of research based on human volunteers, but knowing that the gut microbiota communicate with the central nervous system and influence brain function and behavior may provide new treatment options for anxiety, depression, and other psychiatric disorders. In the study mentioned earlier where mice were fed a high-fat diet, adding probiotics to the diet positively altered the gut microbiota, reduced symptoms of anxiety and depression, and prevented the leaky gut that's often the result of chronic stress.[13]

And more than a decade ago, a landmark study demonstrated that germ-free mice with no gut microbiota had an overactive HPA axis in response to stress. (The HPA axis helps control the stress response and the immune system, and the mice were specially bred in sterile environments to have zero gut microbiota.) But introducing a single probiotic organism, *Bifidobacterium infantis*, reversed this overactivity.[14] *B. infantis* is a common ingredient in most probiotic supplements and in many yogurts. Similarly, another study conducted on mice found that probiotics improved sickness behavior and decreased levels of inflammation.[15] "Sickness behavior" is a set of behavioral changes that come about quickly in response to illness and that closely mirror symptoms of depression, such as fatigue, appetite loss, malaise, and social withdrawal. Evidence shows that people with chronic inflammatory diseases—such as rheumatoid arthritis, chronic liver disease, and inflammatory bowel disease—often develop sickness behavior. We'll look at sickness behavior at greater length in Chapter 8.

This research leads us to the question of whether increasing gut microbial diversity and using probiotics can restore balance and prevent sickness behavior in humans. Could these live organisms be an easy, low-intervention treatment for anxiety and depression and an all-natural stress-buster?

It's very tempting to say yes, but consider a couple of words of caution before we move on. It's difficult to take data from animal studies and draw definitive conclusions for human use. And keep in mind that high quantities of probiotics are needed to gain therapeutic effect, so don't expect an occasional yogurt to keep your stress in check.

That said, there's no doubt that probiotics confer health benefits to their user, usually by enhancing the growth of certain strains of bacteria in the colon. One of their biggest claims to fame is in supporting gut health, and they're thought to do so by multiple mechanisms: (1) enhancing intestinal barrier function (i.e., improving "leaky gut"), (2) tamping down the inflammatory response in the gut, (3) reducing gut hypersensitivity, and (4) promoting a balanced composition of gut microbiota.[16] And with what we know about the connection between the enteric nervous system and the central nervous system, we can begin to see how altering your gut can alter your mood. The potential of probiotics to improve mental health is so strong that some scientists are exploring a whole new field of "psychobiotics" for human use. The aforementioned *B. infantis* is a widely studied (and quite effective) psychobiotic. In addition to alleviating depression and anxiety, psychobiotics have been shown to improve symptoms of irritable bowel syndrome and chronic fatigue syndrome.[17]

One study used brain scans to demonstrate that ingesting a probiotic cocktail alters how the brain processes emotional stimuli. (This particular cocktail contained *Bifidobacterium, Lactobacillus, Lactococcus,* and *Streptococcus* strains.) Researchers assigned healthy women with no GI or psychiatric conditions 4 weeks of a fermented probiotic milk drink, a regular milk drink, or no intervention. The women then looked at pictures of human faces expressing fear or anger or at neutral pictures of geometric forms. MRI scans revealed that the women who had the probiotic drink showed far less reactivity to the negative emotional stimuli. The effect was widespread, affecting areas of the brain that control emotion and sensation, and provided a vivid picture of how the gut can affect brain function.[18] Similarly, in another study, healthy volunteers who took a probiotic cocktail consisting of five common bacterial strains showed significantly reduced reactivity to sad mood compared to those who took a placebo—largely in the form of less rumination and fewer aggressive thoughts. The results of this study are especially important for people with depression or with melancholic tendencies, as heightened reactivity to normal, temporary changes in mood is associated with a heightened risk of depression. Researchers concluded that probiotics provide a noninvasive, low-cost means of reducing negative thoughts associated with sad mood and may help relieve or prevent depression.[19]

In yet another study, a 30-day intervention of a probiotic formula containing strains of *Lactobacillus* and *Bifidobacterium* reduced anxiety in rats and in healthy human volunteers, and it alleviated symptoms such as anxiety, depression, and anger/hostility.[20] Probiotics have also shown promise in treating social anxiety, one of the most common mental health complaints. A study of 710 young adults found that frequent consumption of fermented foods significantly lowered symptoms of social anxiety, especially in those who were prone to neuroticism, which is the general tendency to experience negative emotions such as nervousness, anger, envy, guilt, and depression. [21]

In addition to probiotic supplements, the best way to get probiotics into your system is with fermented foods and beverages. The go-to probiotic food source is of course yogurt; kefir, a fermented milk drink, is its close cousin. These are excellent sources of probiotics and health-promoting nutrients, but keep in mind that the Whole Body Cure Eating Plan requires you to eliminate dairy, at least for a period of time. Dairy products are among the most frequent causes of food sensitivities and food allergies, both of which contribute to gut dysbiosis and chronic inflammation. This plan will first get your system completely calmed down by eliminating dietary triggers of inflammation, and then it will help you identify your unique food sensitivities. Long-term elimination of dairy products may be the best option for some people. So what do you do for probiotics if you go dairy-free, or if you know already that you're lactose intolerant? Fortunately, there are several nondairy fermented food options. Excellent choices include sauerkraut, kimchi, tempeh, miso soup, sour pickles, olives, the fermented tea called kombucha, and even dark chocolate, which has some probiotic content.

Of course, supplements will give you the largest quantities of probiotics. But *add* a probiotic supplement to a healthy diet, rather than substitute it for whole foods. Besides the vitamins, minerals, and polyphenols you'll get from whole foods, there's evidence that the peptides found in fermented foods provide anti-anxiety benefits above and beyond the probiotics found in supplements.[22]

These studies demonstrate that negative changes to the gut microbiome—through stress, antibiotics, inflammation, a poor diet, or food sensitivities we may not be aware of—can affect the way we think and increase the likelihood of psychological disorders. Dysbiosis can also worsen already-existing psychological and GI symptoms. On the other hand, probiotics can positively affect the gut microbiome, leading to a better functioning GI system as well as fewer psychological symptoms. Recognizing that the gut-brain axis is a two-way street, researchers are hopeful that positive changes to one will benefit the other. For example, stress-reducing techniques may lower gut inflammation, while a diverse, well-balanced gut microbiome may lead to less anxiety and depression. Though more research needs to be done, the existing evidence supports this gut-brain strategy for improving health, which is excellent news for the people suffering from our next set of conditions.

Inflammatory Gut Conditions

Inflammatory bowel disease (IBD) is a group of inflammatory conditions of the small intestine and colon that affect over 1 million Americans. The two principal forms of IBD are *Crohn's disease* and *ulcerative colitis (UC)*. Cases of IBD are on the rise, not just in America but worldwide, and like type 2 diabetes, which was once a disease of an older population, IBD is becoming increasingly common in adolescents and children.[23] There is abundant evidence that IBD is associated with the Western diet, which is high in animal protein, highly processed foods, saturated fat, and sugar and low in fiber. (This helps explain why IBD is especially on the rise in countries that follow a Western lifestyle.) A diet that follows the typical Mediterranean pattern, on the other hand, which emphasizes vegetables, fruits, olive oil, fish, legumes, and nuts, seems to decrease the risk of IBD.[24] Let's look at both types of inflammatory bowel disease to see how these eating patterns play out.

Crohn's disease can cause inflammation in any part of the gastrointestinal tract, from the mouth to the anus, but it most often affects the end of the small intestine and the beginning of the large intestine (colon). It can also "skip" areas or attack "in patches," leaving some portions of the GI tract inflamed and others unaffected. Symptoms include diarrhea and bowel urgency, rectal bleeding, abdominal cramps, constipation, the sensation of incomplete bowel movements, loss of appetite, weight loss, fatigue, night sweats, and fever. These symptoms vary in severity from person to person, and they can come and go.

No one knows exactly what triggers Crohn's disease, but we do know that it is a chronic inflammatory condition, that it tends to run in families, that people who live in urban areas are more affected, and that an ailing gut microbiome is a contributing factor. More specifically, dysbiosis, or reduced bacterial diversity, is a characteristic feature of Crohn's. Antibiotics can disturb the gut microbiota, and stress and a poor diet can trigger flare-ups and/or worsen symptoms.[25] Food sensitivities and allergies can have a similar effect on symptoms and flare-ups, and they certainly contribute to gut dysbiosis. Many Crohn's patients have found relief by identifying and eliminating their specific food triggers. One recent study found that the most common food triggers were milk, beef, pork, and eggs; once Crohn's patients eliminated the foods causing the adverse reaction, their symptoms and their overall quality of life improved.[26] Certainly there are other foods that cause adverse reactions, and as mentioned earlier, our eating plan will help you identify your unique food triggers. Crohn's sufferers also have an increased risk of colorectal cancer. Even more frightening, the kind of cancer that develops from either type of IBD is far more lethal than the traditional form of colorectal cancer that develops from a polyp.[27]

Unlike Crohn's, which can affect any part of the GI tract, ulcerative colitis is confined to the colon and rectum. It causes painful inflammation and ulcers on the inner lining of these areas. Symptoms include diarrhea that's sometimes accompanied by blood or mucus, bowel urgency, inability to move the bowels despite urgency, rectal bleeding, abdominal cramps, weight loss, fatigue, and in severe cases, fever. These symptoms vary in severity from person to person, usually depending on how much of the colon is affected, and they can come and go. In severe UC, surgery may be required. Though UC itself isn't fatal, people living with this condition can develop life-threatening complications such as colon perforation, a dangerously swollen colon, severe bleeding, an increased risk of blood clots, and colon cancer, as well as systemic inflammation leading to further complications.

And as with Crohn's, no one knows the exact causes of UC, though there is some evidence that it's an autoimmune disorder in which the immune system mistakenly attacks the cells of the digestive tract. There may be a hereditary component to UC, and UC sufferers do display an altered gut microbiome. Stress and a poor diet can make symptoms worse, as do food sensitivities and allergies.

Drug treatments for Crohn's disease and ulcerative colitis center around medications that reduce inflammation, including corticosteroids, immuno-modulators that trigger or suppress the immune response, and in some cases, a class of drugs called aminosalicylates that specifically decrease inflamma-tion in the lining of the GI tract. Antibiotics are often prescribed in the event of infection, and over-the-counter analgesics are used for pain.

Nondrug treatment options for IBD are all about diet. In fact, diet is such a powerful factor in managing either form of IBD and reducing the possibility of colorectal cancer that many health-care providers emphasize food choices as a first-line treatment. The right diet manages symptoms and prevents their recurrence; eliminates one's unique food triggers; and addresses the malnu-trition that can occur in IBD (especially Crohn's) sufferers because of malab-sorption, loss of appetite, or an overactive metabolic rate. Anti-inflammatory foods (see Chapter 11 for our full anti-inflammatory eating plan) and vitamin- and mineral-rich foods are essential.

As for ulcerative colitis, one study found that a diet high in omega-6 fatty acids, which are proinflammatory, increased the incidence of UC by 30 percent, while consuming the omega-3 fatty acid DHA reduced disease burden by 77 percent.[28] Omega-6, also known as linoleic acid, is found in red meat, vege-table oils, and certain margarines. It's metabolized to arachidonic acid, which causes inflammation and is seen in higher levels in the mucous lining of UC patients. Omega-3s are anti-inflammatory and are found in fatty, cold-water fish; walnuts; and flaxseeds. Probiotics are another option. They've proven more effective in treating UC than Crohn's disease, but research is still in the early stages. Studies have shown, however, that probiotics improve gut micro-biota balance, enhance gut barrier function, and improve immune response, so there is strong potential for probiotics to manage the symptoms of IBD.[29]

Let's now turn our attention to irritable bowel syndrome (IBS). If there is a poster child for a disease of the gut-brain axis, IBS is it. In addition to its GI symptoms—abdominal pain, bloating, gas, nausea, and alternating stool consistency, ranging from diarrhea to constipation—IBS is known for its close links with anxiety and depression. Depression and traumatic life events (in adulthood or childhood) are risk factors for developing IBS. Even short-term episodes of stress are known to trigger IBS and make symptoms worse. Irritable bowel syndrome is very common, affecting almost 2 out of every 10 people worldwide.

Any disturbance along the gut-brain axis could worsen the symptoms of,

NUTRITIONAL MEANS TO SOOTHE AN UNHAPPY GUT

Severe cases of IBD may require a strict diet or in some instances even surgery. To treat mild to moderate flare-ups and to keep periods of remission going longer, talk with your doctor about these strategies.

- Eliminate all meat, at least until your symptoms subside. Studies have shown that animal protein is strongly associated with IBD. Animal protein is inflammatory, and it negatively alters the gut microbiome.

- Eat more fermented foods. Yogurt and kefir are the most well-known fermented foods, but remember that dairy can trigger GI symptoms in many people and is one of the most common sources of food allergies and sensitivities. For nondairy probiotic options, try fermented foods like sauerkraut, kimchi, miso, tempeh, pickles, olives, and kombucha (a fermented tea product). If any of these is on your no-no list, as well, go for a probiotic supplement. The benefits of probiotics are not to be missed.

- Mind your fats. Trans fats and saturated fats are associated with an increased risk of IBD. The same goes for omega-6 fats, commonly found in vegetable oils, shortening, and margarine. However, monounsaturated fats, which can be found in olive oil, nuts, and avocados, have a protective effect.[30]

- Avoid alcohol and caffeine temporarily. Instead, stay hydrated with filtered water or diluted fruit juices. If you feel you just can't tolerate life without caffeine, opt for green tea, which has proven anti-inflammatory benefits.

if not cause, IBS. One especially vexing symptom is the heightened perception of gut pain that is common in IBS patients. Fortunately, probiotics can help. In a study of 362 women with IBS, *B. infantis* improved global IBS symptoms, including pain, by more than 20 percent. Another study found similar effects for *Lactobacillus acidophilus*; abdominal pain and discomfort fell by more than 20 percent.[31]

Studies have also found that IBS patients have significantly less gut microbial diversity compared to healthy people. Some studies have shown a twofold increase in the ratio of Firmicutes to Bacteroidetes in IBS sufferers, and others have found decreased levels of beneficial *Bifidobacterium* strains. Supplementing the diet with bifidobacteria has been shown to improve IBS symptoms like pain, bloating, and bowel urgency.[32]

GI infections could also be to blame in some IBS cases, as various infectious bacteria have been observed in IBS sufferers. The condition known as SIBO, or small intestinal bacterial overgrowth, is implicated in some cases of IBS. While the large intestine is home to trillions of bacteria, under normal circumstances, the small intestine has far fewer bacteria. But sometimes harmful bacteria can multiply quickly in the small intestine, resulting in SIBO. SIBO is more prevalent in those with IBS than in those without,[33] and we also know that SIBO contributes to leaky gut syndrome. Simply put, when infection is present, gut inflammation and an altered gut microbiome occur, both of which increase the chance of IBS. Probiotics can rebalance gut microbiota and enhance intestinal barrier function, helping to keep these other problems at bay.

Weight Management May Begin in the Gut

The newest strategies for weight loss include tending to your gut health in addition to traditional factors such as diet and exercise. Recent evidence suggests that our gut microbiota affect the way we metabolize food, store fat, and regulate blood glucose and how we respond to hormones involved with appetite. Though research is at an early stage, it may very well be that having the

(continued on page 77)

Terry Lipp

AGE: 58

- **Reduced total cholesterol by 42 points to normal range**
- **Blood pressure reduced from stage 1 hypertension to normal range**
- **Mental fatigue, memory lapses, and mood swings eliminated**
- **Daily cough gone**
- **WEIGHT LOST: 22 pounds**
- **INCHES LOST: 15½**

When I joined the test panel, I was at a point where I needed a jump start to get me back on track. I have a young granddaughter, and I want to see her grow up.

During those first 2 weeks, I felt fabulous and was never hungry. You don't think fruits and vegetables will fill you up, but they do. Honestly, I think that was when I felt best, just eating the fruits and vegetables—I could potentially become a vegetarian. The hardest part during that time was going out to dinner, but I found that restaurants could accommodate my requests. We went to an Italian restaurant, but I saw they could steam vegetables or sauté them in olive oil, so I asked them to bring a vegetable plate. They did, and it was gorgeous. At first my friends and family couldn't understand why I wasn't eating garlic bread or a big bowl of pasta. But pretty soon nobody was questioning it because they could see the results.

I lost 22 pounds and 15½ inches on the Whole Body Cure Plan, and my total cholesterol plummeted from 212 to 170. My glucose level dropped 9 points, and my CRP level went from 3.4 to 0.2. I also definitely feel mentally sharper. I have a lot of multitasking to do at my job, and I found that it just came easier to me. I'm a type A personality, a go-getter whose energy level was already at a 9, but it was definitely a 10 by the end of the 12 weeks. And as far as digestive function goes, I've never been so regular or felt so good.

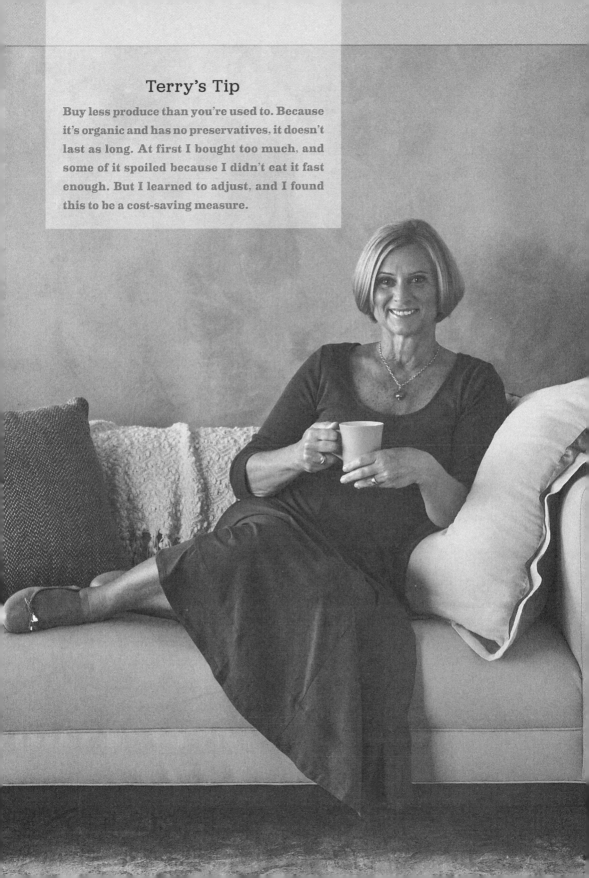

Terry's Tip

Buy less produce than you're used to. Because it's organic and has no preservatives, it doesn't last as long. At first I bought too much, and some of it spoiled because I didn't eat it fast enough. But I learned to adjust, and I found this to be a cost-saving measure.

The other dramatic difference I experienced was with allergies. For years I had a constant dry cough—it was so bad my kids used to joke that I sounded like I had TB. Then during the second week, my husband and I both noticed that I hadn't been coughing. When I reintroduced beef, however, the cough came back. I coughed all 3 days we tested beef, but when I eliminated it, the cough went away. There was just too much of a connection there to be a coincidence! Since then I've had almost no beef, the cough hasn't returned, and my husband says I no longer snore, too.

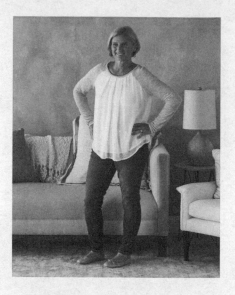

I had such good results on the plan that I told Dr. Kirshner and his staff I could be their poster girl! It's led me to make some permanent lifestyle changes. I've eliminated gluten, for instance. I don't eat any bread at all, actually, and I've eliminated dairy. I drink black coffee now. I used to love ice cream, but I haven't had it once. That's one of the most interesting things to me: I don't even have a desire for those foods anymore. I'm Italian, and I thought I'd really miss bread and pasta—not to mention ice cream and wine. But I don't miss any of it. A glass of wine in the evening was a stress reliever after work, but I found my stress level was better when I was eating healthier. My drinking is almost nonexistent now.

You do have to prepare and plan ahead because you can't grab the quick snacks you were used to. I made sure I always had healthy stuff in the house to grab and snack on. I roasted miniature carrots and kept those as a snack instead of pretzels or potato chips.

Overall I got way more creative with my cooking. One of my new favorites is peas with sautéed mushrooms and onions, and I learned to roast just about any vegetable in olive oil and season it with kosher salt and black pepper. Simple and delicious. That's one of the things I would tell people: Be open to trying new things, and learn from other people's cooking ideas. Be open to the overall program, too. It may sound a little daunting in the beginning, but just give it a try. It can be done, and it really brings major health benefits. ■

right gut bacteria in the right proportions is crucial to having a healthy BMI.

A decade ago, researchers examined the connection between gut microbiota and body fat by randomly assigning obese volunteers either to a fat-restricted diet or a carbohydrate-restricted diet for 1 year. At the outset of the study, the bacterial strain known as Bacteroidetes was far lower in obese people than in lean people who served as controls, while the Firmicutes strain was more abundant in obese people. After a year of following either restricted diet, Bacteroidetes increased and Firmicutes decreased—and the increase in Bacteroidetes correlated with the percentage of body weight lost. (Notably, the same ratio of Bacteroidetes/Firmicutes had previously been observed in obese and lean mice—obese mice had fewer Bacteroidetes and more Firmicutes than their lean siblings.)[34]

But is it the bacterial strain that's contributing to the obesity or the obesity that's altering the gut microbiota? Because the gut-brain axis works in both directions, it may be a bit of both. One study using germ-free mice further supports the connection between gut microbiota and obesity. Researchers fed germ-free mice the gut microbiota of lean and obese mice. The ones who received the "lean microbiota" gained far less fat—20 percent less—than the mice fed the "obese microbiota." The study showed that the obese microbiome (which, again, has too many Firmicutes and too little Bacteroidetes) caused the host to harvest more calories from food and store them as fat—and remarkably, that this trait is transferable.[35]

A few years later, the same group of scientists examined the gut microbiome of twins with similar weights and, when available, their mothers. They found that families had similar gut microbiome compositions and that obesity was closely associated with a lack of diversity of the gut microbiota. And once again, the obese participants had lower amounts of Bacteroidetes and an overabundance of Firmicutes, as well as a strain called Actinobacteria.[36]

Another study transplanted the gut microbiota of twins who were "discordant" for obesity, which means one twin was obese while the other had a normal BMI, into germ-free mice with no gut microbiota. Sure enough, even though all the mice were fed the same diet, only the ones that received the obese twin's gut microbiota gained weight. Researchers then housed both types of mice together so that their gut microbiota would transfer from one group to the other. (Mice, among their many questionable habits, eat each other's waste, effectively performing their own fecal transplants.) The results were very interesting. The microbiota and the weight of the lean mice remained the same, but the obese mice's microbiota began to take on the same profile as the lean mice's—and the obese mice began to lose weight. Guess which bacterial strain from the lean mice was the most successful at "invading" the obese mice? The Bacteroidetes.[37]

Do results like these mean transferring (by the method of your choice!) the gut microbiota of lean folks into overweight folks is a new weight loss method? *Theoretically* the answer is yes—though the time-honored advice of getting sufficient exercise and eating a plant-rich, high-fiber diet still stands. In the last study mentioned, researchers found that part of the reason the lean mice could, in a sense, fend off the obese microbiota is that they were fed a diet high in plant polyphenols and fiber.[38] So in addition to favorably altering your gut microbiome through probiotics, you still need to eat a healthy diet rich in fruits and vegetables.

REDUCE STRESS TO LOSE WEIGHT

There's one more gut-related weight loss tactic to consider, and this one starts with the *brain* part of the gut-brain axis. We're talking about stress management. Have you ever "soothed with food" when you're stressed out? Well that could be because your second brain is subtly suggesting you do so. Stress stimulates the gut to increase the production of ghrelin, a hormone that makes you feel hungry *and* that reduces symptoms of anxiety and depression. Ghrelin stimulates the production of dopamine, which "lights up" the reward and pleasure centers of the brain, so you get a big payoff when you eat.[39] But of course, that effect is temporary, and the health consequences of chronic overeating are extensive. Avoiding sources of stress and learning effective stress-busting techniques can prevent stress-related eating in the first place. For natural means to beat stress, see Chapter 13.

Still, the potential for weight loss by altering the gut microbiome is promising enough that MIT researchers have designed a study testing "poop pills" made from lean donors' gut microbiota in obese subjects (see "The Scoop on Poop: Fecal Transplants" on page 64). We'll have the results by early 2017. But we know already that the disproportionate ratio of Firmicutes to Bacteroidetes contributes to obesity because it inflames existing fat cells and sparks chronic inflammation, increasing the risk not just of obesity but also of insulin resistance and type 2 diabetes.[40] Further, scientists are hopeful that these new developments on healthy and unhealthy microbiota will pave the way for a new generation of probiotics that essentially perform like microbial weight managers. Until then, your best strategy to manage weight with microbes may be to take a probiotic supplement and to eat more fermented foods.

And even if science were to someday create the perfect microbial pill for weight loss, a healthy gut is just one part of an overall lifestyle that keeps weight and inflammation down and disease at bay. (We'll go into greater detail about the interaction between weight and chronic inflammation in the next chapter.) Regular moderate exercise and a diet that emphasizes fresh fruits and vegetables, healthy fats, fiber, and some lean meats and seafood is the best way to keep weight, inflammation, stress, and unhealthy bacteria down, while keeping nutrients, lean muscle, and beneficial bacteria up.

"Rebug" Your Gut

We usually think of *de*bugging as beneficial thanks to the constant presence of computers in our lives, but when it comes to a healthy gut microbiome, the more bugs the merrier. Food and beverages can alter the gut microbiome quickly, so use this fact to your advantage. Reduce items that harm the gut microbiota (such as overuse of antibiotics, artificial ingredients, high-fructose corn syrup and sugar, saturated and trans fats, and fried foods) and rebug your gut by eating a wide variety of foods and increasing probiotic-rich foods. Not only will probiotics increase your microbial diversity, they'll decrease inflammation and boost your immune system.

To supercharge your "rebugging" efforts, don't forget your *pre*biotics.

Prebiotics, those soluble fibers that aid the growth of beneficial bacteria, pass through the GI tract undigested and act like a fertilizer to your gut microbiota. They're available as supplements, but they're essentially fiber, so prebiotics can be found in fiber-rich foods, too. Some top choices on the Whole Body Cure Plan include leafy greens, onions, garlic, Jerusalem artichokes, nectarines, peaches, cashews, and pistachios. Like probiotics, there is evidence that prebiotics confer an antianxiety effect; one study found that 3 weeks of prebiotics resulted in significantly lower salivary cortisol levels, a reliable measurement of the amount of stress hormones circulating in the body.[41] Combined prebiotics and probiotics are already available in supplement form and are sometimes referred to as "synbiotics" in the marketplace.

The future of medicine may have a lot to do with personalized treatments that start at the gut level. Could it be that at some point doctors will be able to prescribe just the right eating plan for each person—based on genetics, family history of illness, metabolic profile, food sensitivities and allergies, where you live, and, who knows, changing life circumstances that affect your mood on a given day? Might this be the wave of the future for maintaining a healthy gut microbiome and whole-body health and wellness?

For now, this idea may be (mostly) entertaining speculation, but that future isn't as far off as you'd think. More long-term studies on the gut microbiome are under way, and personalized medicine is the wave of the future. Further, it's already quite easy to alter your gut microbiome and keep inflammation levels down all on your own, based on what you eat and drink and what you're exposing yourself to, whether that's antibiotics, probiotics, psychobiotics, or environmental toxins. With gut dysbiosis as the source of so many problems, it makes sense to focus the search for solutions there, too. Any long-lasting solution for chronic inflammation and long-term health may very well begin, and end, in the gut.

CHAPTER 5

Metabolic Meltdown

Weight, Diabetes, and Chronic Inflammation

When it comes to weight, many of us have been conditioned to watch the numbers on the scale rather than consider what could be going on internally when our figures change. But it turns out that adipocytes—the technical name for fat cells—are powerhouse generators of chronic inflammation. Ironically, this is the very inflammation that could be making it more difficult to shed those extra pounds. Metabolic conditions—we're talking type 2 diabetes, the constellation of conditions known as metabolic syndrome, and being overweight itself—are primary examples of the vicious cycle of chronic inflammation at work, with inflammation as both cause and consequence of carrying too much weight. If we don't intervene to put those fires out, it's not just our waistlines that will suffer. Being overweight can make us sick.

But on the bright side, when we begin to treat overweight as an inflammatory illness rather than a number to manipulate, we benefit from a whole new way of maintaining health—and a wealth of new opportunities for losing those troublesome pounds.

Those "O" Words

First up, let's discuss what the loaded terms *overweight* and *obesity* mean. These are medical terms based not on pounds or kilograms and certainly not on appearance but on a relatively simple measurement known as body mass index, which is calculated using height and weight. With just a little computation, you can calculate your own BMI, which is your weight in kilograms divided by your height squared in centimeters. Or you can save yourself some time (and possibly stress) and use any of the handy online calculators. The table below defines BMI parameters and what the medical community means by *overweight* and *obesity*, which is the convention we'll be following.

What BMI Means

18.5–24.9	Normal weight
25–29.9	Overweight
30–39.9	Obese
40 and above	Extreme obesity

Source: The National Heart, Lung, and Blood Institute[1]

To translate this into more "real-world" terms, here are a few examples of what these ranges can look like.

- **NORMAL WEIGHT:** An adult who is 5 feet 7 inches and weighs anywhere between 121 and 159 pounds; an adult who is 6 feet 3 inches and weighs between 152 and 200 pounds

- **OVERWEIGHT:** An adult who is 5 feet tall and weighs between 128 and 153 pounds; an adult who is 5 feet 11 inches and weighs between 179 and 215 pounds

- **OBESE:** An adult who is 5 feet 1 inch and weighs between 158 and 211 pounds; an adult who is 5 feet 5 inches and weighs between 180 and 240 pounds

- **EXTREME OBESITY (SOMETIMES REFERRED TO AS MORBIDLY OBESE):** An adult who is 5 feet 2 inches and weighs 220 pounds or more; an adult who is 6 feet tall and weighs 296 pounds or more

Worldwide, a BMI of 30 or above has become so common that obesity is now considered a global epidemic. Statistics from the World Health Organization indicate that as of 2014, 11 percent of men and 15 percent of women are obese, which translates to more than half a billion adults across the globe.[2] In the United States alone, nearly 69 percent of American adults are overweight or obese. Of those, more than one-third are obese, and a little more than 1 in 20 are extremely obese (6.3 percent).[3] With numbers like these, a global health crisis is upon us.

As you can see from the accompanying sidebar, obesity is one of the biggest factors contributing to *preventable* chronic disease, with annual healthcare costs in the United States ranging anywhere from $147 billion to nearly $210 billion.[4] It's difficult to determine the number of lives overweight and obesity claim per year, but we do know that according to 2015 statistics, heart disease, stroke, and diabetes together accounted for nearly 824,000 deaths in the United States.[5]

Now, just in case you hadn't noticed, every condition listed in that sidebar has a strong inflammatory component. Like being overweight itself,

WEIGHT-RELATED CONDITIONS

The health complications that come with being overweight or obese are well known but worth reviewing, if only in brief. They include, but aren't limited to, a greater risk of any of the following conditions.

Arthritis	Heart disease
Asthma	High blood pressure
Certain types of cancer (including breast, esophageal, endometrial, gallbladder, prostate, liver, ovarian, pancreatic, thyroid, and colon cancers)	High cholesterol
	Infertility
	Kidney stones
	Metabolic syndrome
Dementia	Nonalcoholic and alcoholic fatty liver disease
Depression	Osteoporosis
Diabetes	Premature death
Fibromyalgia	Sleep disorders
Gallbladder disease	Stroke
Gastrointestinal disorders	

obesity-related illnesses are inflammatory conditions that are *caused* in part by chronic inflammation, and they all *cause* further inflammation.

But recognizing their strong inflammatory component gives us a powerful tool for prevention, or for reversing the severity of these illnesses if they're already present. In many cases, full recovery is possible. What *is* entirely possible is to step in and interrupt that vicious cycle before you pay the price a high BMI will demand sooner or later. To better understand this opportunity, let's turn back the clock, well before illness sets in, and see how carrying extra pounds jump-starts inflammation and then keeps the heat turned up until you get sick.

Red-Hot-Burning Fat Cells

If you turn the clock *all* the way back—to when a person first starts putting on weight—you'll find something very revealing going on at a cellular level. When fat cells first start to accumulate, guess what happens? The inflammatory army rushes to the scene. Homeostasis has been disturbed, and the body responds to the uptick in fat cells as a threat. Standard operating procedure is for the immune system to send macrophages to the scene of the crime. These white blood cells, whose name literally means "big eaters," defend the body and restore homeostasis by engulfing threatening invaders, which in this case are fat cells. And if the extra fat cells remain, and certainly if more accumulate, more macrophages rush to the scene. In fact, up to 50 percent of the cells present in adipose tissue are actually macrophages, which contribute to and perpetuate the inflammatory nature of fat.

Once those fat-fueled fires get going, it's difficult to put them out because eventually those same inflammation-fighting macrophages accumulate and then transform into a subtype that is highly inflammatory. Technically known as M1 macrophages, these inflammation-promoters are associated with obesity and insulin resistance. And as you might well expect given your emerging familiarity with the pattern of inflammation, as weight increases, so does the production of M1 macrophages, further compounding the problem.[6]

So to review, we've got macrophages kicking off *and* perpetuating the inflammatory nature of fat. Then, in true metabolic meltdown fashion, if the extra weight sticks around, and certainly if it continues to climb, it can lead to other metabolic problems, including insulin resistance, which is the warm-up act for type 2 diabetes. Insulin, a hormone made by the pancreas, enables cells to use glucose (sugar) for energy. When insulin resistance sets in, your body can't respond to insulin as it should, which means cells can't absorb the glucose that's essential for proper function and your blood sugar level remains abnormally high. You can see where we're headed already: Being overweight leads to insulin resistance and significantly increases your chances of developing type 2 diabetes. We'll look at both forms of metabolic meltdown in more detail below.

We used to think that fat cells were merely storehouses for fat, but this type of tissue is so active and so influential in so many physiological functions that it's considered an endocrine organ in its own right. Fat cells pump out a long list of substances, including several proinflammatory cytokines and chemokines (a special type of cytokine involved in cell movement). Together, the cytokines and chemokines secreted from fat cells are known as *adipokines*. Because they act like hormones, adipokines play a huge role in many physiological functions, including homeostasis maintenance, reproduction/fertility, blood pressure regulation, energy use and storage, and the immune response. Adipokines can have proinflammatory or anti-inflammatory effects, just like regular cytokines. In people with a normal BMI, we see a balance of pro- and anti-inflammatory adipokines. But as weight climbs, the balance shifts to proinflammatory, and eventually more fat cells secreting increasing levels of proinflammatory adipokines accumulate.[7] Right here on the cellular level, we see the dangerous cycle set into motion!

This inflammatory cycle that occurs in our cells also explains another troubling aspect to weight gain. Have you ever noticed that once the first 5 unwanted pounds show up, it seems like 10 quickly follow? Well that, too, has something to do with the process of inflammation. Two adipokines called *leptin* and *adiponectin* are involved. Leptin is the "satiety hormone" that inhibits hunger. But once obesity sets in a funny thing happens: Leptin resistance sets in, too. When leptin isn't as effective as it should be, the usual cues to stop eating are blunted, and you're likely to eat more.

There's that vicious cycle, with leptin resistance, increased eating, and weight gain escalating and mutually reinforcing each other. And just as with the proinflammatory M1 macrophages we talked about earlier, the more weight you gain, the more leptin your fat cells produce, which only increases your body's resistance to leptin. As if all this isn't bad enough, leptin also helps produce proinflammatory cytokines. Perhaps it isn't a surprise, then, that several studies have noted that the higher the leptin, the worse the severity of certain diseases, including osteoarthritis, multiple sclerosis, atherosclerosis, and nonalcoholic fatty liver disease.[8]

NOT SO OBVIOUS
WEIGHT LOSS TIPS

The basics of weight loss are tried and true, and they remain the most effective means to get to and maintain a healthy BMI. Don't overeat, don't smoke, be very stingy with sugar, and try to exercise and eat a mostly plant-based diet. But here are a few less obvious tips that can help keep the pounds off for the long term.

- **Get involved in dinner planning and preparation.** Restaurant meals tend to be loaded with extra calories, sodium, saturated fats, and sugars. A traditional eating pattern like the Mediterranean diet makes weight loss and maintenance easier by using fresh ingredients and relying on spices, herbs, and olive oil for additional flavor. A recent study compared 361 people who lost 10 percent or more of their body weight and either kept the pounds off for more than a year or regained them. The "maintainers" ate a Mediterranean-style diet featuring mainly unprocessed grains, fruit, vegetables, olive oil, and low-fat dairy, whereas the "regainers" went back to old eating habits. Men who kept the weight off were more likely to exercise, eat at home, and be involved in meal preparation. For women, eating more slowly and eating smaller, more frequent meals also helped.[10]

- **Enhance the social factor.** A meta-analysis of 27 studies revealed that people who joined weight loss programs featuring supervised attendance and social support were far more likely to stick with their programs and lose the weight (65 percent stayed on track!) than those who chose other methods, such as education, self-monitoring, or individual diet or exercise

Adiponectin, on the other hand, is an anti-inflammatory adipokine that can reverse insulin resistance. You want your adiponectin levels to rise or at least remain steady. Unfortunately, adiponectin *decreases* in response to weight gain, oxidative stress, and the presence of metabolic syndrome or type 2 diabetes. (It also decreases if you smoke.) What are effective ways to boost your adiponectin levels? Number one, lose weight. Adiponectin naturally rises as the pounds come off.[9] Other all-natural adiponectin boosters are exercise, eating high-fiber foods, and eating more omega-3 fatty acids. A metareview of 52 studies found that consuming omega-3s (either through daily consumption of fish or a supplement) increased adiponectin by up to 60 percent. Further, boosting fiber raised levels by up to 115 percent. People who lost

---

regimens. Social support and accountability are powerful factors for behavioral change.[11] Several of our test panelists found that following the Whole Body Cure wellness plan with a friend or spouse helped them stay focused, accountable, and encouraged.

- **Get more sleep.** Many studies have found that insufficient sleep contributes to weight gain. On the other hand, sufficient sleep time and good sleep quality are associated with greater fat loss, greater success at weight loss, fewer cravings for sweet and salty foods, and slower gains in fat mass over time. Seven to 8 hours is the optimal time for most adults.[12]

- **Eat breakfast.** In a study of 388 adults who lost an average of nearly 40 pounds and kept the pounds off for more than 2 years, one of the most frequently cited weight loss and maintenance tactics was to eat breakfast. This is hardly the first study that has found that breakfast helps with weight loss, as skipping breakfast is detrimental for insulin sensitivity and encourages binge-eating later in the day. The other top tactics were keeping healthy foods at home and consuming vegetables regularly.[13] Again, our panelists concurred: Many recommended keeping a supply of healthy snacks at home. Some of the top choices were roasted carrots, roasted asparagus, fresh tomatoes, kale chips, and avocado.

- **Blog about it.** Nearly 200 people who began blogging about their weight loss efforts lost an average of 42.3 pounds since launching their blogs. The longer a person blogged, the greater his or her weight loss tended to be. Most attributed their weight loss success to the sense of community and accountability they gained from the blogosphere.[14]

weight through diet and exercise saw their adiponectin levels rise in the range of 18 to 48 percent.[15]

The Flames Grow Hotter: Insulin Resistance and Type 2 Diabetes

Here's where we must discuss what happens if we *don't* lose weight and if chronic, low-grade inflammation is left unaddressed. The news is stark, but it's also worth pointing out that the outcome is as preventable as it is predictable.

The number-one cause of type 2 diabetes (T2D) is being overweight. Your risk of developing T2D increases sevenfold if you're overweight (a BMI of 25 to 29.9), and a BMI of 30 and above makes you 20 to 40 times more likely to develop T2D than someone with a normal BMI.[16] The World Health Organization estimates that in 2012 diabetes was the direct cause of 1.5 million deaths. By 2030, it's expected to be the seventh leading cause of death.[17] T2D is especially tragic because it's so avoidable. Some sources estimate that 9 out of 10 cases could be prevented with simple lifestyle habits that emphasize exercise and a healthy diet.

We'll look at some ways to manage weight and prevent T2D below, but first, let's start with some diabetes basics. There are two main types of diabetes mellitus, both of which cause blood glucose to rise to unhealthy levels. Type 1 is an autoimmune condition usually diagnosed in children and adolescents, and it comprises no more than 10 percent of diabetes cases. In type 1 diabetes, the pancreas produces very little or no insulin, the hormone that converts sugar into energy. With T2D, the body produces insulin, but muscle, liver, and fat cells can't respond to insulin properly and thus can't absorb glucose from the bloodstream. This condition is known as *insulin resistance*, and it's a precursor to full-blown T2D.

As we've seen, the number-one cause of T2D is being overweight. Other risk factors include a family history of diabetes, lack of exercise, abnormal cholesterol or triglyceride levels, and smoking. T2D is also associated with an increased risk of many serious health conditions—including heart disease, stroke, neuropathy (nerve dysfunction that causes pain and weakness), blindness, and kidney failure—as well as increased risk of infection. In fact, diabetes is the leading cause of blindness and kidney failure in adults.[18]

Excess weight and not exercising are also closely linked with two precursors to T2D, prediabetes and metabolic syndrome. Prediabetes means your blood glucose level is above the normal range, but it's not high enough to warrant a clinical diagnosis of diabetes. Metabolic syndrome is a group of health conditions associated with obesity. It's diagnosed if three or more of the following conditions are present: insulin resistance, excess levels of insulin, impaired glucose tolerance, high cholesterol, high triglycerides, a tendency of the blood to clot too much, high blood pressure, and obesity itself, particularly if excess fat is stored in the belly area, which is even more inflammatory than fat found just under the skin.

Ready for the good news now? Both prediabetes and metabolic syndrome can be reversed. Two of the most effective ways to prevent T2D are losing 10 percent or more of your current body weight and getting at least half an hour of moderate exercise per day. Losing that 10 percent within 6 months of a prediabetes diagnosis dramatically decreases the odds of developing T2D— by as much as 85 percent over the next 3 years. These results are based on a study of adults with prediabetes who lost 10 percent or more of their body weight through diet and exercising at least 150 minutes per week. People who lost 5 to 7 percent of their weight reduced their T2D risk by 54 percent.[19] That 150 minutes of weekly exercise has also been shown to lower insulin resistance and increase insulin sensitivity, regardless of metabolic profile—this applies to people with diabetes, prediabetes, or normal glucose levels.[20]

Better yet, of course, is to avoid weight gain in the first place. The same simple lifestyle measures of regular exercise, not smoking, and eating well are enormously influential. A study of nearly 34,000 people found that the Mediterranean diet, which is anti-inflammatory and strongly associated with heart health and a healthy BMI, is a primary method for preventing metabolic syndrome.[21]

The Whole Body Cure Eating Plan is also based on an overall healthy eating pattern, but it begins with a 2-week elimination period that quickly extinguishes the fires of any existing inflammation and gives you the fresh start needed to regain whole-body health and keep the pounds off permanently. It also helps you identify exactly which foods could be sparking inflammation in your body. Many of our panelists hadn't realized that a particular food was causing their fatigue, brain fog, or GI problems until the eating plan revealed their food sensitivities.

You can also, of course, take measures to reduce inflammation, as both overweight and T2D are inflammatory illnesses. Overeating—when the number of calories consumed exceeds the number of calories the body actually needs—results in a spike in inflammation and compromised glycemic control. In a study of nearly 200 adults with type 2 diabetes, overeating was found to raise hs-CRP and HbA1c levels. High-sensitivity C-reactive protein, you'll remember, is a classic biomarker of systemic inflammation, and HbA1c is a measure of glycated hemoglobin, which can give your doctors a good sense of the stability of your glucose levels over a period of several months. Researchers also found a significant association between overeating and waist circumference, percentage of overall body fat, and the amount of belly fat present. All of these metabolic changes are associated with chronic inflammation and poor blood sugar control.[22]

Now, remember those proinflammatory M1 macrophages that accumulate

Dr. Kirshner's Inflammation Insight

Tom wasn't even a patient of mine. His wife was seeing me for some metabolic issues, and Tom decided to follow the anti-inflammatory eating plan, as well, in support of her. Tom suffered from diabetes and was on four different medications to regulate his blood sugar. When I met him, he had an HbA1c of 8.9 and a fasting blood glucose of 180—and this was while he was on his medications! Two months into following the eating plan, his morning blood sugar had dropped to 70, which was an indication of hypoglycemia, or low blood sugar. With his doctor's recommendation, he cut back on his diabetes medications, and within 4 months, he was off *all* blood sugar medication. His HbA1c dropped to 5.6 and his unmedicated morning glucose was a steady 85 to 95. These results occurred by simply adopting an anti-inflammatory way of eating.

in fat cells and how the adipokines they produce drive up inflammation? Left unchecked, this type of inflammation leads directly to insulin resistance in the liver, muscles, and adipose tissue, and it damages the beta cells in the pancreas that store and release insulin. All of these effects pave the way for prediabetes and eventually full-blown T2D. But that's not all. If and when T2D does set in, these proinflammatory macrophages also contribute to many of the hallmark complications of T2D, including nerve damage, kidney disease, heart disease, and blindness.[23] All of which provides overwhelming motivation to reduce inflammation before it ever gets out of control!

Again, the most effective means to avoid fat-fueled inflammation and its myriad consequences, including prediabetes, metabolic syndrome, and T2D, is to avoid gaining weight in the first place. We know—easier said than done for most of us! If you're already carrying extra weight, the most effective means to prevent a "metabolic meltdown" is to lose weight because less body fat means less inflammation. It's as simple as that. Once again, however, we know this is easier said than done. Be sure and check out our food tips at the end of the chapter to help you lose weight.

But before we plunge ahead, let's consider one more way to cool down fat-generated inflammation—the gut. Gut microbiome dysbiosis—the imbalance that occurs when gut bacteria lack diversity and/or are out of balance—is closely associated with obesity, obesity-related inflammation, and T2D. Thus far, the evidence doesn't suggest that an unhealthy gut microbiome *causes* obesity. But it certainly plays a role. As you'll remember from the previous chapter, the "obese microbiome" is characterized by an overabundance of the bacterial strain Firmicutes and an underrepresentation of Bacteroidetes. (The converse is true: Lean people tend to have more Bacteroidetes and fewer Firmicutes.)[24] Changes to the gut microbiota can happen quickly through what we eat. In one particular study, the gut microbiota of men who were put on a high-calorie diet shifted toward the "obese microbiome" within 3 days—marked by a 20 percent increase in Firmicutes and a 20 percent decrease in Bacteroidetes.[25]

Now consider these gut microbiome changes that can occur in a handful of days and multiply them by months or years of eating a high-fat diet. A steady unhealthy diet, especially if it's high in saturated and/or trans fats, leaves your gut inflamed and your gut microbiome in a regular state of dysbiosis. Beneficial bacteria, like Bacteroidetes and bifidobacteria, decrease in response to a high-fat diet, while strains linked to obesity, such as Firmicutes and Proteobacteria, proliferate. A high-fat diet also increases fat-containing molecules called lipopolysaccharides (LPSs), which are found in the cell membranes of harmful bacteria like *Escherichia coli*. LPSs are no friend to your metabolic health. Once they pour into the bloodstream, they elicit a strong inflammatory response, and they increase oxidative stress, which plays a role in heart disease and cancer. This proinflammatory and prooxidant state is called *metabolic endotoxemia*, and it causes weight gain and insulin resistance.[26] Not surprisingly, LPSs have also been closely linked with type 2 diabetes. In a nutshell, this is the link between a high-fat diet, gut microbiota, inflammation, and insulin resistance, which, if unaddressed, progresses to T2D.

A long-term high-fat diet is also associated with increased intestinal permeability, commonly referred to as leaky gut syndrome. In simplest terms, when the intestine is trying to absorb fat, a temporary injury occurs. You read that correctly—fat absorption injures the intestines, and as you know, any injury provokes the inflammatory response. Though the intestine repairs itself rather quickly, a *steady* high-fat diet will cause repeated injury and can leave the gut barrier regularly compromised. When the gut is "leaky" or thinner than it should be, larger molecules can pass through into the body, including those harmful LPSs we just mentioned. When LPSs pass into the bloodstream, they not only provoke the inflammatory response but also interfere with proper insulin signaling. Elevated blood levels of LPSs have been associated with obesity, T2D, heart disease, and nonalcoholic fatty liver disease.[27]

But the bright side of all this is that positive effects on the microbiome—essentially any measures that preserve or increase bacterial diversity and keep those bacterial strains in balance—have the opposite effect. Unless you want to go the way of the fecal transplant (see the sidebar on page 64), the most palatable means we have of maintaining a healthy gut microbiome—and to enjoy the incredible array of health benefits associated with a healthy gut—is to eat a diverse, plant-based, fiber-rich diet that's rich in probiotics and prebiotics. As mentioned in the previous chapter, probiotics are live organisms that offer benefit to the host, and prebiotics are indigestible fibers that help the probiotics to flourish. Think of prebiotics as fertilizer for the "lawn" of probiotics you want to grow.

Increasing the number of healthy bifidobacteria, for instance, lowers LPS levels, helps heal leaky gut, and prevents metabolic endotoxemia from occurring.[28] Several studies have found that the *Bifidobacterium* and *Lactobacillus* bacterial strains exert several benefits, including an improvement in glucose tolerance, a decline in chronic gut inflammation, a reduction in the amount of fat found deep in the belly, and ultimately weight loss.[29] In one study, subjects with a BMI of between 24.2 and 30.7 (technically overweight people) drank a fermented milk drink containing *Lactobacillus gasseri* or one without *L. gasseri* every day for 12 weeks. In the *L. gasseri* group, belly fat as well as other types of body fat decreased by an average of 4.6 percent, and body weight, BMI, and waist and hip circumference also decreased significantly. The group that did not receive the probiotic drink experienced no significant reductions in any of these same measurements.[30] Another study on *L. gasseri* found that obese adults who added this strain of bacteria to their diets lost an average of more than 8 percent of belly fat over 12 weeks. Regular consumption is needed to maintain these effects.[31]

All of these bacterial strains are common ingredients in probiotic supplements, yogurts with active live cultures, kefir, and other fermented foods, such as tempeh, kimchi, sauerkraut, miso soup, pickles, olives, and natto.

To further stimulate probiotics growth, add a prebiotic like oligofructose,[32] which is available as a prebiotic supplement and can be found in many plant-based foods, including Jerusalem artichoke, chicory and other leafy greens, garlic, onions, nectarines, peaches, cashews, and pistachios. It's not the only prebiotic with positive metabolic effects, though. Alpha-galacto-oligosaccharide, a prebiotic derived from legumes (and also available as a supplement) can reduce appetite, food intake, and inflammation.[33]

All in all, diet has an inestimable impact on any metabolic condition. And this is very good news for us, because that means we have the power to intervene at any point before T2D sets in—from initial weight gain to prediabetes to metabolic syndrome—to better manage our weight and keep our gut microbiota diverse and balanced. Fortunately, healthy eating habits accomplish

(continued on page 97)

Haunani Kekuna

My Transformation

AGE: 65

- Reduced blood sugar 22 points to normal level
- Sed rate lowered 12 points to normal range
- Joint pain relieved
- WEIGHT LOST: 15 pounds
- INCHES LOST: 6½

I have several health conditions—overweight, high blood pressure, hypothyroidism, hyperlipidemia, prediabetes, and psoriasis with the resulting psoriatic arthritis—so I was very interested in making some changes. I had been in an online weight loss program for 2 months and had already lost 12.2 pounds before I switched over to the Whole Body Cure Plan. On this plan, I lost another 15 pounds and 6½ inches, and my triglycerides went down 35 points.

While I'm pleased with the weight loss, what I'm ecstatic about is the change in my HbA1C level. Diabetes runs in my family, and as I'm prediabetic, my doctor has been testing my blood glucose level twice a year for the past 15 years. It has *never*, not even once, been in the normal range, which is 5.7 or lower. But at the end of this plan, it was

5.3! This is all the confirmation I need to know that I have to keep doing this. I can't wait to visit my doctor again and see his reaction and see if he'll adjust my medications accordingly.

The most difficult part of the plan for me was the elimination period. My husband and I walk, and we go to the gym three times a week. During those first 2 weeks, I felt fatigued after a workout, which was unusual for me, and I experienced a bit of minor brain fog, as well. But the detox period is the only way you'll know if you have any food sensitivities, and to what degree.

During the next 10 weeks as we reintroduced new foods, I didn't have any noticeable reactions, and since the program ended, I've reintroduced other foods, like dairy, grains, and legumes, without a problem. But I have chosen to limit those foods. I've mostly eliminated

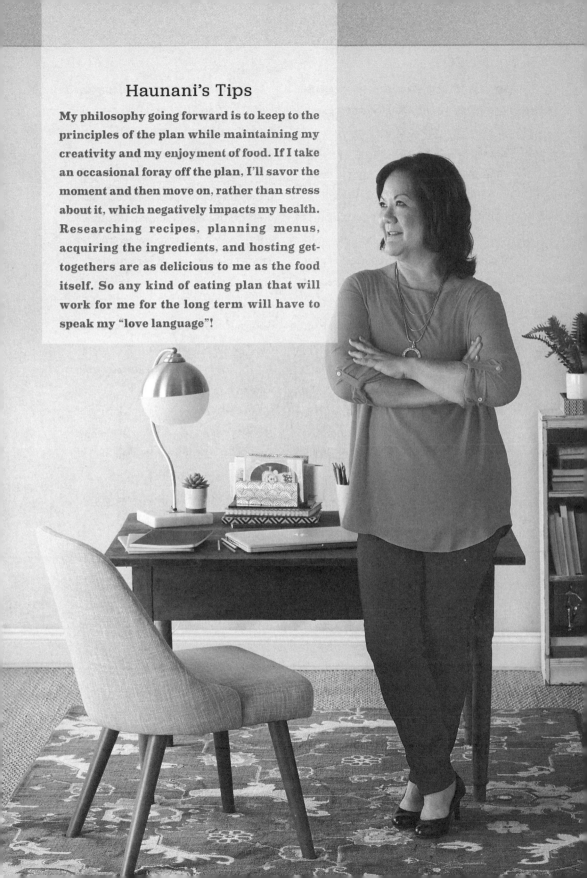

Haunani's Tips

My philosophy going forward is to keep to the principles of the plan while maintaining my creativity and my enjoyment of food. If I take an occasional foray off the plan, I'll savor the moment and then move on, rather than stress about it, which negatively impacts my health. Researching recipes, planning menus, acquiring the ingredients, and hosting get-togethers are as delicious to me as the food itself. So any kind of eating plan that will work for me for the long term will have to speak my "love language"!

dairy, and if I do have cheese, it will be a hard cheese. And though I didn't exhibit any sensitivities to grains or gluten, I've decided to go gluten-free and to eliminate grains—with one exception. I will continue to eat rice. I choose rice because I'm Asian and it's a huge part of our culinary and cultural tradition, and it allows me to have some noodles. I am also limiting my sugar intake and have eliminated refined sugar completely.

Knowing what to eliminate and what to incorporate, and in the right amounts, is still an evolving process for me. I've learned so much more about what foods work for me and why, and I'm able to make conscious choices for Haunani, rather than follow a one-size-fits-all diet. I love that I've learned to pause and think about conscious choices for my body.

I've known for a long time that food is my love language and that I eat with far more than my taste buds. Things like color, texture, and aroma are important to me, and I love any kind of family dinner or special holiday meal. I drew on this insight during the program. Even if it was a simple green salad, I played around with plating and texture and color. Any time I could I'd change a basic recipe and give it a different character. For example, I took a butternut squash soup and made it a Thai curry butternut squash soup. When I had an abundance of zucchini, I made cold or hot zucchini soup. Then if I got a hunger pang, I had half a cup of soup for a snack. I made sure meals were never repetitive or boring, which kept me interested and motivated. ■

these goals simultaneously. Paired with other simple lifestyle habits like regular moderate exercise, not smoking, and most of all, maintaining a healthy BMI, we have the means to stop one of the world's leading causes of death.

What You Gain by Losing Weight

Stories from people who've lost substantial pounds are remarkably consistent: They report having more energy, more mobility, less fatigue, better sleep, and an overall better outlook and quality of life. Many people find that they can quite literally breathe easier (and snore less), that their brain fog clears, and that their joint pain decreases; others find that their doctors say they can safely cut back on or even cease certain medications to control high cholesterol, high blood pressure, arthritis, and diabetes.

But what about clinical and laboratory results? Take a look at what some of the latest evidence reveals about weight loss gains.

- **YOUR LEVEL OF CHRONIC, LOW-GRADE INFLAMMATION FALLS.**
  A metareview of 33 studies found a clear relationship between weight loss and CRP levels: The greater the weight loss, the greater the drop in CRP. Based on an average of all the data, researchers found that for every 2 pounds lost, CRP fell by 0.13 mg/l.[34] (Normal rates are below 3 mg/l.)

- **YOUR RISK OF TYPE 2 DIABETES PLUMMETS.** Body weight loss of just 5 percent improves insulin sensitivity in multiple organ systems simultaneously, including adipose tissue, liver, and muscle. It also improves the function of beta cells, which store and release insulin.[35]

- **YOUR RISK OF HEART DISEASE DECREASES.** A metareview of studies based on data from nearly 9,000 people who lost an average of about 8.5 pounds found that average systolic blood pressure fell by 4.29 mmHg and diastolic pressure by 2.56 mmHg. Total cholesterol dropped more than 5 points, while beneficial HDL cholesterol rose. Fasting blood glucose and glycated hemoglobin (the HbA1c level, used to monitor prediabetes progression) fell, as well.[36] Even modest weight loss pays off big. A study of 401 overweight people who lost just 5 to 10 percent of their body weight showed they experienced significant improvements in triglycerides, total cholesterol, and LDL cholesterol. For patients who lost more than 10 percent, the heart-healthy effects were even greater.[37]

- **YOU'LL SLEEP BETTER.** The National Weight Control Registry (NWCR) is a database of adults who've lost at least 30 pounds and kept it off for a year or more. A survey of 690 NWCR members reported that after their weight loss, they took less time to fall asleep, stayed asleep longer, and had better sleep quality overall.[38]

- **YOU'LL REDUCE YOUR RISK OF CANCER.** Many studies have found that losing weight lowers the risk of cancer. In particular, a healthy weight protects against cancer of the breast, colon, esophagus, stomach, rectum, pancreas, ovaries, liver, prostate, endometrium, gallbladder, and kidneys.[39]

- **YOU MAY EXPERIENCE A BRAIN BOOST.** A study of 75 adults with mild cognitive impairment found that losing weight was associated with improved verbal memory and fluency. These impressive results came with an average weight loss of just 4 pounds.[40] What's more, there is such a strong association between being overweight and Alzheimer's disease that Alzheimer's has been referred to by some experts as "type 3 diabetes." A landmark study based on nearly 1,400 people who were followed an average of almost 14 years found that every unit of increase in BMI at age 50 and above predicts an earlier Alzheimer's onset of 6.7 months. Conversely, a healthy BMI at midlife protects cognitive function and may delay the onset of Alzheimer's disease.[41]

- **YOUR MOOD MAY IMPROVE.** A study of 588 overweight volunteers assigned to a weight loss program for 12 months found that weight loss was associated with lower levels of anxiety and depression and higher levels of self-control, vitality, and overall well-being. Weight loss didn't need to be drastic for these psychological gains: The volunteers in this study lost an average of just 5 pounds.[42]

The Metabolic 5 and 10

Losing just 5 to 10 percent of your current body weight results in huge gains. Here are a "5 and 10" worst and best lists of foods that pack a *double* punch either for or against metabolic health. First up, the worst foods for raising pounds *and* inflammation, followed by the foods that offer the very best weight loss and anti-inflammatory benefits. You'll tame the fires of inflammation *and* supercharge your weight loss efforts if you avoid inflammatory foods and plan your meals around these "best of" foods.

Foods That Increase Inflammation and Promote Weight Gain

1. **SUGAR.** Sugary foods and drinks pack a double punch when it comes to weight gain and systemic inflammation. Top offenders are items like prepackaged desserts, bakery items, frozen meals, breakfast cereals, sodas, and energy drinks. Diets high in refined sugars are known to drive up both weight and proinflammatory cytokine levels.[43] Large metareviews on the effect of sugar intake and weight yield predictable results—reducing sugar intake results in weight loss, while increasing sugar intake results in weight gain. Based on one metareview, which combined results of 68 studies, reducing sugar resulted in an average weight loss of 1.8 pounds, while increased sugar intake resulted in weight gain of 1.7 pounds.[44]

2. **RED MEAT.** A recent study indicated that meat protein has played as prominent a role in the worldwide obesity epidemic as sugar. Meat protein is digested more slowly than fats and carbohydrates, so the excess calories are stored as fat.[45] We know that red meat spikes levels of homocysteine, an inflammatory biomarker that's a risk factor for heart disease, and triggers the production of harmful lipopolysaccharides. The most inflammatory meat of all? Processed red meats, like pastrami, corned beef, hot dogs, and sausage. Red

meat *can* be eaten in small amounts (the American Institute for Cancer Research recommends that you eat no more than 18 ounces per week),[46] and we strongly recommend grass-fed, organic meat. Grass-fed animals aren't raised with food that's been treated with pesticides, fertilizers, and other chemicals, and they tend not to have been treated with antibiotics and other drugs that can be passed on to consumers. Meat from grass-fed animals also tends to have lower saturated fat and cholesterol than conventional meat.

3. **REFINED CARBOHYDRATES.** Grains of any sort elicit an inflammatory response, but as this is a "worst of" list, we can't help but put most of the blame on refined carbohydrates. These products are made with grains that have had all their nutritional value stripped away, offering nothing but empty calories. Refined grain intake has been associated with a rise in an inflammatory protein called PAI-1, which is associated with T2D. Examples of refined grains include white bread, flour and corn tortillas, bakery items (scones, pastries, etc.), and prepared foods such as pizza and burritos.[47] Other sources of refined grains include white flour, white pasta, and many breakfast cereals and prepackaged snack foods.

4. **SATURATED AND TRANS FATS.** We've seen already how high-fat diets drive up inflammation, increase weight gain, and cause a leaky gut. The worst offenders are saturated fats found in red meat and full-fat dairy products, and trans fats, which, in addition to the above effects, are known to increase LDL cholesterol while decreasing healthy HDL cholesterol. Both types of fats also impair glucose tolerance, and worsen insulin resistance and nonalcoholic fatty liver disease.[48]

5. **OMEGA-6 FATTY ACIDS.** While omega-3 fatty acids (see opposite) are anti-inflammatory, omega-6s are proinflammatory. Over the past few decades, the consumption of omega-6s—found in vegetable oils such as sunflower, safflower, and corn—has increased in industrialized countries, while consumption of omega-3s has declined. The optimal ratio of omega-6 to omega-3 should be

anywhere from 1:1 to 4:1, but currently it's in the range of 10:1 to 20:1. Some experts have linked this imbalanced ratio with the rise in inflammatory illnesses such as obesity, T2D, cardiovascular disease, inflammatory bowel disease, Alzheimer's disease, and cancer.[49] Practical ways to reduce your omega-6 intake include switching your cooking and salad dressing oils to healthy, anti-inflammatory oils and avoiding deep-fried and processed foods. The Whole Body Cure Plan encourages the use of extra-virgin olive oil, coconut oil, grape-seed oil, avocado oil, flaxseed oil, and fish oil.

Best Foods for Weight Loss and Lowering Inflammation

1. **OMEGA-3 FATTY ACIDS.** The fats in fish such as salmon, mackerel, tuna, and sardines and in plant sources such as walnuts and flaxseeds are healthy omega-3 polyunsaturated fatty acids, which provide a strong anti-inflammatory effect. Omega-3s can improve obesity-associated metabolic syndrome factors such as insulin resistance, hypertension, and dyslipidemia by reducing triglycerides, a type of fat found in the blood. And their anti-inflammatory and antihypertensive effects can help protect against heart disease.[50] To boost omega-3s, try any of the fish mentioned above (any cooking method except fried is okay); enjoy an ounce (about a handful) of walnuts as a snack; try making salad dressings with flaxseed oil; add ground flaxseeds to any breakfast cereal, cold or hot; or sprinkle flaxseeds on salads or use them as a substitute for bread crumbs in cooking.

2. **OLIVE OIL.** Here is another healthy fat, this time of the monounsaturated variety. Olive oil polyphenols have well-documented anti-inflammatory and antioxidant effects, and they're now emerging as an effective antidiabetic strategy. A 22-year study of over 145,000 women found that substituting olive oil for margarine, butter, or mayonnaise was associated with a

5 percent, 8 percent, and 15 percent lower risk of T2D, respectively.[51] A small study of overweight patients with T2D found that the daily consumption of extra-virgin olive oil for 4 weeks resulted in lower fasting glucose levels, lower glycated hemoglobin levels, lower circulating inflammatory adipokine levels—and lower weight.[52]

3. **NUTS.** Once again, a healthy fat makes all the difference. People who regularly eat nuts tend to have significantly lower weight, BMI, and belly fat than people who say no to nuts—and their heart disease risk factors, including CRP levels, are much lower, too.[53] It seems pistachios have special anti-inflammatory and antidiabetic effects. In one study people with diabetes who snacked on about an ounce of pistachios twice a day experienced a decrease in HbA1c, fasting blood glucose concentrations, systolic blood pressure, BMI, and CRP levels.[54] And in another study, those who ate about 2 ounces of pistachios a day experienced improvements in fasting glucose, insulin resistance, LDL cholesterol, and markers of inflammation.[55]

4. **TART CHERRIES.** High in anthocyanins and other plant chemicals that act as antioxidants and anti-inflammatories, tart cherries and tart cherry juice are known arthritis-fighters. They've been shown to reduce inflammation and oxidative stress, and they can alleviate muscle soreness. They've also been shown to prevent muscle damage for those engaged in rigorous exercise.[56]

5. **PROBIOTIC-RICH FOODS.** As we've already covered the many benefits of probiotics in this chapter and the previous one, here we'll focus on some of the latest findings on one particular bacterial strain, the very common *Lactobacillus*. There are many types of *Lactobacillus*, and it's commonly taken in supplement form to treat a variety of disorders, from GI complaints to yeast infections to canker sores. Now research has shown that *Lactobacillus* provides a host of additional benefits: It can reduce reactive oxygen production, improve gastrointestinal barrier function (i.e., help heal leaky gut), reduce inflammation, and

even provide protection against pesticide exposure by preventing its absorption,[57] making this "friendly" bacteria an anti-inflammatory powerhouse. In addition to supplements, *Lactobacillus* bacteria can be found in pickles, olives, probiotic yogurts, and in especially high concentrations in sauerkraut, which contains lots of vitamin C and virtually no calories.

6. **BERRIES.** A long-term study of over 2,330 men found that berries could protect against the development of T2D by as much as 35 percent.[58] In the short term, eating strawberries increases antioxidant capacity, lowers circulating inflammatory markers, and improves glycemic response after eating. Long-term consumption of strawberries is associated with an improved lipid profile and a reduction of chronic inflammation.[59]

7. **CRUCIFEROUS VEGETABLES.** Known for their anticancer effects, vegetables like broccoli, cauliflower, bok choy, Brussels sprouts, cabbage, and kale have been shown to lower circulating proinflammatory markers, including IL-6 and TNF-α.[60] These vitamin-packed veggies are a time-honored weight loss food, with their high content of fiber and water to help you feel full faster and very low calories.

8. **GREEN TEA.** Numerous studies have demonstrated green tea's anti-inflammatory effects; most of the credit goes to its main polyphenol, epigallocatechin gallate. An analysis based on data from many studies that collectively involved over half a million people found that drinking two cups of tea a day was associated with a 4.6 percent lower risk of type 2 diabetes.[61] Caffeinated green tea plays a special role in counteracting the decrease in metabolic rate that occurs with weight loss—and keeping the weight off once you lose it.[62]

9. **TOMATOES.** Women who ate a raw, ripe tomato every day before lunch for 4 weeks lost an average of more than 2 pounds by the end of the study. Moreover, their body fat decreased by an average of 1.54 percent, and their fasting blood glucose, triglycerides, total

cholesterol, and uric acid levels all decreased, as well.[63] Eating tomatoes can even protect us from some of the negative effects of a high-fat diet. Researchers compared groups who ate a high-fat meal containing a tomato product or a nontomato alternative. They found that tomato significantly prevented the LDL cholesterol oxidation that comes from a high-fat meal and reduced IL-6.[64]

10. **TURMERIC.** No anti-inflammatory list is complete without mentioning turmeric, which is a superfood if there ever was one. Tens of thousands of studies confirm that turmeric and its main compound, curcumin, together make up one of the most powerful anti-inflammatories Mother Nature offers. Whether it's cancer, diabetes, arthritis, high cholesterol, fibromyalgia, asthma, cardiovascular disease, chronic kidney disease, psoriasis, weight management, or even leprosy, turmeric has been shown to play a healing role. Now a new study has revealed why curcumin plays a powerful role in weight loss: It helps to speed up body metabolism and the breakdown of fats.[65]

Turn Down the Heat on Weight and Inflammation

The worldwide epidemic of overweight and obesity constitutes a true public health crisis, with devastating physical, mental, emotional, social, and economic repercussions. But understanding that overweight and obesity are inflammatory conditions provides us with new possibilities for weight loss and for preventing "metabolic meltdown" issues like insulin resistance, metabolic syndrome, and even type 2 diabetes. Given the vicious inflammatory cycle adipose tissue perpetuates, one way to lose the fat that's fueling inflammation is to lose the inflammation fueling the fat.

To effectively break the inflammation cycle, manage weight, improve your metabolic profile, and ward off a host of obesity-related illnesses, following an overall anti-inflammatory lifestyle is key. And that's exactly what we'll show you how to do in Part III.

CHAPTER 6

Five-Alarm Fire

The Role of Chronic Inflammation in Chronic Pain

When it comes to pain, the same dynamic regarding acute versus chronic inflammation is at work. While any amount of pain is never pleasant, an episode of acute (short-term) pain will restore homeostasis and bring your body back to a state of optimal health and wellness. Acute pain is your body's way of getting your attention. The message is often urgent and unmistakable: *Help!* It's a signal to do something, whether it's the shocking pain of a broken bone or the crushing chest pain associated with a heart attack. Or maybe the situation isn't nearly that urgent. That dull headache you've been feeling for the past week could be your body's way of telling you that you are dehydrated or aren't getting enough sleep, or maybe it's time to get your eyeglasses prescription updated.

This messaging system is hardwired into your central nervous system. When you burn your hand, the part of your brain known as the HPA axis triggers a stress response that will temporarily boost your awareness of the situation, get your heart revved up, and activate the inflammatory response. These fast-acting changes enable you to focus and respond quickly to get away from the source of pain, while the acute inflammatory response protects you from infection and jump-starts the healing process. Acute pain, put simply, is a vivid message to take care of yourself.

Chronic pain is an altogether different matter. Chronic pain is pain that persists. The point at which acute pain "officially" becomes chronic pain is a bit of a moving target. Some experts say it's pain that lasts more than 3 months, some say 6 months, some even say 12 months. But this is one of those "you know it when you see it" things—chronic pain is pain that sticks around, and it can make your life miserable.

Generalizations about chronic pain can prove challenging, in part because there are so many different causes of chronic pain, and individual symptoms and experiences vary from person to person. Chronic pain can be an annoying inconvenience or completely debilitating. It can come and go or it can grind on for years, and it can range from mild to utterly excruciating. It can result from injury or illness, and it can be confined to certain areas (for example, lower-back pain, joint pain, abdominal pain, headaches) or experienced systemically in the event of nerve damage or a pain syndrome such as fibromyalgia or central pain syndrome. What's more, chronic pain sufferers respond to treatments in widely different ways. While an opioid such as Percocet may work for one person, a visit with a chiropractor may be better for another, while cognitive-behavioral therapy plus acupuncture may work for yet another. Many people living with chronic pain find they need a combination of interventions to keep their pain in check, and their pain management requirements change over the years. It can become an ongoing quest to find the methods, dosages, and combinations of treatments that work.

Whatever the number, additional statistics about chronic pain present a grim picture. If you combine the health-care costs of chronic pain with the dollars lost to missing work and reduced income, the total cost of chronic pain is estimated at upward of $635 billion a year—more than the costs of heart disease, cancer, and diabetes combined. And this number is far lower than the current reality: Not only are these figures based on 2010 dollars, several significant groups were not included in the analysis, including the prison population, nursing home residents, military personnel, those under 18, and caregivers who lost work due to caring for a chronic pain sufferer.[1] Still, even this partial analysis offers astounding figures that reflect chronic pain's extensive reach.

Other studies reveal the impact of pain on quality of life and general prognosis. Chronic pain sufferers may experience depression, anxiety, chronic stress, neuroticism, sleep disturbances, fatigue, cognitive impairment (including memory loss), weight gain (from reduced physical activity), and even changes to the structure and activity of the brain. These additional problems typically work hand in hand, mutually reinforcing each other. For example, pain interrupts sleep, which leaves you more vulnerable to depression, and depression can interrupt sleep and heighten the sense of pain. Alternately, pain heightens anxiety, which leads to greater cognitive impairment, which can in turn worsen anxiety, and heightened anxiety can increase pain perception. There's that vicious cycle at work again. It's been estimated that up to half of the people living with chronic pain experience symptoms of anxiety and depression; some studies bump this figure up to more than 75 percent.[2]

Further compounding the problem is the plain and simple fact that being in pain can be a profoundly isolating experience—even if you are surrounded by loved ones and caregivers. Chronic pain is so debilitating for some people that they are confined to their homes or even their beds, cutting them off from everyday life and social interactions. According to some estimates, half of chronic pain patients are unable to attend family or social events because of their condition. Further, the understandable emotional consequences of being in chronic pain—irritability, mood swings, anxiety, depression, and anger among them—can strain social activities.[3] Research indicates that people who are socially isolated experience more body-wide inflammation,[4] which can in turn worsen pain. There is also evidence that negative social interactions can contribute to chronic pain. Numerous studies note a higher number of people in chronic pain are also dissatisfied with their jobs or experience significant stress at work. Not coincidentally, these workers also report higher rates of depression.[5]

And as we've already discussed, while pain can lead to depression, it seems the reverse can also prove true. Up to two-thirds of people with major depression experience what's referred to as UPPS, or unexplained painful physical symptoms. People living with depression and UPPS tend to have a poorer response to antidepressant treatment and longer bouts of depression. Because chronic pain and depression so often go hand in hand, brain researchers have begun to investigate whether there is a common cause between the two. Research is ongoing, but science has already turned up some fascinating connections. For example, brain imaging shows that changes in the brain's frontal-limbic system are a common factor between depression and chronic pain. Very generally speaking, the frontal lobes and the limbic system work together to influence behavior, emotions, and thinking. Abnormal

COMMON CONDITIONS ASSOCIATED WITH CHRONIC PAIN

There are many health conditions that are closely associated with ongoing pain. Here are a few.

- AIDS
- Arthritis (osteoarthritis, rheumatoid arthritis)
- Back pain
- Cancer
- Cellulitis
- Central pain syndrome
- Chronic fatigue syndrome
- Chronic pain syndrome
- Crohn's disease
- Depression
- Endometriosis
- Fibromyalgia
- Gallbladder disease
- Headache/migraine

- Injury (especially spinal cord or nerve injuries and injuries resulting in disability)
- Multiple sclerosis
- Musculoskeletal disorders (injuries, carpal tunnel syndrome, tendonitis, etc.)
- Myopathy (muscle disease)
- Neuropathy (nerve damage)
- Repetitive motion syndrome
- Scleroderma (an autoimmune skin disorder)
- Sickle cell anemia
- Temporomandibular joint dysfunction
- Vulvodynia (chronic vulvar pain)

functioning of the prefrontal cortex (part of the frontal lobe) has also been observed in both depression and chronic pain sufferers; this area regulates our ability to think, organize, and plan ahead, as well as our ability to regulate our emotions. Proinflammatory cytokines appear to play a role. Higher levels of proinflammatory cytokines among depressed patients render neurons more sensitive to pain, and over time, this can result in chronic pain. There is also compelling evidence that one cytokine, tumor necrosis factor (TNF), can spark changes in the hippocampus (part of the limbic system) that lead to depression and chronic pain. Elevated TNF also inhibits the brain's ability to control pain, and it leads to an overproduction of cortisol, the stress hormone. The result is hippocampus dysfunction and ultimately hippocampus shrinking, two brain changes that are seen in people with depression and chronic pain.[6]

People with chronic pain even have a higher mortality rate than those without chronic pain. Statistically speaking, part of the reason is due to underlying illness behind the pain, particularly cancer and heart disease.[7] But some deaths linked to chronic pain result from substance abuse disorders and overdose, and some come from suicide. Chronic pain is considered a risk factor for suicide, in fact, because it can lead to feelings of depression and hopelessness and because some people turn to suicide to escape unbearable suffering.[8] One study even suggested that chronic pain *alone* contributes to the higher mortality rate; researchers speculated that in patients with severe chronic pain, regardless of the cause, the high intensity of pain and/or the resulting disability is key to the higher death rate.[9]

How Chronic Inflammation Influences Chronic Pain

If you are in pain, you can bet an inflammatory process is at work. On one level, it's as simple as that. An experience of acute pain is always accompanied by acute inflammation. If you'll recall from Chapter 1, pain, along with redness, heat, and swelling, is one of the primary manifestations of inflammation.

But as we know, any time we move from acute to chronic, we inevitably run into trouble. Besides the obvious trouble of ongoing suffering, pain that becomes chronic can cause a double whammy of hypersensitivity to pain *and* a greater susceptibility to pain. Essentially, ongoing inflammation acts like a megaphone for the pain signals your body generates.

Increased sensitivity to pain, known in medical circles as *hyperalgesia*, occurs when a medley of proinflammatory messengers is released at the site of inflammation, including cytokines, chemokines, neuropeptides, and prostaglandins. This barrage of proinflammatory chemicals renders nerve endings and pain receptors more sensitive.[10] That scenario is bad enough if the inflammation is limited to a specific area of the body, such as at the site of an injury, but imagine the impact if you're in a state of body-wide, chronic inflammation. With hyperalgesia, a bumped knee can feel like a blow from a hammer; a needle prick can feel like a knife wound. Why some people experience hyperalgesia and others don't isn't fully understood. There is also a specific type of hyperalgesia called opioid-induced hyperalgesia that represents a bitter medical irony: Due to changes to the nervous system, some people who are receiving opioids for pain management can develop a greater sensitivity to pain.

A related experience is *allodynia*. Whereas hyperalgesia is an exaggerated pain response to painful stimuli, allodynia is pain that results from normally harmless situations. A shirtsleeve brushing the skin can feel like scratching a sunburn; a simple handshake can feel like a crushing blow. Allodynia is associated with inflammatory conditions such as fibromyalgia, diabetes, central pain syndrome, and various neuropathies (nerve pain disorders). The condition isn't entirely understood, but once again, inflammation is believed to play a major role.

The proinflammatory cytokines that show up again and again in the medical literature on chronic pain are the same ones we see prominently implicated in depression, accelerated aging, kidney disease, and fibromyalgia: IL-6, IL-1β (interleukin-1-beta), and tumor necrosis factor-alpha (TNF-α). These three cytokines are all strongly associated with the initiation and persistence of pain. They trigger pain, and they make it stick around.

Now on the other hand, *anti*-inflammatory cytokines can prevent pain.

The most potent among them is interleukin-10 (IL-10). It can suppress proin-flammatory cytokines, and in experiments using animal models, IL-10 appears to suppress the pain from nerve injuries. Researchers believe that low concentrations of IL-10 and another anti-inflammatory cytokine, IL-4, are at least partially responsible for relieving chronic widespread pain.[11] Fibromyalgia is the classic example of a chronic widespread pain disorder, but others include myopathy, connective tissue disorders, lupus, and osteoarthritis. Let's take a closer look at a couple of these conditions to better understand what's happening when the body is in pain.

Chronic Joint Pain: Arthritis

There are more than 100 types of joint diseases that fall under the general term *arthritis*, and with nearly 23 percent of American adults having received an arthritis diagnosis of some type, this chronic joint condition is the primary cause of disability in the United States. As the population ages, the prevalence of arthritis will rise; it's estimated that by 2040, 26 percent of American adults will have doctor-diagnosed arthritis.[12]

The Arthritis Foundation identifies four main types of arthritis. *Osteoarthritis* is the most common form, and it's what we'll be focusing on

Dr. Kirshner's Inflammation Insight

When patients have a laundry list of complaints, such as constipation, problems with balance, brain fog, and so on, *and* they have joint pain and/or back pain, I usually don't address the musculoskeletal complaint for about 4 weeks. More often than not, these joint and muscle complaints resolve on their own when the patient follows a simple anti-inflammatory diet. This happens so frequently that it's my opinion that allowing the body to heal with a healthy diet serves the patient better than trying to "solve" the issue and possibly causing more harm.

here. It's the general "wear and tear" that happens over time to the cartilage between joints, and it's the type people are most often referring to when they speak of arthritis. *Inflammatory arthritis* is the result of an autoimmune dysfunction in which white blood cells attack the joints and cause inflammation, eroding or even destroying the cartilage. Rheumatoid arthritis is the most well-known type of inflammatory arthritis, and we'll discuss it specifically in the next chapter. *Infectious arthritis* occurs when bacteria, viruses, or fungi enter the joint and trigger inflammation; this type of arthritis requires antibiotics. Finally, *metabolic arthritis* occurs when an excess of uric acid accumulates and forms needlelike crystals in the joint, such as in gout.

No matter the type, the hallmark symptoms of arthritis include joint pain, inflammation, swelling, stiffness (especially in the morning), and decreased range of motion. Symptoms can come and go, and they range from mild discomfort to debilitating pain and disfigurement of the affected joint. If cartilage deterioration progresses, the damage can extend to the underlying bone.

With osteoarthritis (hereafter referred to as "arthritis"), the most commonly affected joints are the neck, hands, lower back, hips, and knees. Though over-the-counter medications (both oral and topical) are commonly used to treat pain, in many cases lifestyle changes can control pain and slow the progression of arthritis. If you're overweight, losing those extra pounds relieves pressure on weight-bearing joints, such as the knees and hips. Obesity (a BMI of 30 and above) is the main modifiable risk factor for arthritis of the knee, and obese patients are more likely to require total knee replacement surgery.[13] But don't assume that it's only weight-bearing joints that are affected if you're overweight. A well-known longitudinal study from the 1990s found that obesity also increases the risk of developing arthritis of the hands—suggesting an underlying systemic inflammatory influence.[14] By now this culprit should be no surprise! But remember, a common culprit leads us to a common cure: Not only will weight loss relieve pressure on joints, it will decrease inflammation by reducing the production of adipokines, special proinflammatory cytokines produced by fat cells.

Exercise, too, can help. It's well known that regular exercise helps protect against joint disorders, but what if you already have arthritis? It's natural to think you should avoid using the affected joints when you're in pain, but research consistently points out that exercise relieves symptoms and improves joint function in cases of knee and hip arthritis. Aerobic, aquatic, and range-of-motion exercises are all excellent options, and programs can be tailored to the individual person's needs. Further, exercises that include a "mind-body" component, such as tai chi, qigong, and yoga, can provide extra benefit by lowering inflammation.[15] For the full qigong sequence our test panelists learned as part of the Whole Body Cure Plan, see Chapter 13.

Nutritional interventions can also play a big role in lowering the underlying inflammation that aggravates arthritis pain. You'll find our full anti-inflammatory eating plan in Chapter 11, but there are a few foods and beverages from the plan that deserve special mention when it comes to targeting arthritis. Turmeric may be at the top of the list for its powerful anti-inflammatory effect. Hundreds of studies have demonstrated the efficacy of curcumin, the active compound in turmeric, in reducing pain, improving function, and improving quality of life in arthritis patients. A recent metareview of 15 studies on curcumin supplements identified a number of improvements, including a decrease in joint pain and tenderness, an increase in pain-free walking time, and a decrease in the need for pain medication. (The dosage of curcumin used in these studies ranged from 180 to 2,000 milligrams daily, and the treatment period ranged from 4 weeks to 8 months.) In addition to lowering inflammation, curcumin may extend the life of cartilage cells and reduce oxidative stress.[16]

To increase the amount of curcumin the body will absorb, don't forget those tips we mentioned before: Combine turmeric with black pepper, which increases curcumin's bioavailability by as much as 2,000 percent,[17] and combine it with a healthy fat like olive oil or coconut oil, which prevents curcumin from being broken down by stomach acids or the liver.[18] Curry dishes provide all of these ingredients, and if your stomach can stand the spice, try boosting the anti-inflammatory effect with hot chile pepper. Capsaicin, the active agent in hot red peppers, has proven anti-inflammatory and analgesic effects, and it is a key ingredient in some topical arthritis creams.[19]

Are you getting thirsty yet? Try green tea. Green tea is bursting with

Dr. Kirshner's Inflammation Insight

Elaine came to see me for a thyroid condition. I started her on an anti-inflammatory eating plan and a few thyroid supplements. Within weeks her thyroid symptoms had cleared up, but 5 weeks into the program, she had another question for me: "Dr. Kirshner, can this diet have any effect on my knees?"

I was a little taken aback by this question because she hadn't related any other symptoms to me except fatigue. She went on to tell me that for the past 8 years she had been dealing with knee pain and had been receiving cortisone injections about every 2 months. On a scale of 1 to 10, her pain would reach an 8 or 9, and then she'd have an injection. The pain would go down to a 2, but over the next few weeks it would slowly creep up to an 8 or 9 again. She'd been managing her pain like this for 8 years!

But the reason she asked me that question that day was that 5 weeks into our program, her pain was gone. None, zero.

I continued to monitor Elaine over the next several weeks and the knee pain never came back, and she had no injections during this time. Then, as we started to reintroduce foods back into her diet, she noticed that whenever she ate bread her knee pain returned. But after eliminating bread and other wheat products, the pain disappeared within 5 days. Elaine had found the hidden cause of her debilitating knee pain.

inflammation-fighting antioxidants, especially catechins, which are flavonoid compounds that stabilize free radicals, but it's the particular catechin known as epigallocatechin-3-gallate, or EGCG, that's especially relevant for arthritis sufferers. Several studies have demonstrated EGCG's ability to slow cartilage deterioration and protect collagen.[20]

Fibromyalgia

We're turning the spotlight onto fibromyalgia now because it's the most common inflammatory chronic pain disorder. The National Fibromyalgia Association estimates that the disease affects about 10 million Americans and 3 to

6 percent of people worldwide.[21] It's no coincidence that fibromyalgia's hallmark symptoms—pain, inflammation, fatigue, sleeping difficulties, mood disturbances, and memory impairment or "brain fog"—echo so many of the symptoms of chronic inflammation.

Fibromyalgia is a complex illness that still isn't fully understood. (In fact, one definition of fibromyalgia is "chronic widespread musculoskeletal pain for which no alternative cause can be identified."[22]) It causes achiness and pain throughout the body that lasts 3 months or more, debilitating fatigue even with proper rest, and swelling and tenderness, and it is often accompanied by anxiety and/or depression. One of fibromyalgia's distinguishing features is tenderness and pain at specific points on the neck, shoulders, back, arms, legs and hips. For unknown reasons, 80 to 90 percent of sufferers are women. Other fibromyalgia symptoms include headaches, dry mouth, hypersensitivity to cold and heat, concentration and/or memory problems, irritable bowel syndrome, an increased severity of PMS, restless leg syndrome, muscle stiffness, and numbness or tingling in the hands and feet.

Ample evidence suggests that chronic inflammation is the underlying factor behind fibromyalgia as well as other chronic pain conditions. People with fibromyalgia show elevated levels of proinflammatory cytokines, which, as we've already discussed, activate and sensitize pain receptors. We also know that being overweight worsens both the physical and mental symptoms of fibromyalgia (remember that body fat is a strong producer of proinflammatory cytokines). Not surprisingly, ample evidence suggests that obese people, regardless of whether they have a fibromyalgia diagnosis, exhibit increased sensitivity to pain.[23]

Studies have also noted that weight gain is directly related to aggravated fibromyalgia symptoms, including higher pain, worse fatigue, poorer sleep quality, and a higher incidence of mood disorders.[24] In one study of 224 people with fibromyalgia, 43.8 percent were obese. Compared to patients of a normal weight, the obese patients had higher depression scores, more physical disability, and more additional illnesses and took more medications for fibromyalgia. Further analysis showed that the higher the BMI, the higher the incidence of disability and depression. These results suggest that inflammatory conditions work hand in hand, each worsening the other. The authors of this study concluded that even if BMI isn't an essential factor in fibromyalgia, it clearly contributes to poor mood and physical dysfunction, and thus, maintaining a normal BMI should be a treatment goal.[25]

Perhaps not surprisingly, this last study also noted that participants who were overweight or obese exercised less than their normal-weight peers. Fibromyalgia patients may be reluctant to engage in exercise for fear of triggering or exacerbating pain, but the evidence shows that regular moderate exercise offers huge benefits. Not only can regular exercise contribute to weight loss and boost mood, it can lower the underlying chronic inflammation that's driving *all* of the symptoms of fibromyalgia. A metastudy based on data from 536 participants found that exercise decreased proinflammatory biomarkers. Exercise also changed levels of the hormone insulin-like growth factor-1, which may help reduce fatigue in obese fibromyalgia patients.[26]

As we all know, exercise isn't the only way to lose weight and reduce inflammation. An anti-inflammatory eating plan like the one we designed for this program can also help reduce symptoms. You'll find the Whole Body Cure Eating Plan in Chapter 11, but for now let's take a closer look at some additives commonly found in the standard American diet that are especially problematic.

Glutamate and aspartate—two amino acids that stimulate the nervous system—are of special significance to people with fibromyalgia. Free forms of glutamate and aspartate are found in the food additives monosodium glutamate (MSG) and the artificial sweetener aspartame, respectively. Studies have linked these amino acids with pain, and diets that eliminate MSG and aspartame appear to reduce many fibromyalgia symptoms.[27] One study found that 84 percent of fibromyalgia patients with irritable bowel syndrome who followed an MSG- and aspartame-free diet for 4 weeks experienced a significant improvement in both fibromyalgia and IBS symptoms. Those who improved were then randomized to a 2-week diet with MSG or a placebo for 3 consecutive days each week. The unlucky folks who ate the diet that included MSG didn't fare well at all. They experienced a return of overall symptoms, an increase in the severity of fibromyalgia, and a decreased quality of life due to IBS symptoms returning.[28]

If you're looking for even more relief, consider boosting your intake of key vitamins and minerals. Low levels of magnesium, zinc, vitamin B_6, and omega-3 fatty acids can make the nervous system more susceptible to overstimulation,[29] so fibromyalgia patients would do well to get adequate levels of these micronutrients. The combination of the first three is found in ZMA supplements, but you can also get all three from a variety of plant-based foods, including nuts, seeds, and dark leafy greens. Omega-3s come from fatty fish, such as salmon, mackerel, herring, and trout, and from walnuts and flaxseeds and their oils.

Another nutrient that shows up repeatedly in fibromyalgia research is vitamin D. A deficiency in vitamin D has been linked to both chronic pain[30] and muscle pain.[31] In one study, 71 percent of chronic pain patients had a vitamin D deficiency, and another 21 percent had insufficient vitamin D.[32] In people with fibromyalgia, low vitamin D also seems to intensify the perception of pain.[33] Because vitamin D levels tend to be significantly lower in people with fibromyalgia, several studies have explored the possibility of reducing pain by boosting vitamin D. In one study, 30 subjects were divided into two groups; one received vitamin D supplements and the other received none. Participants were evaluated at 20 weeks and again in another 24 weeks. Every person in the vitamin D group experienced a significant reduction in pain.[34]

Vitamin D also appears to play a role in the anxiety associated with fibromyalgia: People with fibromyalgia who are also deficient in vitamin D are far more prone to anxiety and depression than those with normal or even insufficient levels of vitamin D.[35] As vitamin D deficiency is one of the most common nutritional deficiencies worldwide, and because boosting vitamin D levels is a low-cost means of treatment, many health-care professionals recommend it for fibromyalgia sufferers. Sunlight exposure is the easiest way to get more vitamin D, though of course, use caution when it comes to direct sun exposure. Food sources of vitamin D include eggs, fish and fish oil, mushrooms, and fortified juices or milks.[36] Use caution here, too: As with any food recommendation, take care to avoid any foods to which you're sensitive or allergic. One survey found that 42 percent of people with fibromyalgia

(continued on page 120)

Ann Michael

AGE: 58

- Constant joint pain, muscle soreness, and a sense of puffiness relieved
- Headaches and dizziness that were experienced daily now occur only rarely
- Reduced total cholesterol by 9 points to almost normal
- Memory problems and mood swings eliminated
- Balance problems relieved
- WEIGHT LOST: 19 pounds
- INCHES LOST: 9¾

I was particularly interested in an anti-inflammatory plan as I have fibromyalgia. Compared to some fibromyalgia patients, my pain levels are fairly low, but in the past, I've had physical therapy and taken large doses of ibuprofen to deal with chronic pain. On a day-to-day basis, I'm more troubled by fatigue than by pain. Before starting the program, I noticed I was getting quite a bit of inflammation. My hands would swell up, for example, and when the swelling and inflammation were at their worst, I often experienced headaches, fatigue, and symptoms of irritable bowel syndrome (IBS).

I started to feel a real difference 3 to 4 weeks into the plan. It was then that I noticed considerably less swelling and less pain generally. I also dropped a lot of weight, even though I didn't need to and wasn't intending to. I'm 5 feet 8 inches and was 148 pounds when the plan began, which was still a size 6. Now I'm down to 129 pounds, and I've kept the weight off. I was surprised at the weight loss, which was almost a side effect of the anti-inflammatory eating, and I was also surprised that I didn't feel hungry. I do feel better at a lower weight. My pain levels decreased, by which I mean the pain is less frequent, and it's less severe when I do get a flare. I was also doing qigong every day during the program, and my sense is that it was extremely soothing to my system. It calmed down whatever it is that kicks up the fibromyalgia pain. Since the plan ended and my job has become more stressful, I haven't practiced qigong as much, and I've experienced some returning pain. I know I need to get the

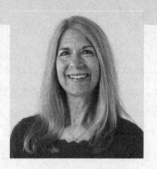

Ann's Tips

Consider getting a group together to follow the plan, or do it with a friend or spouse. For any lifestyle change, moral support helps, and I think it would be helpful for people in the same house to do it together. Then everyone's eating the same meals, and before you begin, you can go through your pantry and get rid of everything that doesn't belong and start from scratch. I'd also encourage people not to look at this as strictly an elimination plan. The way I see it, I'm not eliminating things—I'm just changing what I eat.

qigong routine back into my life. Do I feel more energetic? Yes, but I should mention that fatigue is still one of my symptoms.

I am, however, sticking with the anti-inflammation eating regimen, as one of the biggest improvements for me was in gut health. I didn't have a single recurrence of IBS while I was on the program. I've reintroduced a few things with no problem, such as a small amount of rice. And if I eat oatmeal, instead of flavoring it with brown sugar, I use a bit of local honey, and this switch wasn't difficult at all. I'll continue to limit grains, though, because it seems grains were a contributor to my inflammation. I'm still off soy, I'm still off dairy, and I'm steering clear of sugar. One of these days I may try dairy again—I love cheese—but for now I'm doing well enough that I don't want to rock the boat.

Case in point: I recently tried to reintroduce black beans, and within 12 hours, my IBS kicked up. I hadn't had an IBS symptom in over 4 months, so it was clearly connected to the black beans. The way the plan has you add foods back in one at a time made me far more mindful of what I was putting in my mouth. This was a very valuable aspect of the program—being given 3 months to think about what I eat and noting how I felt the day after. We all have our habits, and we often eat without thinking. I found that when I stopped to think about food and how it affects me, I ended up eating a better diet overall. When you're healthy, that's one thing, but especially when you have an underlying chronic problem, this program forces you to pay attention and to deal with your body. ∎

experienced worse symptoms after they ate certain foods.[37] A more recent survey found that nearly half had a food allergy. Among this group, a little more than half also had gastric reflux symptoms, and nearly 53 percent had gastritis.[38] The foods that tend to cause the most problems among people living with fibromyalgia are gluten, dairy, MSG, aspartame, sugar, and caffeine, though food triggers vary widely from person to person. Our eating plan in Chapter 11 will help you to create the ideal plan by identifying the specific foods that are causing negative reactions and aggravating your symptoms.

Conventional Treatments for Chronic Pain

For a full guide to the latest information on treatments for chronic pain—far more than we can provide here—the American Chronic Pain Association offers an exhaustive list of pharmacological, behavioral, and physical therapies. Check the association's Web site (theacpa.org) for the latest edition of its excellent resource guide.

Chronic pain of any type should be managed under your doctor's care, and it's not unusual to try different combinations of therapies before hitting upon the right course of treatment for you. The following is a brief overview of some of the more common pharmacological treatment options, followed by several all-natural options that can alleviate pain. By following the Whole Body Cure Eating Plan you'll read about in Chapter 11, many of Dr. Kirshner's patients have been able to eliminate most, or in some cases all, of these types of drugs.

TRADITIONAL PAINKILLERS. *Nonsteroidal anti-inflammatory drugs (NSAIDs)* are some of the most well-known and commonly used medications for pain—not to mention fever, which is a consequence of inflammation. Just like their name says, these drugs reduce inflammation, but they're not related to steroids. Chances are you've used NSAIDs dozens, if not hundreds, of times throughout your life. Examples include aspirin, ibuprofen, and naproxen, all of which are widely available over the counter. More potent NSAIDs require a prescription, and examples include diclofenac, oxaprozin, indomethacin, and the COX-2 inhibitor celecoxib.

PREMENSTRUAL PAIN

Growing evidence suggests that premenstrual syndrome (PMS) is an inflammatory condition. PMS symptoms crest monthly as systemic inflammation rises with natural fluctuations in hormones. A recent study of nearly 3,000 women found that elevated CRP levels were linked to an up to 41 percent increase in PMS symptoms, and the higher the CRP level, the more severe the symptoms.[39] And we're betting it's no coincidence that the symptoms of PMS—abdominal pain, back pain, acne breakouts, anxiety, depression, fatigue, GI complaints, headache, mood swings, sleep disturbances, and trouble with memory or concentration—are all associated with chronic inflammation.

Doctors routinely recommend over-the-counter anti-inflammatories such as ibuprofen and aspirin to relieve PMS pain, but they can have many negative side effects. Therefore, it's worth considering whether these nondrug anti-inflammatory remedies may help. Here are a few you might try.

- **Fennel** has an analgesic, anti-inflammatory, and anticramping effect. It may also relieve fatigue and lethargy associated with PMS. Fennel's root, leaves, and fruit can be used, and it's available as an essential oil (for topical use) and a tea.[40]

- **Mint** can help reduce pain, diarrhea, nausea, and vomiting associated with menstruation. A recent study compared the effect of mint (one peppermint oil capsule per day for 3 days after menstruation began) to 250 milligrams of mefenamic acid, a nonsteroidal anti-inflammatory drug. Both were effective in decreasing symptoms, but researchers concluded that mint was superior because it poses no side effects, whereas mefenamic acid causes significant gastrointestinal side effects.[41]

- **Cinnamon** has shown some efficacy in relieving period related pain, though it seems to take several hours for the analgesic effect to kick in.[42]

- **Omega-3 fatty acids** have been shown to reduce period pain.[43] They are available in supplement form but are found naturally in fatty, cold-water fish, such as salmon, mackerel, herring, trout, anchovies, and sardines, and in walnuts and flaxseeds (and their oils). Omega-3s may reduce pain primarily because of their powerful anti-inflammatory effect.

One of the major problems with NSAIDs, however, is that they can pose serious side effects that affect your heart, gastrointestinal system, and kidneys, especially when taken long term, so many health-care providers advise using them only to help control periodic breakthrough pain. NSAIDs are best for mild to moderate pain.

ACETAMINOPHEN (an analgesic in Tylenol and many cold medications) is another common over-the-counter medication used for mild pain and fever. Acetaminophen does not lower inflammation; rather, it reduces pain by inhibiting the synthesis of prostaglandins, which are pain-signaling molecules. Its main side effect is that it can be toxic to the liver when taken at high doses or when taken along with alcohol, so follow dosing directions carefully.

OPIOID MEDICATIONS have been receiving a lot of attention in the news lately for their role in the US opiod epidemic. These are narcotic drugs that alter the pain signals between the brain and the affected area(s). Morphine, codeine, oxycodone, hydrocodone, and fentanyl are all examples, and these medications are commonly prescribed to treat severe pain, including postoperative pain, cancer pain, pain from traumatic injury, as well as chronic pain syndromes, especially when first-line treatments don't work. Opioids are very effective and can improve quality of life in the face of extreme suffering. But because they are so potent and work directly on the body's pain signaling system, they come with serious side effects, including sedation, cognitive impairment, nausea and vomiting, severe constipation, and a high risk of tolerance, dependence, and addiction. And as we mentioned earlier, some people develop the condition called opioid-induced hyperalgesia, which makes pain worse. It's also quite dangerous to stop using opioids cold turkey.

CORTICOSTEROIDS are synthetically produced steroid hormones that can be taken orally or administered by injection at affected sites. They reduce pain and inflammation and are also used to treat allergies and conditions related to immune system dysfunction, such as asthma, bronchitis, colitis, and lupus. Some of the most commonly prescribed corticosteroids are prednisone, cortisone, and hydrocortisone. As with any drug, corticosteroids come with possible side effects and risks, especially with long-term use. Prolonged use can lead to depression, mood swings, insomnia, personality changes, obesity, impaired adrenal gland function, and osteoporosis. Like opioids, corticosteroids should not be stopped suddenly.

ANTIDEPRESSANTS. Because depression and chronic pain are closely linked inflammatory conditions, they can respond to the same modes of treatment. SSRIs and SNRIs—selective serotonin reuptake inhibitors and serotonin-norepinephrine reuptake inhibitors, respectively—are two classes of antidepressants that have shown beneficial effects in pain syndromes. SNRIs, which inhibit the reuptake of the neurotransmitter serotonin and the stress hormone norepinephrine, as opposed to SSRIs, which act on serotonin alone, appear to be better at controlling neuropathic pain and fibromyalgia pain.[44] But that isn't always the case—what works for one person may not work for the next, so some trial and error may be in order. We do know that any type of antidepressant will lower systemic inflammation, so treating the underlying inflammation may decrease pain *and* boost mood. We also know that anxiety and depression play a huge role in the persistence and severity of chronic pain, so treating mood disorders may have the added benefit of providing better, faster pain relief.[45]

The most common side effects of these antidepressants include sexual dysfunction, dry mouth, weight gain, and drowsiness; these side effects also vary greatly from person to person. Like opioids and corticosteroids, antidepressants shouldn't be stopped abruptly.

CYTOKINE THERAPY. Because proinflammatory cytokines are a huge trigger for pain and inflammation, not to mention they can increase the perception of pain, researchers believe there is huge potential to treat chronic pain with anti-inflammatory cytokines or cytokine antagonists. These drugs stop pain at its source rather than dull the symptoms of pain, and unlike opioid drugs, they are nonaddictive.[46]

One recent preclinical trial combined two anti-inflammatory cytokines, IL-4 and IL-10, to create a new drug for pain management. It had excellent results. Two different mouse models with chronic inflammatory pain experienced "full resolution" of pain with this combined therapy.[47] IL-4 and IL-10 are known to downregulate the production of the proinflammatory cytokine TNF-α, and both have been used independently to treat hyperalgesia and nerve pain.[48]

Cytokine antagonists represent another group of drugs that targets specific cytokines and stops them in their tracks. They're used most frequently in treatments for cancer, autoimmune disorders, and various infectious diseases. Anti-TNF-α drugs have been used to treat painful inflammatory conditions such as arthritis, cancer, psoriasis, psoriatic arthritis, Crohn's disease, and the nerve pain associated with herniated discs and sciatica.[49] Anti-TNF-α therapy has been shown to reduce pain-signaling activity in the brain.[50] One of the main side effects of TNF inhibitors is an increased risk of developing serious infections.

OTHER MEDICATIONS. Prescription medications used to prevent seizures (i.e. antiepileptics) have been shown to improve nerve pain. Topical pain relievers are applied to the skin and can also provide temporary relief for mild to moderate pain. They're available as creams and gels and in patch form. Muscle relaxants (prescription only) are short-term means to treat chronic pain, especially flare-ups of back pain. They can make you feel very sleepy and should never be used with opioids.

Natural Treatments for Chronic Pain

The following list describes some of the most widely available nondrug treatments for pain. Most come with no side effects, none present any danger of dependency or addiction, and all can improve overall health and well-being.

EXERCISE. As mentioned earlier in our discussion of fibromyalgia, regular, moderate exercise can reduce pain. Of course, exercise should be undertaken under the guidance of your health-care provider, and when pain is at its worst, exercise simply may not be possible. But if you're able, there are many benefits to regular, moderate exercise and plenty of gentle options that are great for chronic pain sufferers. Examples include aquatic exercise, yoga, qigong, tai chi, walking, and stretching. Regular exercise also provides other important benefits, such as reduced anxiety, depression, and stress and better sleep quality, all of which have a direct impact on chronic pain.

Further, lack of physical activity may worsen some forms of chronic pain, especially back pain, which will affect upward of 80 percent of Western adults at some point in their lives. A meta-analysis of 14 studies found that exercise programs that involve muscle strength, flexibility, and/or aerobic fitness benefit people with chronic lower-back pain and can reduce pain and disability. One word of caution: Rest, rather than exercise, is a standard recommendation in many cases of acute back pain, which will usually resolve on its own within 4 to 6 weeks.[51] If you have any questions, check with your health-care provider.

ACUPUNCTURE. The ancient practice of acupuncture, part of traditional Chinese medicine, involves inserting very thin needles at strategic energy points in the body. Needles can be manipulated by hand or by electrical stimulation. Acupuncture has been used for thousands of years to treat pain, but scientific evidence for its efficacy is quite mixed. Still, more than 3 million Americans a year receive acupuncture, most often for chronic pain, and many insurance policies now cover it. A 2012 meta-analysis published in the highly respected *JAMA Internal Medicine* (formerly *Archives of Internal Medicine*) found that acupuncture was superior to placebo-acupuncture or no acupuncture in controlling back and neck pain, osteoarthritis, chronic headache, and shoulder pain.[52]

CHIROPRACTIC. *Manipulation* and *mobilization techniques* refer to hands-on therapies practiced by chiropractors, osteopathic physicians, physical therapists, and some massage therapists. While there are many different treatment modalities that fall under the broad category of "manipulation and mobilization," they all involve some sort of adjustment of the spinal column. Studies have shown that spinal manipulation can relieve both acute and chronic pain of the neck and lower back. Chiropractors also often perform a type of pain relief called transcutaneous electrical nerve stimulation, or TENS for short (see page 127 for more on this).

BIOFEEDBACK. Through biofeedback, information about various physiological activities—such as brain waves, heart rate, breathing, muscle activity, sweat gland response, and skin temperature—is "fed back" to the individual by instruments that offer very precise measurements. This information allows individuals to learn how to change their bodies' responses at will to affect health and wellness. For example, people can learn to slow breathing and heart rates, decrease the stress response, and lower blood pressure. For chronic pain management, biofeedback helps people learn to lower stress and relax certain muscle groups connected to pain and learn better ways to deal with pain. A recent meta-analysis on biofeedback for chronic back pain found it to be effective not only for reducing pain intensity but also for reducing depression, disability, and muscle tension and in facilitating coping.[53] Biofeedback can be performed at hospitals and medical clinics, but some methods have been created for home use.

NUTRITIONAL INTERVENTIONS. Because we've touched upon this already, here we'll just include the reminder that the typical Western diet—which is characterized by animal sources of protein, highly processed foods, saturated fats, sugar, and refined carbohydrates—is highly inflammatory. Poor nutrition increases body-wide inflammation, which in turn delays recovery as well as heightens sensitivity to pain. On the bright side, dietary changes quickly reduce inflammation, and by following an overall anti-inflammatory approach to eating and eliminating food triggers that may cause pain or make it worse, many people have experienced significant reductions in pain and improved quality of life.

PSYCHOLOGICAL INTERVENTIONS. *Cognitive-behavioral therapy (CBT)* may be an important tool to decrease the habit of catastrophizing and to introduce better pain management options. "Catastrophizing" is a common pattern that refers to a set of exaggerated and repetitive thoughts and feelings about any number of things, but it can cause real problems regarding the perception of pain. Pain catastrophizing is an independent risk factor for predicting chronic pain and poorer outcomes.[54] Here's one interesting side note: A recent study found that people with chronic pain who had higher baseline levels of the proinflammatory cytokines TNF-α and IL-6 did not experience any improvements from behavioral interventions, but CBT strategies did work for those with lower levels of TNF-α and IL-6. This latter group experienced less pain as well as greater psychological measures of wellness.[55] This was a small study based on only 41 participants, but it does showcase the potential of CBT as a tool to fight inflammation-related pain.

One type of cognitive-behavioral therapy known as acceptance and commitment therapy (ACT) is a particularly effective way to treat some of the effects of chronic pain, including anxiety, depression, and addiction. With ACT, the aim is not to eliminate or deny the negative thought, sensation, or feeling—in this case, the pain itself—but to notice and accept it, affording an opportunity to clarify one's perception of the experience and then pursue actions that will help. Participants in studies who employed this technique experienced significant improvements in pain acceptance, psychological flexibility, and depression.[56]

MEDITATION. Studies of mindfulness meditation and its close cousin mindfulness-based stress reduction indicate meditation is a useful way to treat many types of chronic pain. It's important to remember any measures that reduce stress have huge potential to reduce pain because stress worsens the perception of pain. We'll talk about mindfulness practices in greater detail in Chapter 13 and the complementary approaches to lowering inflammation, but here's just one study that may entice you to give meditation a try. Researchers examined the effects of a brief mindfulness meditation training program on pain levels in 22 healthy volunteers. On the first day, volunteers received electrical pulses in their arms and then reported their pain intensity levels. Over the next 3 days, the volunteers, none of whom had any previous meditation experience, were given 20 minutes of mindfulness meditation instruction each day. The following day, researchers subjected volunteers to the same painful stimulus, but this time, they did so once while volunteers were meditating and once while they were not. Compared to Day 1, volunteers reported less pain to both low and high intensities of electrical stimulation while meditating and less anxiety overall after each meditation session. One of the most remarkable observations from this study is how quickly meditation worked to lower pain. Even these meditation beginners experienced significantly lower pain after only 3 days of instruction.[57]

ELECTRICAL STIMULATION. Transcutaneous electrotherapy is the most common form of electrotherapy. A form of electrotherapy called TENS has been around since the 1960s. A practitioner places electrodes on the surface of the skin and sends a mild current to the area that's in pain. It works by stimulating nerves in the affected area and "scrambling" the pain signals sent to the brain. TENS therapy is best for superficial pain (as opposed to deep, visceral pain) and offers short-term relief.

In a newer form of electrical stimulation called interferential current stimulation, the electrical current goes deeper into the tissue and provides less stimulation to the skin than TENS. It has been most commonly used for back pain but has also been shown to reduce the pain of arthritis, shingles, interstitial cystitis, degenerative joint disease, joint injuries, and neuropathy.

Intradiscal electrothermal therapy, another form of electrical stimulation, helps lower-back pain resulting from disc problems, and it works in an altogether different manner. This outpatient procedure is performed while the patient is under local anesthesia, and it involves inserting a slim electrothermal catheter into the disc and delivering electrical current and heat. It reduces pain by destroying pain receptors in the affected discs, and it provides an excellent alternative to opioid medications and invasive surgery.

SPINAL CORD STIMULATION. Spinal cord stimulation addresses chronic, intractable pain that hasn't responded to other therapies. In this technique, thin, flexible wires with electrical leads are inserted with a needle in the epidural space within the spinal canal (surgery is not required). The patient controls the electrical current with an adjustable remote control device, which makes it ideal for fluctuating levels of pain. Permanent implantation is possible.

Whole-Body Relief

Though any experience of pain is obviously unpleasant, acute, short-term pain can help return us to an optimal state of health and wellness. It's the body's signal that something is amiss and needs attention.

But there is *zero* physical or mental benefit to chronic pain, which is a disorder unto itself, regardless of the cause. Given the many effects chronic pain has on our physical function, mental health, social life, work life, and, indeed, our overall quality of life, managing this debilitating condition is a top priority. Often pain relief requires a multidisciplinary approach. Fortunately, there have been great advances in the field of pain management, and many health-care providers welcome the use of complementary therapies, which carry little to no side effects and potential for addiction. Nonpharmacological interventions may just provide the hidden key to getting relief when other methods haven't worked. If you have an unknown food sensitivity, for example, identifying and eliminating that trigger can sometimes stop pain in its tracks. Mindfulness-based techniques can help decrease the experience of pain and leave you better equipped to deal with pain when it does flare. And certainly, any means we take to reduce inflammation will have a positive effect on pain—from its root causes to how we perceive and experience pain. As we will continue to see throughout the book, putting out the fire of the underlying inflammation is half the battle.

CHAPTER 7

Accidental Arson

Autoimmune Disorders, Allergies, and Chronic Inflammation

The connection between seasonal hay fever or a peanut allergy with diseases like lupus, type 1 diabetes, or multiple sclerosis is hardly obvious, but the reality is that such conditions result when the immune system malfunctions. The two types of conditions we're referring to—allergies and autoimmune disorders—are both chronic inflammatory conditions, and they arise when the immune system makes a serious mistake.

In the case of allergies, the immune system perceives a substance that's usually harmless (such as eggs, nuts, or latex) as a threat. In the case of autoimmune disorders, the immune system mistakes the body's own tissues as a threat and attacks itself accordingly. In both conditions, the inflammation army is sent out to attack and neutralize benign threats, and the consequences can range from irritating to debilitating to life-threatening. In the general population, allergies and autoimmune disorders are on the rise and both involve some connections to the gut microbiome that might surprise you.

Welcome to the strange world of allergies and autoimmune disorders, run by a trigger-happy inflammation army bent on self-sabotage.

Autoimmunity:
When the Body Attacks Itself

The word *autoimmunity* simply means an immune response directed toward the self. (*Auto* is one of the Greek terms for "self.") Autoimmune disorders constitute a true hodgepodge of illnesses, spanning the gamut in terms of severity, organs affected, impact on health, rate of progression, treatment, and prognosis. They can attack any part of the body and can alternate between periods of remission and incapacitating flare-ups, and it's not uncommon for more than one autoimmune disorder to strike at a time. Common examples include rheumatoid arthritis, lupus, celiac disease, type 1 diabetes, multiple sclerosis, psoriasis, inflammatory bowel disease, the thyroid disorders Graves' disease and Hashimoto's thyroiditis, the skin disorders vitiligo and scleroderma, and the blood disorder pernicious anemia. This list is just a small handful of the 80 or more known autoimmune disorders.

While researchers continue to make great strides in understanding autoimmunity and the disorders it spawns, autoimmune diseases remain a medical mystery. For unknown reasons, they're far more common in women than in men; roughly three-quarters of sufferers are female. Their wide-ranging symptoms can make diagnosis difficult. People with the same autoimmune condition can have quite different symptoms, and some symptoms, like joint pain or fatigue, can be present in any number of illnesses. Moreover, because more than one autoimmune disorder can develop at the same time, symptoms of one condition can mask symptoms of the other. It's not uncommon for people with autoimmune diseases to see multiple doctors and specialists before receiving the correct diagnosis.

The causes of autoimmune disorders—and thus, any possible ways to prevent them—are also something of a mystery. But experts believe a combination of factors rather than just one thing usually initiates the disease. Overall, most theories boil down to two overarching factors—genetic susceptibility and an environmental trigger. When *both* are present, conditions are ripe for autoimmunity. Let's look at both.

Dr. Kirshner's Inflammation Insight

Mary was 22 when I met her at one of my educational thyroid meetings. Her mother had brought her out of concern for her daughter's health, and indeed Mary looked gray and "out of it."

Her mom related that Mary's health had been declining over a 3-year period. She had been a competitive swimmer in high school and began college as a high achiever. But beginning her sophomore year, her concentration and her energy levels had begun to decline. She graduated, and when I met her, she was a schoolteacher. She could get through the day, but she was asleep by 4:30 p.m. every day, utterly exhausted. She tried energy drinks, coffee, and over-the-counter stimulants. When she tried to exercise, she became even more exhausted. She also noticed that in high-stress situations, her speech became soft and a little garbled.

My clinic ran several tests and discovered that Mary's underlying condition was an autoimmune condition called Hashimoto's thyroiditis. This is a condition that's becoming increasingly prevalent. We put her on an anti-inflammatory diet and the right supplements to support gut health, and within 2 weeks, Mary noticed her energy picking up. Six weeks into the program, she started exercising again, but now the exercise energized her. Within 3 months, she was working a full schedule, exercising an hour after work, and socializing. With her condition under control through an anti-inflammatory way of eating, this 22-year-old reengaged with life.

First up, genetics. While autoimmune diseases aren't passed down genetically like hemophilia or sickle-cell anemia, they do tend to run in families. They also tend to afflict African Americans, Hispanics, and Native Americans more than other ethnic groups. Oddly, family members won't necessarily develop the same autoimmune condition. Your mother may have Graves' disease, while you may have lupus, and Uncle Bob comes down with Crohn's. What we do know is that some people are born with a genetic propensity for autoimmune disease and then something happens to activate the gene.

And that "something" is where the environmental trigger comes into play.

There are potentially dozens of environmental triggers that can spark autoimmunity in genetically susceptible people, but some of the most common ones include infection, toxins (like chemicals or pollution), sunlight, stress, certain foods, and some medications. Other triggers include trauma, surgery, childbirth, and menopause. Some triggers are associated with certain autoimmune disorders more than others. Lupus, for example, is especially associated with sunlight and certain medications, and silica dust (released when construction materials such as bricks, tile, concrete, and mortar are cut, ground, or drilled) has been linked with scleroderma. Smoking is a major risk factor for rheumatoid arthritis, and once the disease is present, smoking worsens symptoms, increases inflammation, and lowers the rate of remission.[1]

There's also evidence that gut dysbiosis contributes to autoimmune disorders. Gut dysbiosis, which we covered at length in Chapter 4, occurs when the bacteria in the gut are out of balance and/or lacking diversity. Often caused by an unhealthy diet and food sensitivities or allergies, dysbiosis increases the likelihood of leaky gut syndrome (intestinal permeability), which allows pathogens and toxins to pass through the gut membrane and into the bloodstream, triggering the inflammatory response. In genetically susceptible individuals, this state of imbalance can be enough to launch autoimmune disease.[2] Gut dysbiosis has been linked to the autoimmune disorders inflammatory bowel disease (Crohn's disease and ulcerative colitis), rheumatoid arthritis, lupus, type 1 diabetes, celiac disease and other food allergies, and multiple sclerosis.[3]

Environmental factors may explain why the number of people with autoimmune disorders has risen so sharply. The latest estimates regarding the prevalence of autoimmune disorders worldwide indicate an increase by more than 12 percent over the past three decades, with the most rapid rise occurring in industrialized countries that follow a Western lifestyle. (By the way, allergy and cancer rates are rising in these areas, as well.) Rheumatoid arthritis and lupus saw the biggest increases, followed by endocrine disorders such as type 1 diabetes and Graves' disease and gastrointestinal disorders such as celiac disease and Crohn's disease.[4]

What's so unhealthy about an industrialized Western lifestyle? It is associated with more toxic pollution and a wider use of chemicals; an inflammation-inducing diet that features processed foods, unhealthy fats, high sugar and sodium, and exposure to pesticides and food additives; higher stress; and excessive hygiene habits that may disrupt the balance and composition of gut bacteria. (Now, just for kicks, turn back to the primary causes of chronic inflammation listed on page 15. Do you see the similarities? With such an inflammatory lifestyle, it's no wonder rates of autoimmune disorders and allergies are skyrocketing.)

A recent study found a direct link between processed foods and the risk of autoimmune diseases. It seems that eating processed foods can damage the "tight junctions" of the intestines that form a protective barrier against toxins, harmful disease-causing pathogens, allergens, and carcinogens. Once again, we're talking about leaky gut. When these harmful substances enter the bloodstream through a small intestine that inflammation has rendered more permeable, a cascade of side effects may trigger the immune system to attack otherwise healthy parts of the body. This study identified seven common food additives that contribute to leaky gut: (1) sugars, (2) sodium, (3) emulsifiers (food "stabilizers"), (4) solvents used to extract oil from oil seeds (hexane, benzene, methyl/ethyl acetates, etc.), (5) gluten, a protein found in wheat and other grains that is hard to digest, (6) microbial transglutaminase (a food enzyme that is added to many bakery products to act as a "glue"), and (7) engineered nanoparticles used to improve taste, texture, or color of food or to keep food fresh longer.[5] Clearly, processed foods aren't healthy choices for anyone, but this study makes clear that *especially* if you have a family history of autoimmune illness, you should remove processed foods from your diet. Remember, it's genetics plus an environmental trigger that causes autoimmunity.

Because autoimmune diseases don't yet have a cure, treatments are usually designed to prevent flare-ups and prolong periods of remission. Drug treatments center around, not surprisingly, anti-inflammatories and immune-suppressing drugs. Corticosteroids (like prednisone), nonsteroidal anti-inflammatories (like aspirin and ibuprofen), and tumor necrosis factor blockers are common medications. Their goal is to reduce the abnormal immune response—essentially, to stop the body from attacking itself. Many of these drugs have serious side effects. The earlier the disease is detected and treated, the better the outcome. Other appropriate healthy lifestyle habits includes plenty of sleep, good nutrition, the elimination of food triggers, regular moderate exercise, and stress management.

Now that you've got some background on autoimmune disorders, and since we've covered inflammatory bowel disease in Chapter 4, let's go a little more in depth with four of the most common conditions: rheumatoid arthritis, lupus, psoriasis, and celiac disease.

Rheumatoid Arthritis

More than 1.3 million Americans are living with rheumatoid arthritis (RA), and like other autoimmune conditions, it affects women more often than men. RA can occur in any joint, but most often it's seen in the joints of the fingers, hands, and wrists. Unlike most other forms of arthritis, RA occurs symmetrically, affecting both sides of the body equally. RA causes pain, inflammation, swelling, stiffness, impaired function, and disfigurement. One of the telltale signs of RA is stiffness of the joints that occurs in the morning and lasts for an hour or more. (Morning joint stiffness from the "wear-and-tear" degeneration of osteoarthritis usually clears up within a half hour.)

But unlike osteoarthritis, which affects joints only, RA is far more than a joint problem. A systemic inflammatory illness, RA can affect the lungs, kidneys, liver, bones, skin, gums, nerves, eyes, heart, and blood vessels. People with RA also face a higher risk of developing non-Hodgkin's lymphoma. What's behind these complications? Chronic inflammation.

Some of the most dangerous RA-related complications are cardiovascular in nature—especially as the odds of sudden cardiac death are twice that of the general population—and half of the premature deaths in RA patients can be attributed to heart disease. Exactly why RA so drastically raises the risk of heart disease is still under investigation, but the underlying systemic, low-grade inflammation deserves some of the credit. Chronic inflammation accelerates the progression of congestive heart failure and atherosclerosis, leading to reduced bloodflow and abnormal thickening and stiffening of heart tissue (a condition known as cardiac fibrosis). Inflammation, along with these changes to the heart, can affect the electrical impulses that govern the heartbeat and a key measurement of heart health known as heart rate variability (HRV),[6] which is the variation in time between one heartbeat and the next. Low HRV levels can indicate stress and are associated with heart disease. One study of 101 RA patients found that elevated CRP levels were directly correlated with reduced HRV and a longer QT interval, a measure of the electrical activity in the heart's lower chambers, the ventricles. (A long QT interval is associated with a higher risk of irregular heart rhythms, known as cardiac arrhythmia.) This study demonstrates that rising inflammation increases the risk of potentially deadly heartbeat irregularities.[7]

Fortunately, RA patients can reduce their risk of many heart problems when inflammation is kept under control. Immunosuppressive drugs are one option. One study, for example, examined the effectiveness of tocilizumab, a medication that targets the infamous proinflammatory cytokine IL-6. At the outset of the study, participants had high levels of inflammation, and 76 percent exhibited a long QT interval. After receiving the immunosuppressive drug, patients' QT intervals fell to a normal rate within 3 months. As inflammation levels continued to fall throughout the study, QT intervals continued to normalize.[8]

Other treatment options for rheumatoid arthritis include over-the-counter and prescription-strength nonsteroidal anti-inflammatory drugs, which reduce pain and inflammation but do not alter the course of RA, and corticosteroids, which can reduce inflammation quickly. But the main drug treatments for RA are DMARDs, or disease-modifying antirheumatic drugs, which slow progression of the disease, and biologic DMARDs, which are usually prescribed when regular DMARDs don't work. Biologic DMARDs (tocilizumab, mentioned above, is one) act directly on proinflammatory cytokines and can be used in combination with regular DMARDs. These medications can help, but they come with a long list of serious side effects, so regular monitoring is essential.

Of course, some nondrug options can improve the problems associated with rheumatoid arthritis, too. Any lifestyle measures to control chronic inflammation—not smoking, getting regular moderate exercise, getting adequate sleep, and keeping stress levels in check—will help.

And certainly, anti-inflammatory eating has a huge positive effect, especially on some of the heart complications we've been discussing. Because chronic inflammation decreases beneficial HDL cholesterol and increases the risk of atherosclerosis,[9] anti-inflammatory *and* HDL-boosting measures are recommended. One of the best ways to boost HDL is exercise, but some foods help, too. Here are some anti-inflammatory, HDL-boosting, and heart-healthy foods to enjoy that are included in the Whole Body Cure Eating Plan: extra-virgin olive oil, avocado, cold-water fatty fish (salmon, mackerel, herring, etc.), flaxseeds and flaxseed oil, nuts, chia seeds and chia oil, and fresh fruits and vegetables. You may notice that this list is similar to the traditional Mediterranean diet, and in fact, long-term adherence to the Mediterranean diet has been shown to significantly boost HDL cholesterol and lower proinflammatory cytokine levels. Other cardiovascular risk factors fall, too, including total and LDL cholesterol, blood pressure, and triglyceride concentrations.[10] Any overall healthy eating plan is an excellent place to start, but our plan also includes an effective way to first detox your system and then identify any food sensitivities and allergies that are keeping you sick and inflamed. Many people find that their autoimmune and allergy symptoms decrease or even fully disappear after adopting the Whole Body Cure way of eating.

The next treatment tactic takes us back to the gut, where the goal is to restore the diversity of the microbiome. Rheumatoid arthritis patients consistently show an imbalance not only of the bacteria in the gut but also of the bacteria that live in the mouth.[11] So eat to restore balance to and increase the microbial diversity of your microbiome. This means eating a greater diversity of foods, upping your fiber intake, and eating more probiotic-rich fermented foods that won't aggravate your food triggers. Choose from sauerkraut, kombucha, olives, and sour pickles. For an even higher level of probiotics, add a supplement.

Finally, there is evidence that lower vitamin D levels can play a role in some of the more severe symptoms of rheumatoid arthritis, and we know that vitamin D can reduce inflammation and help maintain proper immune system function.[12] Accordingly, vitamin D supplementation may be appropriate for people with RA. For vitamin-D-rich foods, along with other healing foods for autoimmune conditions, see "Nutrition Check for Autoimmune Disease" on page 144.

Lupus

There are four main types of lupus and several subtypes, but what we'll be addressing here, systemic lupus erythematosus, is the most common form of the disease and thus known simply as lupus. Like other autoimmune disorders, the exact cause of lupus is unknown, but a combination of genetic, environmental, and hormonal factors is at play. The most commonly cited environmental factors are sunlight, infections, certain medications, and exposure to silica dust, which is often found in new building construction. Lupus can run in families, and even if there is no family history of lupus, it's more likely to develop when family members have other autoimmune disorders. Lupus also occurs more frequently in women, and symptoms tend to be worse during pregnancy or just before menstruation, when estrogen levels are high.

No two cases of lupus are exactly alike, but the most common symptoms are joint pain and swelling; fatigue; chest pain; low-grade fever; shortness of breath; a red, butterfly-shaped facial rash; dry eyes; hair loss; edema; and headaches. Many people with lupus develop photosensitivity, and skin lesions can appear and/or worsen after exposure to sunlight. Sunlight can also trigger flare-ups in some people.

Lupus, like other autoimmune disorders, exhibits alternating periods of flare-ups and remission, and it carries potentially life-threatening complications. The major complications include kidney damage; brain and/or central nervous system problems (such as memory loss, seizures, or behavioral changes); damage to the heart and blood vessels; increased susceptibility to infection and lung inflammation; a greater risk of cancer; bone tissue damage; and pregnancy complications like preterm birth, preeclampsia, and miscarriage. Kidney damage and cardiovascular damage, the most pressing concerns, are among the leading causes of death for lupus sufferers. As dire as all of this sounds, it's worth remembering that most cases of lupus are mild and that proper treatment greatly improves the chances of living a normal life span with a good quality of life. To that end, sufficient rest and healthy nutrition are essential.

Anti-inflammatory eating benefits people with lupus because of its heart-healthy and inflammation-lowering effects. Omega-3 fatty acids, for example, provide multiple benefits. These polyunsaturated fatty acids lower triglycerides, a type of fat found in the blood and an important measure of heart health. Omega-3s also reduce protein in the urine and protect the kidneys against the effect of free radicals, unstable molecules that can speed the progress of chronic kidney disease. Flaxseed oil alone may preserve kidney function by reducing protein being passed into the urine and inhibiting platelet-activating factor, which at high levels causes inflammation and increases the chance of blood clots.[13] A study comparing 114 lupus patients with 122 healthy controls found that higher levels of DHA and EPA—both long-chain omega-3 fatty acids found in fish, fish oils, flaxseeds, flaxseed oil, walnuts, and walnut oil—decreased disease activity and reduced atherosclerotic plaques. Conversely, higher omega-6s, which are found primarily in vegetable oils, had the opposite effect.[14] Another study compared fish oil supplementation (six capsules a day equaling 2.25 grams EPA and 2.25 grams DHA) with an olive oil placebo in patients with lupus. Those receiving fish oil reduced inflammation and improved energy levels and emotional well-being.[15]

Vitamin D, which as we've mentioned plays an important role in rheumatoid arthritis treatment, may also prove helpful for people with lupus. In a study of 177 lupus patients, 82 percent had low vitamin D, and this deficiency was associated with elevated markers of antibodies that attack DNA. Low vitamin D levels are also associated with heart disease in lupus patients.[16] And in one study, researchers divided 267 lupus patients into two random groups. One group received a vitamin D supplement of 2,000 IU/day for 12 months, and the other a placebo. At the start of the study, 39 percent of the participants were deficient in vitamin D, and 69 percent had suboptimal levels. Those who had lower vitamin D levels also had higher inflammation levels and more lupus symptoms. After 12 months of treatment, participants receiving the vitamin D supplements experienced a significant reduction in inflammation levels and symptoms compared to the placebo group.[17]

People living with lupus should also aim to get enough calcium because they are at greater risk for developing osteoporosis and tend to have decreased bone mineral density. One study found that women with lupus are five times more likely to suffer fractures than healthy women of the same age.[18] For a list of calcium-rich foods, see "Nutrition Check for Autoimmune Disease" on page 144.

Finally, one other food deserves special mention when it comes to lupus, and that's turmeric. Multiple studies have demonstrated the healing effects of this aromatic spice, which is known for its powerful anti-inflammatory abilities. Patients with lupus nephritis, a painful kidney inflammation that can cause weight gain and swelling, received turmeric supplements with each meal for 3 months, while a control group received a placebo. Researchers assessed the volunteers at the beginning of the study and again in monthly intervals for 3 months. Those in the turmeric group had significantly lower protein levels in their urine at each assessment. By the end of the study, blood pressure and the presence of blood in the urine had also significantly decreased.[19] Curcumin is the active compound in turmeric, and it's been shown to inhibit autoimmune diseases by regulating proinflammatory cytokines.[20]

Psoriasis

Psoriasis is a chronic, autoimmune skin disease that causes skin cells to build up rapidly, resulting in redness, scaling, itchiness, dry skin, and pain. These patches of inflamed skin are known as psoriasis lesions. They can appear anywhere on the surface of the body, though most often they show up on the scalp, knees, and elbows. Like the other autoimmune conditions, the causes of psoriasis aren't entirely clear but experts believe a combination of genetic predisposition and environmental trigger is in play.

Psoriasis can have a profound negative impact on quality of life not only because of its physical symptoms but also because lesions can be disfiguring.

In a review of over 500 psoriasis patients, 73 percent reported that they felt stigmatized in some way because of their appearance.[21] Psoriasis patients also report higher levels of anxiety, depression, and suicidal thoughts than the general population,[22] and the worse the severity of their psoriasis, the greater the burden on self-esteem, body image, psychological health, social life, and overall quality of life.[23]

Sadly, the emotional toll of psoriasis is only one aspect of its challenges. Psoriasis patients are also at greater risk of additional autoimmune illnesses, including rheumatoid arthritis, another form of arthritis known as psoriatic arthritis, and inflammatory bowel disease. But on top of it all, the risk of yet another autoimmune condition, celiac disease, is especially severe. Research suggests that having psoriasis roughly *doubles* the odds of being diagnosed with celiac disease. (Another study found the converse to be true, too: Having celiac disease significantly raises the risk of developing psoriasis.[24]) On a happier note, one study found that 42 percent of psoriasis in patients with celiac disease could be attributed to the underlying celiac disease, suggesting that for psoriasis patients with a gluten sensitivity, adopting a gluten-free diet may improve psoriasis symptoms.[25] This is yet another instance of the healing power of eating for your particular body and your particular health profile. Many foods have different effects on different people. Use this knowledge to heal, rather than harm. We'll show you how in Chapter 11.

Another way people with psoriasis may better control their symptoms is to lose any extra weight. That's right—losing weight can improve your psoriasis *and* improve how you respond to medications.[26] In one study, 60 obese patients with psoriasis were divided into either a weight loss group that ate 800 to 1,000 calories a day for 8 weeks, followed by 8 weeks of no more than 1,200 calories a day, or a control group. After 16 weeks, the weight loss group lost an average of nearly 34 pounds, compared to less than 1 pound in the control group. Those in the intervention group also experienced an average change of −2.3 points in their Psoriasis Area and Severity Index (PASI) scores, a standard assessment of psoriasis activity, as opposed to just −0.3 in the control group. Researchers also noted that the greatest reduction in psoriasis severity occurred in the first half of the study, when the greatest weight loss occurred.[27] Researchers later conducted a follow-up study of this same group to observe the long-term effects of weight reduction, following the participants for an additional 48 weeks. Of the 32 people who completed the full course, average weight loss compared to original weight was just over 22 pounds and PASI scores were 2.9 points lower compared to the baseline. According to these results, long-term weight loss appears to keep psoriasis severity down for the long term.[28]

Psoriasis is also associated with an increased risk of metabolic syndrome, high cholesterol, high blood pressure, and type 2 diabetes—conditions that help explain why psoriasis is strongly associated with a higher risk of heart attack and stroke. The association is so strong, in fact, that psoriasis is now classified as an independent risk factor for heart disease, as dangerous as smoking, excess weight, and diabetes.[29]

What's going on here? By now you won't be surprised to hear that *all* of the coexisting conditions in psoriasis, from depression to celiac disease to cardiovascular illness, are linked by chronic inflammation. In study after study, researchers have observed that people with celiac disease and psoriasis also display signs of a leaky gut (intestinal permeability) brought about by inflammation. Obesity alone promotes a chronic inflammatory state and can lead to metabolic syndrome, as fat cells continually release a special type of cytokine known as adipokines and affect levels of leptin, the hormone that plays a role in controlling hunger.[30] It seems that psoriasis is associated with inflammation above and beyond other heart disease risk factors, and the worse the psoriasis, the worse the inflammation. Once you add depression into the mix (and remember, psoriasis patients have a higher risk of depression), the risk of heart disease rises. Psoriasis patients with a history of depression have higher inflammation and more plaque deposits in their arteries than those with no depression.[31]

As inflammation is the common factor behind all these complications, taking measures to lower chronic inflammation can improve psoriasis symptoms and its complications. To this end, the National Psoriasis Foundation recommends an anti-inflammatory diet. More specifically, it cautions people living with psoriasis to avoid fatty red meats, dairy products, processed foods, refined sugars, and nightshade vegetables, such as peppers, white potatoes, eggplants, and tomatoes, as some people have found that these foods can trigger flares. Meanwhile, the foundation advises enjoying a variety of anti-inflammatory foods, specifically those rich in omega-3s, and colorful fruits and vegetables. For additional specific recommendations, see the "Nutrition Check for Autoimmune Disease" sidebar on page 144, and take note that the anti-inflammatory whole-body eating plan that starts on page 214 will help you reach many of these goals.[32]

Celiac Disease

Celiac disease (CD) is a chronic autoimmune and digestive disorder that causes an abnormal immune response to gluten, a protein found in grains like wheat, rye, and barley. Gluten triggers serious intestinal inflammation and if left untreated, CD can cause permanent damage. Symptoms include abdominal bloating and pain, constipation, diarrhea, flatulence, weight loss, nausea, and vomiting. Celiac disease can also lead to malnutrition because the inflamed small intestine is unable to properly absorb nutrients. But the symptoms aren't confined to GI problems. Other problems include anemia, canker sores, fatigue, headache, infertility and/or recurrent miscarriages, missed menstrual periods, skin rash, tingling in the hands or feet, and weak or brittle bones. Currently there is no known cure for CD, and the only available treatment is a strict gluten-free diet. Fortunately, going "g-free" can quickly and effectively eliminate symptoms.

Like other autoimmune disorders, CD is on the rise: The Celiac Disease Foundation estimates that it may affect 1 in every 100 people worldwide, and many cases go misdiagnosed. As with other autoimmune diseases, the exact cause of CD remains under investigation, but research indicates that a combination of genetic and environmental factors is to blame. Because celiac disease runs in families, people who have a first-degree relative (a parent, sibling, or child) with CD stand a 1 in 10 chance of developing it,[33] and those with severe food allergies are five times more likely to develop CD.[34] The risk of developing inflammatory bowel disease is 10 times higher in celiac patients than in the general population.[35] Analysis of large sets of data from similar studies points to a connection, though not direct, between viral infections and CD. Studies have noted a higher risk of CD in infants who contract infections in the first month of life, and the common childhood virus rotavirus is associated with early-onset CD. It is interesting to note that the body responds to both CD and viral infections by overproducing a proinflammatory cytokine called interferon alpha. Further demonstrating the interferon-CD

NUTRITION CHECK FOR AUTOIMMUNE DISEASE

Given the enormous diversity of autoimmune diseases, not to mention individual differences when it comes to food allergies and sensitivities, there is no single "anti-autoimmune diet" that will help address every condition. However, certain foods do seem to trigger flare-ups, and there is clinical evidence that additives in processed foods can cause the bacterial imbalance in the gut that allows an autoimmune condition to take hold. Drawing on the principles of anti-inflammatory eating, here are some general guidelines to help prevent autoimmunity and autoimmune flare-ups. Feel free to adapt these guidelines to your individual needs, such as avoiding any foods to which you're sensitive or allergic or that have triggered a flare-up in the past.

Foods to Definitely Avoid

- Trans fats (and keep saturated fat intake as low as possible)
- Processed foods (processed meats, bakery items, convenience foods, etc.)
- Artificial ingredients (avoiding any ingredient you can't pronounce is usually a safe bet)
- High amounts of sugar and sodium (eliminating processed foods will go a long way in avoiding these two)
- Sodas

Foods to Consider Avoiding or Taking a Break From

- Dairy
- Meat, especially conventionally or industrially produced meat

connection, some patients who've received interferon alpha as part of a treatment regimen for leukemia or hepatitis have developed CD.[36]

Many people wonder if there is a way to prevent CD. There is some evidence that infants who are breastfed for more than 1 year have a lower risk of CD, especially when they are introduced to gluten-containing foods slowly.[37] This information could make a big difference in the lives of children with a genetic predisposition, but other studies have disputed this finding[38] and

- Gluten

- Alcohol

- Nightshades (this plant group triggers autoimmune flare-ups in some people; it includes tomatoes, eggplants, peppers, white potatoes)

Foods to Enjoy to Your Immune System's Content

- Overall, concentrate on fresh, whole foods (see Chapter 11 for our full anti-inflammatory approach to eating)

- Fresh fruits and vegetables (organic is best to avoid pesticides)

- Dark leafy greens (these fiber-rich, calcium-rich veggies are important enough to highlight separately, and examples include collards, broccoli, broccoli rabe, kale, spinach, bok choy, turnip greens, mustard greens, arugula, Swiss or rainbow chard, watercress, cabbage, and chicory)

- Foods containing vitamin D: fortified beverages (dairy or plant milks, orange juice), mushrooms, eggs, fish, and fish oil (vitamin D supplementation may likely be recommended, as well)

- Calcium-rich foods (but make sure to avoid food triggers): fortified beverages (dairy or plant milks, orange juice), dairy products, tofu, sardines, shrimp, soybeans, okra, white beans, black-eyed peas, and dark leafy greens

- Foods that are rich in omega-3s: salmon, mackerel, herring, albacore tuna, walnuts, walnut oil, flaxseeds, flaxseed oil, olive oil, and pumpkin seeds

- Probiotic-rich foods: fermented foods like sauerkraut, kimchi, buttermilk, and kefir (to get far larger quantities of probiotics, add a supplement)

- Spices with an anti-inflammatory effect: turmeric, ginger, garlic, and black pepper concluded that primary prevention of celiac disease is simply not possible. Instead, they advocate for prevention through mass screening of the general population; if celiac disease is detected at an early age, even before the onset of symptoms, a gluten-free diet can prevent nutrition problems that may delay growth and reduce bone mineral density.[39]

Research on celiac disease is ongoing, and some of the newer studies have revealed severe gut dysbiosis in those with CD. (A gluten-free diet does improve the imbalance in bacterial strains, but it doesn't completely restore a healthy gut microbiome.) As dysbiosis, inflammation, and leaky gut have been definitively linked, probiotics that reduce the inflammatory response and reverse gut dysbiosis could help treat CD patients, along with a gluten-free diet. More randomized, controlled trials are needed.[40]

Allergies

Allergies are among the most common chronic inflammatory conditions in the world. They're different from autoimmune conditions but closely linked, as both result from a similar malfunction in the immune system. In the case of allergies, the immune system goes in attack mode to fight what's normally a harmless substance (rather than other parts of the body, as with autoimmune conditions). The most common triggers (known as *allergens*) are pollen, dust, animal dander, mold, insect bites or stings, medications, latex, and many common foods. While there are at least 190 known food allergens, 90 percent of food allergies fall into eight food groups: peanuts, tree nuts (almonds, walnuts, cashews, Brazil nuts), dairy, eggs, wheat, soy, shellfish (shrimp, crab, lobster), and "finned" fish (salmon, tuna, halibut).

Essentially, when the body encounters an allergen, the immune system overreacts and produces an antibody called immunoglobulin E (IgE), which triggers a very powerful inflammatory reaction. IgE also triggers the production of histamine and other chemicals, such as interleukins. It's histamine and these other chemicals that produce allergic symptoms, which vary based on the type of allergy, though nearly all allergic reactions will produce inflammation, itching, a rash or hives, and irritation. Additionally, allergic rhinitis, or hay fever, will result in watery, bloodshot eyes, sneezing, a headache, allergy "shiners" (dark circles under the eyes), and a runny nose. Asthma and sometimes mold allergies can produce airway constriction and wheezing. Food allergies can also produce digestive problems and sometimes breathing

FOOD SENSITIVITIES VERSUS FOOD ALLERGIES

Food sensitivities are also known as food intolerances. While similar to food allergies because they can produce many of the same unpleasant signs and symptoms, there are crucial differences between the two. First, while food sensitivities can make you feel miserable, they don't have the potential to produce life-threatening anaphylaxis. Second, food sensitivity symptoms tend to show up more slowly than symptoms of food allergies. This is partly because food sensitivities are often a response to intestinal permeability (leaky gut), or put another way, it's the inflamed and leaky intestinal lining that results in a person being sensitive to certain foods. In contrast, a food allergy is an immune reaction to a specific food (like peanuts), and it'll show up quickly after eating the allergenic food. Third, while food allergies produce symptoms throughout the body—for example, diarrhea, hives, and a runny nose—food sensitivities predominantly cause gastrointestinal symptoms. That said, some people with food sensitivities do experience symptoms such as a headache, a rash or hives, a feeling of "spaciness," and a runny nose.

Because they share many of the same signs and symptoms, it can be difficult to determine if a reaction is a food sensitivity or an allergy. Skin-prick tests and blood tests to measure the level of IgE (immunoglobulin E) antibodies can help identify an allergy, but the best way to identify a food intolerance is through an elimination diet. In most elimination diets, any foods that are suspected of causing the trouble are initially excluded to see if the symptoms resolve. If symptoms disappear, and certainly if the food is reintroduced and symptoms return, you've found your culprit. These diets can take time, and keeping a food diary helps. Our Whole Body Cure Eating Plan begins with eliminating all of the most common food triggers, which quickly cuts down on inflammation. After this whole-body "reset," foods are reintroduced individually. With this method, you'll be able to identify your unique food triggers while healing your gut and reducing inflammation.

problems. The most severe allergic reaction is called anaphylactic shock, a potentially lethal reaction in which inflammation runs rampant very quickly. Anaphylaxis can cause nausea, vomiting, breathing difficulty, swelling, rapidly falling blood pressure, dizziness, and shock, and it always requires immediate medical treatment. The most common triggers of anaphylaxis are food, latex, insect bites or stings, and medications.

When most of us think about allergies, hay fever and hives or maybe a certain food allergy usually comes to mind; however, allergists and other specialists think more in terms of *allergic diseases*. These diseases are identified as anaphylaxis, insect allergies, drug allergies, food allergies, certain forms of asthma, hay fever, pinkeye, eczema, hives, angioedema (rapid swelling of the skin and underlying tissue), and eosinophilic disorders, which can occur in any part of the body when a type of white blood cell known as eosinophils plays a role in allergic reactions and becomes overabundant.[41] Other sources add occupational allergies as a separate category, and these are considered *preventable* allergies that occur because of contact with an allergen at work. Common examples are occupational asthma caused by inhaling fumes, gases, or dust or allergic contact dermatitis caused by latex or chemical exposure.

Like autoimmune diseases, allergic diseases have been on the rise over the past few decades, and their severity and complexity are increasing, as well. It's not uncommon for two or more allergies to occur concurrently. For example, there is a strong association between asthma, hay fever, and eczema. The latest statistics from the World Allergy Organization, an international organization that compiles data and provides resources, paint a troubling picture.

Overall, allergies affect more than 20 percent of the world's population.

- Hay fever, which affects up to 30 percent of people globally, is on the rise and is a risk factor for asthma.
- Since the 1960s, the prevalence of asthma and deaths due to asthma in countries with an industrialized, Western lifestyle is rising. According to the World Health Organization, an estimated 300 million people suffer from asthma, and that number is expected to grow to 400 million by 2025.

- Globally, up to 550 million people may suffer from food allergies.

- Hives are a common occurrence; the probability of experiencing hives at least once in your life is more than 20 percent. Chronic hives impairs productivity by up to 30 percent due to missed workdays and lower job performance.

- Adverse drug reactions affect up to a tenth of the world's population and up to 20 percent of hospitalized patients. Drug allergies may be responsible for up to 20 percent of deaths due to anaphylaxis.[42]

Clearly, there is an urgent need for prevention and treatment strategies for a wide range of allergic reactions and allergic diseases. Currently there is no cure for allergies, and complete avoidance of the allergen may be necessary. This can create a significant burden on allergy sufferers who must scrutinize food labels for even trace amounts of allergens like peanuts, tree nuts, wheat, or egg, for example. (To learn the differences between a food sensitivity and a true food allergy, see the sidebar on page 147.) Others must avoid any contact with something that will trigger their eczema, or avoid environments with pets, or feel like they're confined indoors during pollen season—and good luck avoiding dust! Avoiding all allergens simply isn't feasible in many cases.

Drug therapies for allergies depend on the type and severity. Antihistamines reduce or block the body's production of histamines and thus prevent allergy symptoms, steroid medications reduce inflammation, bronchodilators open airways, anti-IgE medications bring down high serum levels of IgE, decongestants can clear blocked nasal passages, and emergency epinephrine is necessary when anaphylaxis occurs. In addition, allergen-specific immunotherapy can be used for respiratory allergies, hay fever, and insect bite allergies; it's delivered by injection or under the tongue. Researchers are investigating the possibility of new forms of immunotherapy for food allergies and eczema. Other more recent therapies include a class of drugs known as immunomodulators that target proinflammatory cytokines. Many of these drugs are still being investigated.

As for prevention, some of the most innovative research points to therapies that teach the immune system to tolerate a wider diversity of substances. Noting the sharp rise in allergic diseases that has occurred alongside the increased use of antibiotics and antibacterial products, some scientists concluded that excessive hygiene was playing a role in the increase in allergies. According to this theory, a lack of early exposure to infectious agents leads to an untested, weakened immune system. However, based on the latest evidence, a growing number of researchers are urging the abandonment of the "hygiene hypothesis."

The better metaphor, these experts suggest, is to think of a baby's immune system as a computer with hardware and software but very little data. If data isn't "uploaded" over the years in the form of microbes from other humans and the natural environment, the regulatory mechanisms of the immune system fail, leading to attacks on harmless substances like pollen, dust, or foods. Increasing exposure to a wide variety of microbes supplies the immune system with more "data" and teaches it to tolerate a wider array of substances. Allergic and infectious disease experts recommend a combination of strategies throughout one's life span to restore a diverse microbiome and reduce the risk of allergic diseases, including vaginal childbirth, breastfeeding, increased social exposure through sports and other outdoor activities, less time spent indoors, a varied diet that includes fiber and plenty of colorful fruits and vegetables, and avoiding the unnecessary use of antibiotics.[43]

Is there still a place for personal hygiene? Absolutely. Regular handwashing and cleaning the places hands regularly touch, such as bathrooms, utensils, and food preparation surfaces, are still the best ways to prevent infectious diseases. Such "targeted hygiene" maximizes protection against pathogens while preserving the spread of essential microbes.[44]

As for nutrition interventions, we know already that the Western diet is associated with allergy risk and with worse symptoms. An Australian study of over 156,000 adults examined dietary patterns and occurrence of asthma as well as a dual diagnosis of asthma and hay fever. Researchers found that a diet high in meat—especially processed meat and red meat—was a risk factor for asthma and hay fever.[45] A study based on nearly 60,500 women found that

POSSIBLE CAUSES OF THE RISE IN ALLERGIES

Allergies of all types are on the rise. Here are some possible causes.

- Increasing outdoor pollution (smog, automobile fumes, etc.)

- Increased smoking (globally)

- Climate change (shorter growing times and higher temperatures mean more pollen; higher temperatures also exacerbate breathing problems)

- Gut microbiome dysbiosis (less microbial diversity; less exposure to microbes that can teach the immune system greater tolerance)

- An increase in caesarean births and a decrease in breastfeeding (both interfere with a newborn receiving a mother's microbes)

- Increased migration (moving to a new area exposes one to a new set of pollutants and allergens)

- The rising proliferation of the Western diet, which contains processed foods with harmful additives, less diversity of foods, fewer plant polyphenols, and less fiber[46, 47, 48]

drinking artificially sweetened sodas while pregnant resulted in a greater chance of having a child develop asthma or hay fever during his or her first 7 years.[49]

Nutrition may also be the way to treat or even prevent food allergies. Some promising advancements in our understanding of peanut allergy have been made through the landmark Learning Early about Peanut Allergy (LEAP) study. Researchers demonstrated that introducing peanuts to infants who are at high risk of peanut allergy can prevent the development of the allergy. Over 600 babies between 4 and 11 months with severe eczema, egg allergy, or both were put into two groups based on a preexisting sensitivity to peanuts: one group with a positive reaction to a skin-prick test, the other with no measurable reaction. They were then randomized either to consume a peanut-containing snack at least three times a week up until the age of 5 or to avoid peanuts altogether. Of the 530 children who initially had a negative reaction to the skin-prick test and avoided peanuts, 13.7 percent went on to develop a peanut allergy

(continued on page 154)

Terri Bortz

AGE: 47

- Reduced total cholesterol by 25 points
- Eliminated severe joint pain
- WEIGHT LOST: 18 pounds
- INCHES LOST: 12½

I was skeptical at first about what this plan could do for me. I was already a healthy eater—I've never been a soda drinker, and I've cooked from scratch and avoided processed foods for years. I've also tried different diets all my life. I lost weight on each one, but I never found anything I'd stick with permanently, and the weight would always come back. This is the first plan I've found that I'm going to continue to use. This plan forces you to pay attention to what you're eating and to how food is affecting you. If you're incorporating a food back in after the elimination period and you suddenly experience a symptom that hadn't been there for weeks, you know there's a connection. They say diets don't work unless you make serious life changes in the way you eat and the way you cook, and the Whole Body Cure Plan breaks it down for you and guides you in doing that.

I lost 18 pounds in 12 weeks, and my cholesterol level fell tremendously. The cholesterol was an especially big deal in my case because I have Graves' disease and my cholesterol is always on the high side. But one of the biggest benefits I experienced was relief from joint pain. For the past 5 years, I've had horrible joint pain in my knees and my hips. It was severe enough that it would wake me out of a sound sleep. It hurt just to put my feet on the floor in the morning, and lying down was horrible. But as the first 2 weeks progressed, I realized my knees didn't hurt anymore. I didn't put two and two together until I transitioned to the egg test in Week 3. Before the plan, it wasn't unusual for me to eat three eggs a day. But the first day I added the eggs back, I developed a headache, I had heartburn, and my joint pain returned. When the symptoms continued the next day, my husband pointed out that eggs were not agreeing with me. So I stopped eating eggs, and within half a day, my symptoms were gone. My knees and hips are fine.

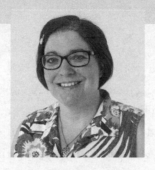

Terri's Tip

During the elimination period, don't skip the protein shake in the afternoon. I was cranky from not eating, mostly from craving protein. In retrospect, if I'd had half a protein shake later in the day I think I would've been okay.

I thought a food intolerance would only cause GI issues or maybe allergy symptoms like hives, and it does for some people. But I did some research on my own and found out that the exact symptoms I was having—headache, heartburn, and joint pain—were classic symptoms of a food intolerance. I've since followed up with my own doctor, and I've learned that I have an intolerance to albumin, which is found in egg whites.

If I use eggs at all now, it's very sparingly, like in an egg bath for zucchini chips. I've also permanently eliminated cow's milk because this helped bring my cholesterol down. I drink almond or cashew milk instead. I've drastically cut back on snacking, and I always think about what I'm eating before I eat it. If I have something I consider a "cheat"— like a little goat cheese for a treat—I'll

keep that in my mind and know that I've had my treat so I won't have one later. We forget about the "everything in moderation" rule, but it makes sense.

I also continue to have the protein shakes every morning, and I make the smoothies, which are good! I've learned a lot of new ways to be creative with vegetables. My new best friend is cauliflower! I rice it in my food processor and use it anywhere I once used regular rice. I made stuffed peppers with the riced cauliflower, and my husband thought they were the best he'd ever had. Another new favorite for us is spaghetti squash.

Overall, I have lots more energy now, and I want to use it. I enjoy biking, walking, and yoga, and my goal is to lose a few more pounds, and then my daughter and I are going to do a 5-K together. I haven't felt this good in 15 years. ■

by the time they were 5. But of the children who were exposed to peanuts early, only 1.9 percent developed a peanut allergy. Among the 98 children who initially had positive test results, the prevalence of peanut allergy was 35.3 percent in the avoidance group and only 10.6 percent in the consumption group. These are extraordinary results with life-changing potential—especially considering that peanut allergy is the leading cause of anaphylaxis and death associated with food allergy.[50] Based on the LEAP data, the American Academy of Pediatrics now recommends that high-risk infants should be exposed to peanuts between 4 and 11 months of age. Parents should consult an allergist or physician with training in allergic diseases for help implementing these recommendations and monitoring the child.[51] There is also evidence suggesting that taking probiotics and prebiotics during pregnancy and offering a child supplementation up to the age of 2 offer some protection against food allergy and eczema. A study found that giving probiotic and prebiotic supplements to children up to age 4 is effective for preventing eczema in those at high risk of allergy, and that *Lactobacillus rhamnosus* was most effective.[52] Of course, talk with your pediatrician first before starting any supplements for your child.

Probiotics can also help with the symptoms of hay fever. In one small study, researchers exposed volunteers with a history of hay fever to grass pollen and then gave them a probiotic preparation consisting of the common bacterial strains *Lactobacillus acidophilus* and *Bifidobacterium lactis*. The treatment significantly reduced nasal itching and the percentage of white blood cells in nasal fluid.[53] Yet another study compared 8 weeks of the *Bifidobacterium lactis* strain versus a placebo on people with a history of hay fever—right in the midst of pollen season. Concentrations of proinflammatory cytokines were significantly lower in the probiotic group at the end of the study, and nasal symptom scores and markers of allergic activity were far lower in the probiotic group in the second month.[54]

Accidental Arson

The contradictory term *accidental arson* refers to the paradox of what's going on with autoimmune disorders and allergies. When the inflammation army attacks the wrong enemy, the ultimate outcome is misplaced harm. With autoimmunity, the body attacks itself. With allergies, it attacks a substance that usually wouldn't be dangerous. Both disorders can have dire consequences.

Immune system disorders are incredibly complex, and they require a multifaceted approach to medical care as they inevitably have system-wide effects and many potential complications. Further, these conditions are highly individual, affecting no two people in the exact same way. There is no cure for autoimmune disorders, and there is no definitive "cure" for allergies other than strict avoidance of all allergens. Working regularly with your primary care physician and a rheumatologist and/or allergist, as well as additional specialists as needed if complications arise, is essential.

All of this said, there are still plenty of ways to maintain periods of remission and avoid allergy attacks and to get relief when symptoms occur. Medications can treat symptoms, but living an anti-inflammatory lifestyle is the best way to get at the root of the problem. When your body is chronically inflamed, your immune system can easily become hyperreactive. Adopting an anti-inflammatory lifestyle can reduce systemic sensitivity and calm the allergic response, which can improve quality of life overall.

CHAPTER 8

The Inflamed Brain

The Surprising Effects of Chronic Inflammation on Memory and Mood

Scientists have known for a while now that neuroinflammation—inflammation that occurs in brain cells and tissues—plays a key role in diseases such as Alzheimer's and Parkinson's. But accumulating evidence reveals that chronic neuroinflammation plays a starring role in the development of a far wider range of conditions than we once thought. Not only dementia but also milder forms of memory loss, depression, anxiety, and even bipolar disorder and schizophrenia are directly linked to "the inflamed brain."

If you're wondering how it's possible that neuroinflammation is implicated in so many diverse conditions, remember that the brain and the central nervous system are no more immune to chronic inflammation than any other organ or system. And with the 100 billion neurons (nerve cells) in the brain, controlling everything from memory to mood to appetite to cognitive function to sex drive, along with the incredibly complex network of blood vessels supplying oxygen and nutrients to brain cells, the stage is set for a vast set of potential outcomes when chronic inflammation is at work.

Brain on Fire

At its most basic level, neuroinflammation operates just like inflammation anywhere else in the body. In short doses—when neuroinflammation is acute, in other words—it can be a good thing. The acute inflammatory response can fight off an infection that attacks the brain, or it can start the healing process in the event of a head injury. With short-term neuroinflammation, the body is often able to return to optimum health and wellness. But when neuroinflammation sticks around, it starts to degrade and destroy healthy neurons, interfering with healthy brain function. Unlike, say, the inflammation that occurs when you injure your knee, leaving you unable to walk for a few days, the effects of neuroinflammation can be nothing short of devastating because your central command center is under attack. Depending on the area of the brain most affected, dramatic changes in physical functioning, speech, thinking, mood, memory, and even personality can occur. To cite just one all too familiar example, think of the drastic changes in cognitive function, personality, physical ability, and mood that occur to a person as Alzheimer's disease progresses.

Because the stakes are high, our bodies have built-in means of protection that, nine times out of ten, work beautifully to protect our brains. The skull, meninges (membranes that surround the brain), and the cerebrospinal fluid between the brain and skull protect the brain from injury. Meanwhile, the blood-brain barrier keeps harmful pathogens and toxins from entering the brain, allowing only the molecules it needs to function, such as hormones, water, glucose, and amino acids, to pass. The blood-brain barrier works because the layer of cells that line the blood vessels supplying the brain are very tightly packed together. If you're of a certain age, you may remember a game called Red Rover. Two groups of kids line up side by side on opposing sides of the field and tightly link arms. One team calls for a runner to sprint across the space between them—"Red Rover, Red Rover, send Kevin right over!"—and try to break through the line. The blood-brain barrier functions something like those lines of kids. If the links between them are strong, nothing is getting through the line. But if there is a weak link, then a runner can break through.

In the case of the brain, guess what creates a weak link? Or to leave our metaphor behind, guess what weakens the blood-brain barrier? Inflammation. More specifically, neuroinflammation makes the blood-brain barrier more permeable—not unlike how inflammation makes the gut barrier more permeable! When neuroinflammation sticks around, more molecules can pass through the blood-brain barrier and gain access to the protected space of the brain—including harmful pathogens. When the blood-brain barrier is too permeable, it can't do its job effectively, leaving the brain vulnerable to infection and, over time, to any number of neurodegenerative disorders, from mild cognitive impairment to Alzheimer's disease. We'll look at some specific conditions below.

By now you're probably wondering what can cause neuroinflammation. On one level the answer is very simple—any of the things that can cause general inflammation. (For a full list, see Chapter 2.) But some of the most common causes of neuroinflammation are an infection, exposure to pollutants and toxins, smoking, aging, an autoimmune condition, or a traumatic brain injury. Other causes include poor diet, chronic stress, and insufficient sleep. Let's take a closer look at what can happen when inflammation of the brain becomes chronic.

How Neuroinflammation Can Rob You of Memory

There is a whole spectrum of memory loss, from the annoying but harmless forgetfulness that accompanies aging, to the occasional brain fog that leaves us feeling like we're not firing on all cylinders, all the way to the ruinous effects of dementia. Somewhere in the middle of that spectrum is the condition known as mild cognitive impairment (MCI). Some doctors see MCI as the intermediary stage between normal age-related memory loss and dementia; others consider it a very early form of Alzheimer's. With MCI, there is definite memory impairment that can be observed by others as well as the sufferer, but it hasn't yet progressed to dementia. A person with MCI is chronically forgetful but retains general cognitive function.

Here's the thing: At any point on the spectrum, from age-related memory loss to MCI to Alzheimer's, neuroinflammation is working behind the scenes. We know that neuroinflammation alone—without the presence of injury, stroke, infection, or other obvious insult to the brain, that is—can cause memory loss. Studies have found that brain inflammation impairs the function of the hippocampus, an area involved in memory, cognition, and behavior—so much so that the hippocampus can shrink in the presence of long-term inflammation! When hippocampal volume decreases, the growth of new neurons slows while brain cells degrade and die faster.[1] (This is the familiar pattern we see with chronic inflammation: It always degrades cells and tissues, and it always interferes with normal function.) Studies have also found elevated biomarkers of inflammation in patients with reduced hippocampal volume. In one study, healthy adults with detectable CRP levels were found to have smaller medial temporal lobes, the area where the hippocampus is found, than those who had undetectable levels of CRP, and they performed worse on memory tests.[2]

Now, how about *brain fog*? This term is popping up in headlines everywhere. People use it informally to describe being unable to focus or concentrate, feeling confused, or being unable to think clearly. But it's also a medical term that refers to a constellation of symptoms, including short- and long-term memory loss, inability to concentrate, inability to multitask, and generally reduced cognition. Brain fog has been associated with many diverse conditions; a partial list includes celiac disease, PMS, menopause, chronic fatigue syndrome, fibromyalgia, multiple sclerosis, leaky gut syndrome, exposure to toxins (especially mold), thyroid problems, obesity, yeast infections, chronic stress, and allergies. Do you notice the common component here? All of these are inflammatory conditions. The connection makes sense because research has shown that spikes in inflammation trigger brain fog. The triggers behind those spikes are, again, any of the triggers of chronic inflammation. But some research places much of the blame for brain fog on two culprits: stress and exposure to mold. Certainly both of these causes trigger acute inflammation, and if they're not stopped, the inflammation can become chronic.[3]

Countless studies have illustrated the harmful effects of stress on memory loss—and the effects can occur very quickly. In one recent study, researchers had mice learn a maze with an escape hole, and then they gave the mice a big-time stressor: They placed a larger, aggressive mouse in the maze. The mice that repeatedly had to face the intruder became quite stressed and, though they'd previously memorized the maze, had trouble remembering where to find the escape hole. They also displayed social avoidance behavior, a clinical measure of depression. Confirming the stress-inflammation connection, researchers also found markers of neuroinflammation in the brains of the stressed mice. They concluded that stress-induced neuroinflammation impairs function of the hippocampus. But happily, this wasn't the last word of this study—when another group of mice received anti-inflammatory treatment, they displayed no signs of stress-induced memory loss.[4]

There is also evidence that age-related memory loss occurs because of free radical damage to neurons. Again, chronic inflammation is a key causal factor. Free radicals are the normal by-product of cell metabolism, but harmful agents such as inflammation, UV radiation, toxins, stress, and nutritional deficiencies can stimulate free radical production, too. When there are too many free radicals circulating in the body, they can damage DNA, cell membranes, and tissues. As free radicals cause more and more damage, cells become progressively unable to take in nutrients and get waste out. And as they falter, they produce more inflammation, triggering that vicious cycle that we've previously discussed. Free radicals are both a cause and an effect of inflammation. It's this damage and eventual dying off of brain cells over time that causes neurodegenerative diseases. And without a doubt, one of the consequences of free radical damage to neurons is memory loss.

What combats free radicals? Antioxidants. Antioxidants scavenge free radicals, *and* they have a powerful anti-inflammatory effect. Thus, eating a diet rich in antioxidants is one of the very best ways to prevent memory loss by warding off chronic neuroinflammation before it ever catches fire. In a study of 2,574 middle-aged men and women, a higher flavonoid intake was associated with better verbal and episodic memory, the ability to recall autobiographical events.[5] Flavonoids are a class of antioxidants that are especially effective when it comes to protecting memory; they're found in abundance in fruits, vegetables, and tea. Berries in particular are highly recommended because they're rich in a class of flavonoid called anthocyanins, which can cross the blood-brain barrier and directly affect the hippocampus.[6] Resveratrol, a phytonutrient found in grape juice and red wine, and pterostilbene, a phytonutrient found in grapes, blueberries, and both their juices, also protect memory by activating signaling pathways that protect the brain against free radical damage and inflammation.[7] We'll give you our full anti-inflammatory approach to eating in Chapter 11, and for a quick guide to memory-boosting phytonutrients, take a look at the sidebar on page 172.

Further Down the Spectrum of Memory Loss

Now let's move a little further down the line—past misplacing the car keys and occasionally forgetting names, past brain fog and mild cognitive impairment, and into the territory of dementia. For the record, dementia isn't a single disease. It's a general term that covers several types of dementia, any of which doesn't come into play until memory loss has become so severe that it impairs daily functioning.

According to the latest estimates, 47 million people worldwide currently live with some form of dementia, and the number is expected to rise to 131.5 million by 2050.[8] Alzheimer's disease is the most common form, accounting for between 60 and 80 percent of all dementia cases.[9] Other forms include Parkinson's disease, vascular dementia (which results from damage to blood vessels, including stroke), Huntington's disease, frontotemporal dementia, and dementia with Lewy bodies. Each of these conditions is extremely complex and multifaceted, requiring highly specialized long-term care, but for the purposes of our discussion, there are a few key traits that we can identify.

- Any type of dementia is a neurodegenerative disorder that results in a decline in mental function severe enough to compromise everyday life. Most commonly, the decline manifests as a progressive loss of memory, impaired reasoning, and personality changes.

- Most forms of dementia are irreversible.

- Dementia results from damage to neurons and brain tissue.

- One of the top causes of damage to neurons and brain tissue is neuroinflammation.

That dementia and inflammation are closely linked makes sense. Chronic inflammation *always* damages cells and tissues and impairs function—and here we're talking about chronic inflammation of the brain's cells and tissues. Results from a recent metastudy based on more than 5,700 participants found that an increased level of CRP was associated with a 45 percent increased risk of developing dementia of any type. A higher level of inflammatory biomarker IL-6 was associated with a 32 percent increased risk.[10]

Studies that examine the individual causes of chronic inflammation find this same pattern at work. A metareview that examined the link between smoking and dementia, for instance, concluded that smoking dramatically increases the risk of dementia of any type, including Alzheimer's. (As you'll remember from Chapter 2, smoking is one of the most damaging causes of chronic inflammation, for the smoker as well as anyone exposed to second-hand smoke.) For every 20 cigarettes smoked per day, the risk of dementia increases by 34 percent. This study, which was based on data from over 960,000 people, also provided some good news: Once people quit smoking, their risk of dementia fell to that of nonsmokers.[11] We also know that high blood pressure and stroke, both of which have strong inflammatory components, are risk factors for cognitive impairment and dementia, especially vascular dementia and Alzheimer's disease.[12]

Further confirmation of the inflammation-dementia link comes from nutritional studies. In one, researchers compared a "prudent" diet to the typical Western diet, which is highly inflammatory. A total of 2,223 participants who were dementia-free at the outset of the study were followed for up to 6 years. Those who best kept to the prudent diet experienced the lowest levels of mental decline, and those who opted for the Western diet showed the highest levels of mental decline. The prudent diet was characterized by fruits, vegetables, legumes, low-fat dairy products, whole grains, fish, lean poultry, and water, while the Western diet was high in fruit juice, potatoes, trans fats, medium- or high-fat dairy products, red meat, sweets, sodas, and beer.[13] These results offer a compelling snapshot of the effects of an anti-inflammatory approach to eating versus an inflammatory diet. An unhealthy, high-fat diet has in fact been linked with several neurological problems, including decreased hippocampal volume, impaired memory and cognition, reduced attention, and an increased vulnerability to depression and anxiety. Certainly, this is due in large degree to the rise in inflammation that comes from a long-term high-fat diet, not to mention the inflammatory conditions (heart disease, obesity, type 2 diabetes, metabolic syndrome) this type of diet can cause.[14]

Once again, there are no real surprises, right? Chronic inflammation undermines whole-body health and wellness, and the brain and its 100 billion neurons are no more immune to the effects of inflammation than any other organ system.

The story gets even more interesting when we look at the role of inflammation in specific neurodegenerative disorders. Alzheimer's disease, the most common form of dementia and the sixth leading cause of death in the United States, has an indisputable inflammatory component. Very briefly, it works like this. Alzheimer's is characterized by the accumulation of plaques and tangles in the brain, by the progressive loss of connections between neurons, and by the eventual death of neurons. The plaques we're referring to are called amyloid plaques, and they accumulate in the spaces between neurons. Amyloid plaques are composed mainly of beta-amyloid (often written as Aβ), a toxic protein. Tangles, meanwhile, are twisted protein threads that accumulate inside neurons; their chief component is called tau. So we've got amyloid plaques choking off connections between neurons and tangles choking off neurons from the inside. As plaques and tangles accumulate over time, they damage neurons to the point that they cannot function properly; when the neurons eventually die, serious neurodegeneration results.

Does this process sound familiar? This is very much the way chronic inflammation works. That is, over time, chronic inflammation destroys cells and tissues, resulting in impaired functioning and eventually disease and death.

But the similarities go further. Just as acute inflammation can be helpful (including the acute neuroinflammation that would occur after a stroke or brain injury, for example), there is now evidence to suggest that beta-amyloid plaques *in the short term* help protect the brain against infection. New research has found that infection triggers the production of Aβ, which acts as a natural antibiotic, protecting the brain from infection. Put another way, Aβ is part of the natural inflammatory response. As with chronic inflammation, when Aβ *persists and accumulates* devastating tissue damage results. Researchers demonstrated this connection by infecting the brains of normal mice and mice that had been genetically altered to express human Aβ with a *Salmonella* bacterium. The mice with the Aβ alteration survived far longer than the control mice. How did Aβ work? By the very characteristic that makes it so deadly in Alzheimer's disease: by clumping together and forming plaques. The Aβ "clumps" banded together to trap and imprison the bacteria.[15, 16] This action is reminiscent of the work of macrophages in surrounding and engulfing invading pathogens. And again, it illustrates the beneficial effect of acute inflammation—and the guaranteed harm of chronic inflammation.

Now, if you feel like you still don't know a plaque from a tangle, just focus on this study's takeaway: Drugs that target the inflammatory pathways of our natural immune system offer new avenues for Alzheimer's prevention and treatment. If researchers can identify which pathogens trigger the inflammatory response and resulting production of Aβ plaques, they may be able to target those pathogens specifically.[17] Thus they could arrest the inflammatory response well before it becomes chronic and harmful.[18]

Whether chronic neuroinflammation is a cause or a result of Alzheimer's— or, as we see so often with chronic inflammation, *both*—is still being worked out. But we do know that proinflammatory cytokines are found at high levels in people with Alzheimer's, and it appears that TNF-α plays an especially prominent role in tipping the scales from MCI to full-blown dementia. One study compared blood levels of TNF-α in patients with MCI, Alzheimer's disease, and healthy controls over 18 months or longer. In those who progressed from MCI to Alzheimer's, levels of a TNF-α soluble receptor were significantly higher. Researchers concluded that the abnormal activation of the TNF-α signaling system is linked to a higher risk of progressing from MCI to Alzheimer's disease.[19] What's behind that abnormal activation is quite complex, but part of the answer lies in TNF-α's role in initiating chronic inflammation and perpetuating it. (In other words, it both kindles the fire and keeps it burning.) We also know that TNF-α contributes to the formation of amyloid plaques[20] and that drugs that inhibit TNF-α may decrease amyloid plaques and inhibit changes to tau proteins that lead to dementia.[21]

Likewise, research is under way to evaluate anti-inflammatory medications to prevent and treat Alzheimer's. The results are mixed. People who use NSAIDs (nonsteroidal anti-inflammatory drugs) for the long term *do* have a reduced risk of developing Alzheimer's disease. It would be wonderful if preventing dementia was as simple as taking ibuprofen every day, but alas, the full picture is more complicated than that. For one thing, the neuroprotective effect only seems to come with long-term use—as in 2 years or more—and long-term NSAID use comes with the risk of serious side effects for the gastrointestinal tract, heart, and kidneys. Further, the correct NSAID seems to be key, and it must be taken well before symptoms are present. In the later stages of Alzheimer's, NSAIDs may have an adverse effect. But a daily naproxen given to people who had a family history of Alzheimer's (but no symptoms) resulted in a reduced incidence of the disease—but only after 2 to 3 years of use.[22, 23]

What's the bottom-line takeaway? Your best bet for keeping your brain healthy and preserving cognitive function—thinking, decision-making, planning, organizing, remembering—is to prevent neuroinflammation before it sparks. And the best way to do that is to live a full anti-inflammatory lifestyle. By now you know the drill: Don't smoke, get enough exercise (which includes intentional moderate exercise as well as moving regularly), take an anti-inflammatory approach to eating, keep stress in check, maintain a healthy BMI, avoid exposure to toxins, and get sufficient sleep.

Additionally, you might consider taking folic acid supplements. This B vitamin helps produce new, healthy brain cells. Low folate levels impair vitamin B_{12}

absorption, which leads to systemic inflammation. A recent trial that gave newly diagnosed Alzheimer's patients 1.25 milligrams of folic acid a day for 6 months found that biomarkers of inflammation fell and levels of SAM and SAH, two compounds that reduce inflammation, rose. Participants who took folic acid also scored better on cognitive function tests compared to a control group.[24]

"Inflammood": An Introduction

You may not think of psychiatric conditions as inflammatory illnesses like arthritis or sinusitis, but studies have established a firm connection between chronic inflammation and mental health. Most of the research focuses on anxiety and especially depression (and that's where we'll spend most of our time), but let's first examine some of the evidence that establishes mood disorders and psychiatric conditions as inflammatory illnesses.

A small but fascinating study conducted back in the early 2000s vividly demonstrates the impact of even a short-term spike in inflammation on mood. Researchers injected healthy volunteers with a low dose of a *Salmonella* endotoxin. The toxin had no effect on physical sickness symptoms, heart rate, or blood pressure. But it did spark an inflammatory response. Volunteers experienced a mild increase in temperature and significantly increased levels of inflammatory biomarkers, as well as an increase in the stress hormone cortisol. Even more fascinating? Volunteers became depressed and anxious, and they performed worse on tests of verbal and nonverbal memory. In other words, though volunteers had no outward symptoms of illness, the natural inflammatory response and subsequent proinflammatory cytokine release dramatically affected their mood and their cognitive abilities. Thankfully the effects were temporary. Once the inflammation subsided, mood and memory returned to baseline levels.[25]

And ladies, even the moodiness that accompanies your menstrual cycle—and we're talking from that very first period all the way to menopause—is due in part to cyclic rises in inflammation. Elevated CRP levels have been associated with premenstrual cramping, bloating/weight gain, appetite cravings, moodiness, and breast pain,[26] and high levels of IL-6 have been associated with hot flashes and night sweats in peri- and postmenopausal women.[27]

It seems that any time there's a disturbance in mood, inflammation is at work. Chronic stress, which can be counted on to spark neuroinflammation and worse, keeps the flames burning. Chronic stress also raises the risk of developing any anxiety disorder, in part because it increases neuroinflammatory signaling. Once an anxiety disorder has taken hold, it raises inflammation levels, and then anxiety and inflammation engage in that constant feedback loop, mutually reinforcing and worsening each other. And once again, don't discount the power of a poor diet in contributing to neuroinflammation and poor mood.

The Inflammation Blues

Now as for depression, which affects some 350 million people across the globe, research reveals that proinflammatory cytokines are higher in depressed people—especially IL-6, IL-1β, and TNF-α. At the same time, depressed people have lower levels of the *anti*-inflammatory cytokine IL-10, leading to a double-jeopardy, proinflammatory state. Further, scientists have noted that depression is more prevalent in people with chronic inflammatory diseases, such as heart disease, rheumatoid arthritis, and diabetes, and in those who experience an acute inflammatory event, such as a stroke or surgery.[28] We also know that antidepressants have an anti-inflammatory effect, and that anti-inflammatory medications can decrease symptoms of depression. This latter effect seems to be more prevalent in people who have higher levels of inflammation. Any way you slice it, inflammation and depression work hand in hand.[29]

The strong correlation between chronic inflammation and depression has given rise to the highly influential "cytokine hypothesis of depression." In brief, the hypothesis suggests that high proinflammatory cytokine levels and an increased immune response are associated with the development of depression, its symptoms, and its severity.[30] Results from a population-based study using data from more than 14,000 participants found that the CRP levels of depressed people were, on average, 31 percent higher than of nondepressed people. Further, their FeNO levels—a marker of airway inflammation that's typically *lower* in depressed people—were indeed 10.7 percent lower than in people with no depression.[31] Another recent study found that people with major depressive disorder (MDD) and suicidal thoughts had significantly higher inflammatory index scores than those with MDD and little to no suicidal thoughts or those who weren't depressed.[32]

Further support for the cytokine hypothesis for depression came from the experience of patients on interferon therapy. Interferons are a special type of cytokine made by the immune system. There are more than 20 types, but all interferons help govern the immune system in some way, and they all have anti-viral effects. (Their name comes from their ability to *interfere* with viruses reproducing.) Scientists began to produce interferons synthetically in the 1980s, and interferon therapy is now widely used to treat inflammatory disorders such as hepatitis, multiple sclerosis, and some cancers, including skin cancer and leukemia. Interferon therapy is a powerful healer, but it has serious side effects—and one of them is depression. In fact, depression has been so severe in some patients on interferon therapy that they have committed suicide. Depending on the dose, as much as 50 percent of patients who receive interferon for hepatitis C or melanoma develop major depression, and as much as 80 percent experience depressive symptoms such as fatigue, lack of energy, and the type of slower movement and thinking that's commonly seen in neuropsychiatric disorders, including depression. A previous history of depression or anxiety,

INFLAMMATION AND DEPRESSION, BY THE NUMBERS

- Nearly one in five people with heart disease experiences major depressive disorder.

- A diabetes diagnosis doubles the odds of having depression.

- Up to 70 percent of patients with autoimmune diseases, such as rheumatoid arthritis, celiac disease, psoriasis, or lupus, experience depression.

- Fifteen percent to 25 percent of cancer patients experience depression, compared to 9 percent of the general population.[33]

being female, and high doses of interferon increase the risk of interferon-induced depression.[34]

There is also a connection between inflammation and what's come to be called sickness behavior, which occurs in humans as well as in animals. Think of the last time you had the flu. You probably felt weak, tired, uninterested in food, and listless. Your sleep was probably disrupted, maybe you felt irritable or depressed, and maybe you couldn't think clearly. *Sickness behavior* is the term used to describe these dramatic, short-term changes that occur when you're under the weather—and they're uncannily not unlike the symptoms of depression. (In fact, antidepressants have been observed to decrease sickness behavior.)

The inner event that's giving rise to these exterior changes is none other than a dramatic uptick in proinflammatory cytokines, especially IL-1β and TNF-α. These cytokines are released in response to illness, and some scientists believe the resulting sickness behavior is a built-in response that forces us to "lie low" and conserve energy until we're better.

A study conducted with mice highlighted the powerful connection between proinflammatory cytokines and sickness behavior. When scientists injected healthy mice with IL-1β and TNF-α, the mice sequestered themselves in a corner of their cage, didn't socialize, ate and drank less, and experienced sleep and cognitive disturbances—again, their sickness behavior mirrored classic depressive behavior. But when the mice were treated with anti-inflammatory IL-10 or insulin-like growth factor 1, all signs of their sickness behavior disappeared.[35]

There is also a connection between inflammation and the cognitive dysfunction that so often accompanies depression and sickness behavior. One study assessed the CRP and IL-6 levels in 112 people with a diagnosis of MDD and in 57 healthy controls. As expected, CRP and IL-6 levels were higher in those with depression. But researchers also found that people who had high CRP levels also had poor cognitive function. Further, a high hs-CRP level (a more sensitive test of CRP) was associated with greater impairments in executive function, a set of mental skills that help us plan, organize, and store information. The higher the inflammation, the worse the symptoms—of depression *and* of cognitive impairment.[36]

A BROKEN HEART

There is a strong connection between depression and heart disease, two inflammatory illnesses that mutually reinforce one another. People with major depressive disorder (MDD) are more likely than nondepressed people to develop heart disease and to have worse outcomes once diagnosed. They're also at higher risk of developing major risk factors for heart disease, including overweight and obesity, metabolic syndrome, reduced heart rate variability, impaired vascular function, and chronic inflammation. Heart patients with depression even have a higher incidence of mortality than those who aren't depressed.[37] Research from longitudinal studies found that MDD increases the risk of illness and death from heart disease as much as 80 percent.[38]

Inflammation's undisputed role in depression has led some to investigate the potential of anti-inflammatories for treating it. A recent metareview of 14 clinical trials examining data from 6,262 depressed patients focused on exactly this question. Ten of the studies used nonsteroidal anti-inflammatory drugs, and four used cytokine inhibitors (such as infliximab and etanercept). The pooled results indicated that anti-inflammatory treatment was superior to a placebo for reducing depressive symptoms and for the rate of remission—and that the higher a person's inflammatory marker levels, the more effective anti-inflammatory therapies were at treating the depressive symptoms.[39]

The beneficial effect of anti-inflammatories on depression is a welcome development for a condition that is notoriously difficult to treat. Up to 30 percent of people don't respond to antidepressants, and even many who do still experience symptoms such as fatigue, anhedonia (the inability to experience pleasure), and a pattern of slower thinking and physical movement that is characteristic of depression.[40] However, studies have shown that anti-inflammatory medications can enhance the effect of antidepressants. COX-2 inhibitors, TNF inhibitors, and even plain aspirin have all demonstrated some success in improving depressive symptoms when added to an antidepressant therapy. It's still unclear why this method helps some people and not others, but higher baseline levels of inflammation play some role.[41]

There are also many nondrug interventions to consider, especially when it comes to nutrition. For example, curcumin, the active agent in the spice turmeric, has shown strong antidepressant and antianxiety potential—in large part because it is so effective at lowering inflammation.[42] In addition to whole turmeric, you can get curcumin through turmeric tea or in supplement form.

There is also a link between vitamin D and depression. A deficiency in vitamin D has been observed in people who attempted suicide—along with high levels of proinflammatory cytokines. It seems that low levels of vitamin D contribute to higher inflammation, which in turn may contribute to the worsening of depression. Experts recommend routine testing of vitamin D levels in patients with suicidal symptoms, with supplementation for those who are low.[43] Food sources of vitamin D include fortified dairy or plant milks, fortified juice, mushrooms, eggs, and fatty fish.

Speaking of fatty fish, a metastudy of omega-3 polyunsaturated fatty acid (PUFA) supplementation found beneficial clinical effects for people with MDD, bipolar disorder, and depressive symptoms.[44] Not surprisingly, PUFAs have strong anti-inflammatory effects, too. Whole foods sources of PUFAs are salmon, mackerel, herring, trout, sardines, walnuts, walnut oil, flaxseeds, and flaxseed oil.

Just as with memory loss, it seems that any intervention to lower inflammation may have a positive effect on depressive symptoms. One recent study found fascinating connections between shorter telomere length, an inflammation related sign of cellular aging, which is often inflammation driven, and both anxiety and depressive disorders. Based on data from 2,750 participants, researchers found that short telomeres were related to both psychiatric illness and the severity of symptoms. The most significant factors associated with the psychiatric illness and short telomeres were elevated levels of IL-6 and CRP, cigarette smoking, and metabolic problems such as high LDL cholesterol and high triglycerides. In other words, chronic inflammation and the lifestyle habits that cause it are associated with a higher risk of anxiety and depression *and* with more severe symptoms.[45]

Conversely, we can help protect ourselves against anxiety and depression by keeping inflammation as low as we can and relying on a few strategies that are relatively straightforward: Don't smoke, enjoy an anti-inflammatory diet, and get plenty of exercise and sleep. Another study found that 1,283 people with an active anxiety disorder had significantly shorter telomeres than a control group (582 people), indicating that their cells were aging more quickly than those without anxiety. Even more interesting, they also had significantly shorter telomeres than 459 people whose anxiety disorder was in remission. These very encouraging results illustrate that accelerated cellular aging caused by anxiety is *reversible*.[46]

Keep a Cool Head

We know that chronic inflammation has long-term effects on all body systems, and certainly the brain and central nervous system are no different. But because the brain is our central command center, any inflammation

---

FIGHT MEMORY LOSS AND STABILIZE MOOD WITH PHYTONUTRIENTS

Here's a quick-reference list of several powerful phytonutrients that can help protect against inflammation and chronic illness, preserve memory, and boost mood. These are health-promoting compounds found only in plant sources. So "eat the rainbow" and enjoy a cornucopia of brightly colored fruits and vegetables, a variety of teas, and every now and again, a treat of dark chocolate.

- Anthocyanins are flavonoids that give fruits their red, purple, blue, or black color. They can cross the blood-brain barrier and have shown special efficacy when it comes to preserving cognitive function.
  - *Found in . . .* acai berries, blueberries, blackberries, goji berries, raspberries, mulberries, and strawberries
- Catechins are flavonoid antioxidants that have demonstrated memory-preserving, mood-boosting, and even antiviral effects.
  - *Found in . . .* peaches, prunes, cocoa, acai oil, and especially green tea
- Theaflavins are antioxidant polyphenols with anti-inflammatory, antioxidant, anticancer, and cholesterol-lowering effects.
  - *Found in . . .* black tea
- Curcumin is the active compound in turmeric. It seems that there's little that "the golden spice" can't do: It's been shown to have anticancer, anti-

---

occurring there has the potential to affect multiple systems at once, with not just physical effects but mental and emotional effects, as well. With so much at stake, it's in our best interests to "keep a cool head" by keeping inflammation levels as low as possible throughout our lives.

Fortunately, many lifestyle habits support brain health, such as eating a diet rich in antioxidants and phytonutrients, getting in some exercise every day, getting sufficient sleep every night, and keeping stress in check. Anti-inflammatory living can often make the difference between the blues and depression, a normal lapse in memory and cognitive impairment, or temporary stress and full-blown anxiety. And for many of us, that's *all* the difference.

---

inflammatory, antidepressant, antiviral, antifungal, antiparasitic, antibacterial, and cognitive-preserving effects.

> ○ *Found in . . .* turmeric

- Flavonoids have a powerful antioxidant effect and can improve vascular function and increase cerebral bloodflow.

  > ○ *Found in . . .* a wide variety of fruits and vegetables, teas, red wine, and dark chocolate

- Flavonols include myricetin, kaempferol, and quercetin. These compounds reduce systemic inflammation and lower proinflammatory cytokines. One study of over 10,000 middle-aged adults found that low flavonol consumption was associated with cognitive decline—and the less participants ate, the faster the rate of decline.[47]

  > ○ *Found in . . .* yellow onions, scallions, kale, broccoli, apples, berries, teas, dark chocolate, and guava

- Luteolin is a flavone that has exhibited antioxidant, anti-inflammatory, neuroprotective, and memory-preserving effects. An olive extract of luteolin has been shown to improve attention and decrease brain fog.[48]

  > ○ *Found in . . .* broccoli, celery, green pepper, parsley, thyme, olives, olive oil, rosemary, oregano, peppermint, and chamomile tea

- Resveratrol is mainly known for its cardioprotective benefits, which are due in large part to its anti-inflammatory activity, but it's also been shown to delay the onset of neurodegenerative diseases.

  > ○ *Found in . . .* grapes, red wine, peanuts, blueberries, raspberries, and mulberries

CHAPTER 9

The Slow Burn

Cardiovascular Disease and Chronic Inflammation

For years, health experts considered a high level of cholesterol in the blood to be the primary cause of heart disease, the world's number-one killer. This theory makes sense because cholesterol—a waxy, fatty substance—is one of the main components of the plaques that accumulate within blood vessels, and these plaques can lead to atherosclerosis, blood clots, heart attack, and stroke. It's also true that the higher your blood level of the "bad" type of cholesterol (low-density lipoprotein, or LDL, cholesterol), the greater your chance of developing heart disease. But while it's clear that cholesterol levels play some role—and that we should avoid any lifestyle habits that drive them higher, such as eating saturated and trans fats—we now know that cholesterol is simply one part of the story. It's what the body does in *response* to the presence of elevated cholesterol that's a key instigator of heart disease. And we know that response well by now: the inflammatory response.

To understand how this story unfolds, let's start with a closer look at how inflammation affects the cardiovascular system. Remember that the body will launch an inflammatory response in the presence of anything it considers a threat—an injury, a pathogen, or an irritant. So what would constitute a threat to the cardiovascular system? That is, what would cause damage or injury to the heart or the blood vessels—and especially to the highly sensitive inner lining of the blood vessels known as the endothelium? Some of the top offenders are tobacco smoke, high blood pressure, high triglycerides, being overweight, chronic stress, a sedentary lifestyle (especially when that involves prolonged periods of sitting), poor sleep habits (either too much or too little sleep), and a poor diet. In the presence of any of these threats—every one of which is an independent risk factor for heart disease—the immune system kicks into gear and launches an inflammatory response. The greater the number of threats, the more pronounced the immune response. And as it's quite common to experience several threats at the same time (for example, high blood pressure, overweight, and a sedentary lifestyle), it's easy to see why heart disease is so prevalent, claiming more lives globally per year than all forms of cancer combined.[1]

To get a better understanding of the process, let's look at what happens in the acute phase of the inflammatory response when the body encounters one of these cardiovascular threats. We'll use tobacco smoke as an example because it is one of the top risk factors for heart disease and affects both smokers as well as nonsmokers in the form of secondhand smoke.

With each cigarette, a smoker immediately experiences its stimulant effects, namely higher blood pressure, an increase in heart rate, less oxygen delivered to the entire body, and reduced bloodflow to the heart. (And while less pronounced, these effects occur with secondhand smoke, as well.) On top of those reactions, the smoke itself causes inflammation. Even brief exposure to tobacco smoke irritates the mucous membranes in the mouth, nasal cavity, and lungs. In response, the inflammation army mounts a defensive attack, sending immune cells to the irritated membranes and triggering inflammation.[2] Further, with each tobacco smoke encounter, the body is exposed to an enormous array of toxins and chemicals—many of them carcinogenic and *all* of them proinflammatory. If the exposure is a one-time occurrence, the inflammation army easily handles the threat and then goes back to the barracks, if you will, to rest up for the next assignment.

But when exposure to cigarette smoke is chronic—either through regular secondhand smoke or a primary smoking habit—the inflammation army is constantly on the attack and the immune system is perpetually revved. What would have been a helpful, short burst of acute inflammation has become chronic, low-grade inflammation whose effects extend well beyond irritated mucous membranes. Smoking affects every organ and tissue. Over time, irritated, constricted blood vessels that see no relief give rise to chronic high blood pressure and higher risk of blood clots—both major contributors to atherosclerosis. Smokers are also known to be more susceptible to and have worse outcomes with pneumonia, bronchitis, influenza, tuberculosis, and chronic obstructive pulmonary disease. And smokers have increased

YOUR SKIN AND HEART HEALTH

Did you know that your skin may reveal things about your health that are more than skin deep? Psoriasis, an autoimmune disease that causes dry, red, raised patches on the skin, is associated with an increased risk of heart attack and stroke, and it has even been classified as an independent risk factor for heart disease. This means it's right up there with smoking, excess weight, and diabetes for raising the risk of heart disease.[3] A recent study found that the severity of psoriasis was linked to the amount of inflammation in the blood vessels. To measure this type of inflammation, researchers injected study participants with a mildly radioactive agent that caused areas of inflammation to light up on a PET/CT scan. They found that the higher the inflammation in the blood vessels, the more severe the psoriasis. They also found higher levels of a type of white blood cell called neutrophils in those with more severe cases of psoriasis.[4] Neutrophils always show up when the immune response is triggered.

Likewise, a study of more than 61,000 adults found that eczema, which causes itchy, dry, red skin, is also a marker of heart disease risk. Based on this population, those with eczema were 48 percent more likely to have high blood pressure, 35 percent more likely to have adult-onset type 2 diabetes, and 29 percent more likely to have high cholesterol, as well as overall have higher odds of smoking and lower odds of daily vigorous activity.[5]

Results from these studies provide dramatic evidence that what's happening on our outsides gives a vivid indication of what's happening on our insides.

susceptibility to rheumatoid arthritis, gum disease, and infections from *Escherichia coli* and *Candida albicans*, the most common cause of gastrointestinal infections and yeast infections, respectively.[6]

What's the common denominator among these diverse disorders? Immune dysfunction and chronic inflammation.[7]

Chronic Inflammation: Cause and Effect in Atherosclerosis

If inflammation is the major culprit behind heart disease, then atherosclerosis, or what's commonly known as hardening of the arteries, is its chief accomplice. However, what's interesting about the relationship between heart disease and inflammation is that in some situations the immune system may help fight the progression of heart disease instead of advance it. But before we get to that twist in our plotline, let's begin with a quick overview of why atherosclerosis takes center stage in the first place.

Atherosclerosis is a chronic inflammatory disease. It can affect arteries anywhere in the body, including those of the heart, brain, pelvis, kidneys, arms, or legs. The disease progresses as plaques that travel through the bloodstream—made up of lipids (fats), cholesterol, calcium, and other substances—adhere to and settle within artery walls. As these plaques accumulate over the years, the arteries thicken and become less flexible (i.e., they become sclerotic). Eventually, bloodflow slows and may become cut off, resulting in disease and dysfunction, such as peripheral artery disease or chronic kidney disease. Atherosclerosis can also cause a heart attack or stroke if a piece of plaque breaks off and blocks an artery or if a blood clot forms and blocks an artery.

Like many inflammatory diseases, atherosclerosis can progress for years without producing symptoms (it can begin as early as childhood), but the final outcome is usually swift and deadly in the form of heart attack or stroke. There are many risk factors for atherosclerosis, including advancing age, family history, and lifestyle factors such as smoking and physical inactivity.[8] An unhealthy diet is also a huge contributing factor, as a diet high in saturated and trans fats and processed foods drives up cholesterol levels and contributes to weight gain, high blood pressure, and diabetes, which also raise the risk of atherosclerosis. Other emerging risk factors are sleep apnea, chronic stress, and excessive alcohol consumption.[9]

What's the common denominator in every one of these situations? Each triggers the immune response and causes inflammation. We know this because these risk factors have been shown to raise CRP levels. Elevated CRP has long been associated with heart disease and has been observed at all stages of atherosclerosis, even before symptoms are present.[10]

The trouble begins when the endothelium incurs damage. What can cause damage to this highly sensitive inner lining of the blood vessels? Any lifestyle risk factors that trigger the inflammatory response set the stage for chronic inflammation. Then the accumulating fatty plaques progressively block bloodflow and cause further damage.

The body reacts to the accumulating plaque as it would to any foreign invader: It mounts an inflammatory response to try and rid the body of the threat. More specifically, the immune system sends white blood cells known as macrophages to storm the affected areas and destroy harmful plaques. At this point a lot of things are happening at once. The immune system is revved up, steadily sending out its foot soldiers to neutralize the threat and prevent more endothelial damage. And as with any action of the immune system, inflammation occurs. It's here that things get interesting with our old friends the cytokines, the cell-signaling messengers of the immune system. Depending on the type, cytokines can contribute to plaque progression *or* plaque regression. Proinflammatory cytokines *promote* the progression of atherosclerosis. But there are also anti-inflammatory cytokines that protect arteries by reducing macrophage recruitment and inflammation. The balance between these two camps—the anti-inflammatory cytokines versus. the proinflammatory cytokines—dictates the progression of atherosclerosis.[11]

Meanwhile, as the macrophages are busy with their job of engulfing more and more lipids and fatty plaques, they become stuffed with lipid deposits. The resulting cells are called foam cells, due to their foamy appearance after engulfing LDL cholesterol and lipids, and these lipid-laden foam cells play a major role in the progression of atherosclerosis. Foam cells hang out in the arteries and secrete proinflammatory cytokines that trigger *more*

BOOSTING ANTI-INFLAMMATORY COMPOUNDS

With all this talk of proinflammatory cytokines and how to lower them, we know some of you are wondering if it's possible to raise the level of heart-protective anti-inflammatory cytokines circulating in the body. The short answer is yes, and you do so by living an anti-inflammatory lifestyle. There is no better way to maintain heart health, as well as whole-body health, than to avoid chronic inflammation and to embrace anti-inflammatory living. If you're eating well, getting exercise and sufficient sleep, not smoking, and keeping stress in check, those pro- and anti-inflammatory cytokines will remain in balance.

That said, there *are* a few compounds found in plant foods that have been shown to increase the ranks of important anti-inflammatory cytokines like IL-4 and IL-10, and one of them is a natural antioxidant found in abundance in green tea called epigallocatechin gallate (EGCG).[12] Another is curcumin, the active compound in turmeric.[13] Other 1L-10 boosters are probiotic supplements containing the strain *Lactobacillus salivarius*,[14] and exercise works both ways by lowering proinflammatory cytokines and boosting anti-inflammatory ones.

inflammation, and they help produce new plaque and can make existing plaque unstable, causing it to break off and potentially block an artery. Foam cells even promote further inflammation as they die off.[15] Boosting HDL cholesterol through exercise, a healthy diet, and/or medication can also interrupt the vicious cycle of endothelial damage and the resulting inflammation.[16]

Inflammatory Markers and Cardiovascular Disease

Many tests can determine the levels of inflammatory biomarkers circulating in your blood. Doctors can use this information to help determine heart disease risk and progression. The most extensively studied and commonly used diagnostic tool for detecting inflammation *and* determining cardiovascular disease risk is the CRP test. An overwhelming number of studies have shown an association between elevated C-reactive protein levels and heart attack, stroke, peripheral artery disease, and sudden cardiac death. In fact, elevated CRP is an even stronger predictor of heart disease than elevated LDL cholesterol.[17] CRP levels can also indicate the progression of atherosclerosis: the higher the levels, the more advanced the disease.[18]

As discussed in Chapter 1, CRP is a substance the liver produces when inflammation occurs—more specifically, it's produced in the presence of proinflammatory cytokines, especially IL-6. CRP levels are determined by a blood draw; levels above 3 mg/l indicate a high risk of cardiovascular disease. High-sensitivity C-reactive protein is a more sensitive test and allows doctors to detect inflammation down to 0.04 mg/l.

CRP levels rise in the presence of any risk factors for heart disease—and they increase as the risk factor worsens. For example, increased hs-CRP levels are associated with smoking (in some studies the numbers rose according to how many cigarettes were smoked per day), diabetes, and higher fasting glucose levels.[19] One particularly fascinating study revealed just how powerful CRP is as a predictor of heart disease by assessing CRP levels in people with one of the most harmful risk factors, obesity. In this study, researchers compared data collected over 4 years from nearly 7,300 metabolically healthy obese and nonobese people. They found that obese people with low CRP levels had a heart disease risk comparable to that of nonobese people. In other words, even when a person was obese, a low CRP level rendered the risk of coronary heart disease as low as that of a person with a healthy BMI. Obese or not, it was the CRP level that made the difference.[20]

How do we reduce CRP levels? By reducing inflammation. And how do we do *that*? In brief, the first lines of defense are exercising regularly, avoiding cigarette smoke, maintaining a healthy weight, and eating a healthy diet. There is also evidence that intermittent fasting can promote weight loss, increase insulin sensitivity, improve blood pressure, lower cholesterol and triglycerides, *and* reduce systemic inflammation—all major risk factors for heart disease. Intermittent fasting can be done several ways, but the basic format is to alternate days of eating normally with days of calorie restriction. Some people alternate every other day, but more recently, the 5:2 formulation, in which you fast for 2 nonconsecutive days a week (on Mondays and

Thursdays, for example) and eat normally for 5, has proved popular. On fasting days, men should eat fewer than 600 calories per day, and women, fewer than 500.[21] Some people use the 5:2 plan to achieve weight loss goals, but many enjoy the long-term health benefits so much they adopt it for the long term.

Aside from CRP, another important way to assess inflammation is by measuring homocysteine levels. Elevated homocysteine is an independent risk factor for heart disease and, like CRP, increasing levels can also indicate the progression of heart disease.[22] Blood levels above 15 μmol/l are considered high.

Homocysteine is an amino acid that the body produces naturally when it breaks down methionine, an amino acid found in abundance in animal protein. High homocysteine levels can result from genetic factors or a deficiency in certain B vitamins, but many cases are due to eating a diet high in animal protein. Elevated homocysteine has been noted in several diseases, including kidney and thyroid dysfunction, cancer, psoriasis, and diabetes. More recent research has established a connection between high homocysteine levels and neurodegenerative disorders such as dementia, Alzheimer's, and Parkinson's, and psychological conditions such as depression. Of course, it's not hard to notice that these diseases are also associated with chronic inflammation.[23]

So why exactly is elevated homocysteine so dangerous? In part because it can make blood vessels less flexible and because it can trigger an inflammatory response in the smooth muscle cells that line the endothelium, which is the first stage in atherosclerosis. It can also increase the risk of blood clots. Furthermore, elevated homocysteine raises cholesterol and blood pressure. Given these combined effects, high levels of homocysteine constitute a recipe for disaster when it comes to heart health.[24]

Anti-Inflammatory Therapies for Cardiovascular Health

Given the outsize role of chronic inflammation in heart disease, many researchers have focused on the practical question of how to quench the fires

(continued on page 184)

Donna Mallard

AGE: 60

- Energy level doubled
- High blood pressure reduced to normal
- CRP reduced from high to normal
- Joint pain and a sense of puffiness eliminated
- Irritability, mood swings, and mental fatigue reduced from daily to rarely
- WEIGHT LOST: 26 pounds
- INCHES LOST: 12

I've been overweight most of my life. I've tried every diet known to man or woman, and I have lost weight on each of them but have never kept it off. The Whole Body Cure Plan suited my metabolism and my digestive tract. I lost more than 25 pounds over the 12 weeks, as well as 12 inches, mostly from my waist and hips. I feel healthier, and I don't have heartburn anymore. If I've learned anything from this plan, it's that I don't have heartburn when I eat healthy! I once had pizza after the plan was over, and my system immediately rebelled. Pizza is good, but it's not worth feeling that uncomfortable anymore. I'm okay without it.

I admit I was nervous about the first phase, the detox part of the plan. There were a few times I was ready to pack it up and give in. I was irritable and hungry. I think this was mostly because of my weight. I know some of the other people who didn't weigh as much to begin with didn't get as hungry, but for me the 2 weeks of detox translated to a lot fewer calories than I was used to. But once I started losing weight, which was within that first week, I felt better about it. Losing weight is a motivator, always has been.

I work full-time and am usually pretty tired when I come home, so one thing that was important for me was finding quick and easy recipes with fruits and vegetables. That was a challenge at first, but I did find that I really liked roasted vegetables. I'd never roasted so many different vegetables, and I also tried different spices. Roasted carrots are delicious all on their own, and one new favorite is roasted asparagus and garlic. If you want to give it some variety in terms of taste and texture, you can

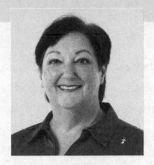

Donna's Tips

Get yourself in the right frame of mind before you begin. If you know in advance that you're going to be eating fruits and vegetables for all three meals during that first 2 weeks, and you know that you'll probably be hungry part of that time, you'll be in the right mind-set. Then get your herbs and spices ahead of time, and do some research on recipes. I found that searching Pinterest for paleo recipes helped a lot. Go in with that positive attitude, and remember that the first 2 weeks is a finite period, and you can get through it. We all did, and it was worth it.

include toasted almonds or other nuts after Week 5. I didn't necessarily come up with all new recipes, but I did things I normally wouldn't have done, and I added some variety in my overall diet.

Since completing the plan, I've added a few things back in, like dairy. But I'm swapping out things that aren't as healthy. For example, I was a very big cereal eater for breakfast, and now I have Greek yogurt with fruit. I also still have salads for lunch, and that's new for me—I was never a salad-for-lunch person! My normal lunch was a burger or a sandwich, or maybe leftovers from the night before. But now I find that I'm not turning to the simple sugars and carbs anymore, and I don't miss them. This new eating pattern

is fitting my life, and I'm maintaining my weight loss. I know that I'll lose more because I know I can limit myself and I have a better attitude about food.

One of the best things about the plan is its flexibility. It *is* restrictive in the first 2 weeks, but even within that framework, you can choose from lots of fruits and vegetables. I personally think that the overall flexibility is what helps people stay with it. I've tried so many diets, and my mind-set is that if you tell people they absolutely cannot have certain foods or absolutely cannot go over a certain calorie limit, it makes them not want to be on the diet. I want to keep with this plan. It worked, and I know I can make my own modifications here and there. ■

of inflammation before they can do irreversible damage. As covered earlier, the very best way to keep not just your heart but your whole body healthy is to keep inflammation low throughout your life through simple lifestyle measures. We'll discuss those in more detail below, but here, let us mention a couple of drug therapies doctors turn to when inflammation is already present and causing damage.

The most commonly prescribed medications to address heart disease risk factors are statins. These well-known drugs lower blood levels of cholesterol in two ways: (1) by stopping the production of cholesterol by blocking the enzyme that creates it and (2) by reabsorbing existing cholesterol. In this latter way, statin drugs work a bit like macrophages, and indeed they can absorb the cholesterol in the fatty plaques that are already present in arteries. There are many pros and cons to statins, so let's take a closer look. In addition to reducing cholesterol, statins reduce inflammation generally (as indicated by lower CRP and other proinflammatory cytokine levels), improve endothelial function, make atherosclerotic plaques more stable (thus helping to prevent a plaque from rupturing and blocking a blood vessel), and keep blood platelets from clumping together.[25] According to a large study known as JUPITER (the name is short for Justification for the Use of Statins in Primary Prevention: An Intervention Trial Evaluating Rosuvastatin), statins were shown to reduce the rate of first heart attacks, stroke, or cardiovascular death by 47 percent in patients with LDL cholesterol levels of less than 130 mg/dl and hs-CRP levels greater than 2 mg/l.[26] A recent meta-analysis based on 9,369 coronary bypass patients found that when statins were used before and after surgery, patients had a lower risk of atrial fibrillation after surgery. Statin users (5,598 of the total patients) also experienced lower systemic inflammation and shorter hospital stays after surgery.[27] Similarly, a meta-analysis of cardiac surgery patients—18,684 statin users and 24,033 nonusers—found that statin use protected against acute kidney injury and decreased the chance of death if kidney injury did occur.[28] Other recent studies have found that statin therapy can slow and even reverse mild noncalcified plaque,[29] and statins appear to have a protective effect against new-onset Crohn's disease and ulcerative colitis, the two main forms of inflammatory bowel disease.[30]

EAT YOUR WAY TO LOWER HOMOCYSTEINE LEVELS

One of the most effective ways to keep your homocysteine level in the normal range is to alter what you eat. First and foremost, you'll need to decrease your intake of animal protein. At the same time, increase your intake of folate, also known as vitamin B_9, by eating more citrus fruits, green leafy vegetables, and nuts. Folic acid is the synthetic form of folate and can be taken as a supplement. A folic acid supplement, or foods that are fortified with folic acid, have been shown to be more effective at lowering homocysteine than eating folate-rich foods alone,[31] so if you have any heart disease risk factors, check with your doctor about adding a folic acid supplement. Vitamins B_6 and B_{12} can also help lower homocysteine. Vitamin B_6 can be found in poultry, fish, citrus fruits, dark leafy greens, papaya, and cantaloupe. Vitamin B_{12} is found only in animal products (meat or dairy) or in fortified foods, such as cereals. The one vegetarian exception is seaweed, especially the variety known as nori.

Statins, however, are not without risks. The preeminent medical journal the *Lancet* just released a review detailing the benefits and risks of statin therapy. The authors found that large-scale evidence from randomized trials showed that statins can lower cholesterol and reduce the risk of major vascular events (such as heart attack or stroke) by about 25 percent for each millimole per liter (mmol/l) reduction in LDL cholesterol after the first year they're taken. On the other hand, statins are associated with a higher risk of new-onset diabetes, muscle pain, and hemorrhagic stroke. Treatment of 10,000 patients for 5 years with a standard statin would be expected to cause around 5 cases of muscle pain, 50 to 100 new cases of diabetes, and 5 to 10 hemorrhagic strokes.[32] Results from a newly released meta-analysis based on nearly 94,000 participants found that it was two statins in particular—atorvastatin and rosuvastatin—that increased the risk of diabetes in people with high cholesterol.[33] Complaints of statin-associated muscle pain are common, and in rare cases, patients can develop a painful, very serious condition called rhabdomyolysis, which can cause muscle pain and damage, liver damage, kidney failure, and even death. Some people have also reported memory loss and mental confusion while on statin therapy.

With the potential for such serious side effects, it's important to talk with your doctor about your medical history to better understand the benefits versus the risks of long-term statin use. Many physicians are moving away from automatically prescribing statins as a preventive measure for people with high cholesterol who do not have a history of heart disease. Instead, they believe that statins are best indicated for people who are at high risk of developing a cardiovascular disease (such as patients with diabetes or a family history of high cholesterol) or who have already experienced a cardiac event.

The other main anti-inflammatory medication is the class of drugs known as nonsteroidal anti-inflammatory drugs, which includes the common over-the-counter medications ibuprofen, naproxen, and aspirin. Their main therapeutic effects are to reduce inflammation, reduce pain, and lower body temperature. But it's aspirin we want to focus on here, as it's become a go-to preventive means to avoid heart attack and stroke.

Daily low-dose aspirin protects cardiovascular health by preventing blood platelets from clumping together and forming a clot. Many people think of daily aspirin as an easy, perfectly harmless way to protect their health and "prescribe" this treatment for themselves. But as with statins, daily aspirin is not without risk, most notably the increased risk of bleeding. The American Heart Association and the Food and Drug Administration in fact do *not* recommend daily aspirin for those with no history of cardiovascular risk. Daily aspirin is best indicated for those who have suffered a cardiac event such as heart attack or stroke in the past—in these cases, the benefits outweigh the risks.[34] As with any drug, only use daily aspirin under the guidance of your health-care provider.

All-Natural Ways to Protect Your Heart from Inflammation

Because heart disease is typically a product of certain lifestyle choices, there are plenty of simple, noninvasive, commonsense strategies that can help prevent and reverse the inflammation that leads to heart disease—and without the risk of side effects that come with medications. That means the power to keep our hearts healthy is largely under our control. Don't be fooled by the simplicity of these recommendations! There are no more powerful means to maintain heart health.

DO NOT SMOKE. Smoking harms every organ in the body and is the main preventable cause of death and illness in the United States. One out of every five deaths is linked to smoking. Long-term smoking (or long-term exposure to secondhand smoke) doubles the chance of stroke and vastly increases the chance of coronary artery disease.[35] Exposure to tobacco smoke and chronic inflammation go hand in hand—you don't have one without the other. So don't smoke, and as much as possible, avoid secondhand exposure to smoke.

EAT TO COOL THE BURN. We'll be going over all the details of an anti-inflammatory approach to eating and enjoying food in Chapter 11, so here we'll just offer a few brief highlights that have special relevance to heart health. First, do your best to avoid any processed or refined foods, which tend to be higher in sodium, sugar, saturated and trans fats, preservatives, additives, and other chemicals that weren't meant to be in the human body. There is *no* safe amount of trans fats, and high amounts of sodium, saturated fats, and sugar cause an inflammatory response and free radical damage, thus accelerating disease. Moreover, these foods can contribute to a high LDL cholesterol level, which, as we saw, triggers further inflammation and puts us on the fast track for atherosclerosis.

On the other hand, do eat whole, unprocessed foods that are rich in antioxidants and polyphenols, which limit free radical damage and counteract inflammation. To get sufficient antioxidants and polyphenols, many nutrition experts suggest that you "eat the rainbow"—that is, eat any brightly colored fruit or vegetable. Other anti-inflammatory favorites are foods rich in omega-3 fatty acids, such as wild-caught salmon, mackerel, and herring, and healthy fats that come from nuts, avocados, flaxseeds, and extra-virgin olive oil. These foods will also help to boost your HDL levels (the "good" cholesterol), which will keep your unhealthy LDL levels in check. Finally, spice it up: Some of Mother Nature's most powerful anti-inflammatories include some undeniably tasty spices, such as turmeric, ginger, garlic, and ground red pepper.

LIGHTEN UP. At one point, adipocytes—fat cells—were thought to be little more than storehouses for fat, but more recent research has shown that body fat is also a metabolically active endocrine organ. As a person becomes heavier and adipocytes enlarge, inflammation rises. Moreover, those macrophages that do such damage during the development of atherosclerosis increase in number as weight increases, resulting in *more* inflammation and insulin resistance.[36] This combination of chronic inflammation and metabolic dysfunction sets the stage for any number of negative health effects, including hypertension, impaired glucose metabolism—and eventually, full-blown chronic inflammatory diseases such as type 2 diabetes and atherosclerosis.[37]

And as always, when it comes to chronic inflammation, nothing occurs in a vacuum. One recent study demonstrated a link between high BMI, stress, and a type of blockage called myocardial ischemia, which can lead to a heart attack. Essentially, myocardial ischemia occurs when bloodflow to the heart is reduced by a partial or complete blockage of the coronary arteries. In this study, researchers assessed participants' bloodflow at rest and during a period of stress. They found that BMI was an independent risk factor for stress-induced myocardial ischemia. And the greater the person's weight, the greater the risk. Even with modest increases in BMI, researchers observed a marked increase in inflammation and endothelial dysfunction, one of the earliest signs of atherosclerosis.[38]

CHILL OUT. Chronic psychological stress is so harmful that many doctors and researchers consider it an independent risk factor for heart disease, just as dangerous as high BMI, tobacco use, a sedentary lifestyle, high blood pressure, or diabetes. Chronic stress keeps adrenaline flowing, raises cortisol (a major stress hormone), raises blood pressure, interferes with sleep, and contributes to anxiety, depression, and other mood disorders. In fact, any sort of unresolved negative mood state, from stress to worry to hostility to depression, *causes* chronic, low-grade inflammation. Once the fires of chronic inflammation start burning, they spark the vicious cycle: Stress causes inflammation, which causes more stress, which causes more inflammation. And when you combine any of these "inflammatory emotions" with any of the other cardiovascular risk factors, you're increasing your risk of myocardial ischemia, abnormal heart rhythm, and heart attack.

GET SOME EXERCISE. Your heart is a muscle, and it flourishes with a workout just like the rest of your muscles do. Without regular exercise, beneficial HDL cholesterol levels fall and harmful LDL cholesterol levels rise. A sedentary lifestyle also contributes to weight gain, the accumulation of belly fat, insulin resistance, and every other risk factor for cardiovascular disease. Belly fat is especially dangerous to your health because this kind of fat stores and produces proinflammatory factors known as adipokines. Further, sitting for prolonged periods of time—even if you're perfectly healthy—is associated with higher levels of the inflammatory biomarkers CRP and fibrinogen,[39] and it has been shown many times to be an independent risk factor for increased cardiometabolic risk and all-cause mortality.[40]

On the positive side, regular exercise has been shown to decrease inflammation by, among other factors, reducing deep, visceral fat (thus preventing the release of proinflammatory adipokines), increasing anti-inflammatory cytokines, and reducing the number of proinflammatory monocytes (these are the white blood cells that can become LDL-hungry macrophages).[41] Exercise also reduces CRP levels irrespective of health status. A metareview of several studies involving 3,575 participants showed that exercise lowered CRP levels in healthy adults as well as in those with heart disease.[42]

To Your Heart's Content

You can achieve optimal health and wellness for your heart and your whole body without drugs, without invasive procedures, and without complicated fitness or eating regimens. Heart disease is largely a condition of lifestyle, which means our own choices influence our level of health and wellness.

As elevated inflammation combined with high cholesterol is known to be a deadly combination, live to keep both inflammation and total cholesterol down. This means avoiding the well-known triggers of chronic inflammation and, on the other hand, embracing healthy lifestyle habits such as getting regular exercise, keeping stress in check, getting enough sleep, and taking an anti-inflammatory approach to eating. So enjoy fresh fruits and vegetables, healthy fats, aromatic spices, and delicious green tea—all to your heart's content! We have the power to live a vibrant, healthy life for many years to come.

CHAPTER 10

Like a House Afire

The Connections between Cancer and Chronic Inflammation

For over 150 years, scientists have known about a link between inflammation and cancer thanks to German pathologist Rudolf Virchow, who first observed that cancer arose from inflammatory sites. And now, just a mere century and a half later, we find ourselves in an exciting area of rapidly expanding research. We now understand that inflammation and the immune system are involved at every stage of cancer development, from the time chronic inflammation creates conditions in our cells that render them ripe for mutations, to the uncontrolled growth that gives rise to tumors, all the way to the time cancer metastasizes and becomes life-threatening.

But as we've seen so many times, where there's a dark side to inflammation, there is also a light. Scientists are harnessing the innate power of the immune system to create cancer therapies that just a few decades ago seemed like science fiction. Just as the final chapter of this book was being completed, for instance, news broke of a new immunotherapy intervention that extended the lives of patients with metastatic pancreatic cancer. Though these are early results based on a clinical trial with a relatively small sample size (110 people), there is plenty to celebrate. Pancreatic cancer is one of the most lethal forms of cancer, with a mortality rate nearly equal to its incidence rate—only 18 percent of patients survive a year after diagnosis, and just 4 percent are alive after 5 years. If pancreatic cancer has metastasized, the average survival rate from diagnosis is just 4.6 months. In this study, patients with metastatic pancreatic cancer who received immunotherapy lived an average of 2.6 extra months. A few lived beyond a year, and one lived nearly 3 years.[1] Given pancreatic cancer's grim survival rates, these are extremely encouraging results.

We'll cover all the details of this study as well as other immunotherapy drugs later in the chapter. For now, rest assured that it's just one of hundreds of clinical trials that are currently investigating how to harness the power of our own immune systems to beat deadly forms of cancer. By the time this book is in your hands, there will likely be even more medical breakthroughs because this field is advancing so rapidly. That's news we're happy to live with.

The Inflammation-Cancer Connection

If we could look through a microscope and watch how normal cells become cancerous cells—a process known as *carcinogenesis*—we'd see that inflammation occurs at every stage. In fact, chronic inflammation is at work even before cancerous cells exist because it creates the right conditions for cancer to form. This should be a wake-up call for everyone because so many of us are chronically inflamed. Maybe it's because we have a chronic infection like Epstein-Barr virus or a chronic inflammatory condition like ulcerative colitis. Or maybe it's because we engage in inflammatory lifestyle habits such as smoking, eating an inflammatory diet, letting our stress levels go unchecked, or being overweight. Whatever the cause, when the immune response remains in overdrive, we produce an abundance of cytokines, chemokines, growth factors, and harmful reactive oxygen species. And *that's* where the potential for cancer arises: The combined effect of these bioactive substances coupled with chronic inflammation creates a perfect storm on a cellular level, raising the potential for DNA damage and other mutations that can lead to cancer. To further complicate the problem, all the extra growth factors and nutrients generated by the inflammatory response—which were intended for healing and tissue repair—provide the fledgling tumor with everything it needs to grow rapidly.

So instead of eliminating the threat, chronic inflammation creates the ideal conditions for cancer and can accelerate tumor growth.[2]

And really, this is just the tip of the iceberg. There are other ways that chronic inflammation and carcinogenesis work hand in hand—in fact, up to 90 percent of cancers are inflammation-related. When chronic inflammation exists, a malignancy can hijack the immune system and cause cancerous cells to divide more rapidly. Chronic inflammation is also directly involved in the growth of new blood vessels that support a tumor's survival, a process known as *angiogenesis*. It can suppress the immune system's response to abnormal cells, allowing rogue cells to escape detection. And even if abnormal cells are detected, chronic inflammation may inhibit or delay their eventual demise. If a tumor forms, it has the power to release its own cytokines and chemokines, further enhancing its own growth. A protein known as nuclear factor kappa B (NF-κB), which controls the production of cytokines, has been called the "matchmaker" between inflammation and cancer. When NF-κB is activated during an inflammatory disease, it leads to more aggressive cancers.[3]

Bottom line? Chronic inflammation is at work in every step of cancer development. It heightens the risk of cancer, helps perpetuate cancerous cells, and fuels tumor growth, and it's directly involved in tumor invasion and eventually metastasis. Chronic inflammation can even interfere with how our bodies respond to cancer treatments and may make us resistant to chemotherapy drugs.[4]

Of course, there's still a lot we need to learn about cancer and chronic inflammation, and scientists continue to find new links. One study conducted with specially engineered mice involved exposing them to a substance that's known to cause pancreatic inflammation. The researchers found that if the inflammation was acute (short lived) and the mice were given time to recover, there was no evidence of the type of increased mutations that can give rise to cancer. But if inflammation occurred frequently, thus limiting the opportunity for DNA repair, there was a significant increase in mutations. While DNA damage occurs quickly, inflammation doesn't provoke faster cell division for several days, which means that if another round of inflammation occurs as cells are dividing because of a previous bout of inflammation, even more mutations are bound to appear. In other words, chronic inflammation creates an environment that encourages potentially cancerous mutations at accelerating rates. This finding translates to big news for people who are often chronically inflamed for months or years at a time.[5] Controlling inflammation may indeed be one of our biggest tools for cancer prevention.

Other research supports this idea. Take, for example, the results of a new study that examined the association between cancer risk and an inflammatory score based on blood levels of three inflammatory biomarkers: CRP, fibrinogen, and white blood cell count. Using data from 84,000 people followed an average of 4.8 years, researchers found that high inflammation levels corresponded to an increased risk of colorectal, lung, breast, and prostate cancers. Compared to people with no indication of chronic inflammation, people who had high levels of all three inflammatory biomarkers had more than double the risk of colorectal cancer, three times the risk of lung cancer, and 1.4 times the risk of breast cancer. Researchers also found an elevated risk of oral, pharynx, kidney, and esophageal cancers in those with chronic inflammation. They noted that cancers of the lung, oral cavity, pharynx, and esophagus are all smoking-related cancers, underscoring the connection between chronic, system-wide inflammation and smoking.[6] Indeed, the Centers for Disease Control and Prevention reminds us that tobacco smoke doesn't just cause cancers of the lungs, mouth, and nasal passages—in addition to the types listed above, it also causes cancers of the kidney, bladder, liver, pancreas, stomach, cervix, colon, and rectum, as well as acute myeloid leukemia.[7] Not surprisingly, all of these cancers are inflammation-mediated illnesses.

So if you're looking for ways to avoid cancer of any type, all of the traditional advice still applies: Don't smoke or use other tobacco products, maintain a healthy BMI, eat a healthy diet, stay physically active, avoid environmental pollutants and other carcinogens, and use a sunscreen to prevent too much UV radiation exposure. But now we know to add "prevent the onset of chronic inflammation" to that list.

The Infection-Cancer Connection

By some estimates, as much as 20 percent of all cancers are linked with infections. At first glance this may seem like a strange concept since it's not like you

CANCER: A SNAPSHOT

Here are some quick facts and statistics about cancer. As you read, note all the ways inflammation is lurking in the background.

Up to one-third of cancer deaths are due to five dietary and behavioral risks: (1) tobacco use, (2) high BMI, (3) low intake of fruits and vegetables, (4) lack of exercise, and (5) overconsumption of alcohol.[8]

- The American Institute for Cancer Research estimates that eating a healthy diet, staying active, and maintaining a healthy weight could prevent roughly one-third of cancers in the United States, or 340,000 cases a year.[9]

- In 2017, 1,688,780 Americans are expected to be newly diagnosed with cancer. An estimated 600,920 will die from cancer, which makes for about 1,650 deaths per day.[10]

- In the United States, the 5-year survival rate for all cancers combined has increased 20 percent for whites and 24 percent for blacks.[11]

- In the United States, the lifetime probability of developing cancer is 40.8 percent for men and 37.5 percent for women.[12]

- Based on figures through the year 2014, the cancer death rate in the United States has dropped 25 percent since 1991. That's 2.1 million lives saved.[13]

- Lung cancer claims more lives per year than any other type of cancer. It accounts for 26 percent of all cancer in the United States in 2016. The runner-up is colon cancer, with 49,190 deaths.[14]

- Lung and colon cancer are two of the most preventable forms of cancer.

- Lung cancer death rates declined 43 percent from 1990 to 2014 among men and 17 percent from 2002 to 2014 among women, large because of reduced tobacco use.[15]

- Smoking increases the risk of colorectal cancer, as does being overweight, having type 2 diabetes, being physically inactive, engaging in heavy alcohol consumption, and eating a diet that's high in red meat, processed meat, and/or meats cooked at very high temperatures.[16]

- Bizarre cancer fact: Greater height is associated with a higher risk of cancer and death from cancer for both men and women. Scientists think hormonal and genetic factors related to greater height can also stimulate cancer development and progression.[17]

can "catch" cancer like you'd catch a cold from a rhinovirus or strep throat from streptococcus bacteria. And certainly, cancer isn't contagious—it can't be passed from one person to another.

But there are some cancers that are clearly connected to infections from certain viruses, bacteria, and parasites. Stomach cancer, for instance, is linked with previous exposure to *Helicobacter pylori* bacteria, cervical cancer is largely caused by several types of human papillomavirus (HPV), and, less commonly, a waterborne parasite known as *Schistosoma haematobium* has been linked with bladder cancer and a parasite known as liver flukes with liver cancer. The table below provides a list of some of the common infections and their associated cancers.

BACTERIA	LINKED WITH...
Helicobacter pylori	Stomach cancer MALT (mucosa-associated lymphoid tissue) lymphoma
Chlamydia pneumoniae	Lung cancer
Chlamydia trachomatis	Cervical cancer
Escherichia coli (recurrent infections of localized tissues, such as the bladder)	Occasionally, affected tissues may become cancerous, such as the prostate, bladder, or colon
VIRUSES	**LINKED WITH...**
Human papillomavirus	Cervical cancer (most common) Also linked with vulvar, vaginal, penile, anal, mouth, and throat cancers
Hepatitis B and C viruses	Liver cancer Hepatitis C may also be linked with non-Hodgkin's lymphoma and T-cell leukemias
Human immunodeficiency virus	Kaposi sarcoma Cervical cancer Non-Hodgkin's lymphoma Also linked with anus, mouth, throat, liver, lung, and skin cancers and Hodgkin's lymphoma
Epstein-Barr virus	Nasopharyngeal cancer Burkitt lymphoma Hodgkin's lymphoma Stomach cancer
Human T-lymphotropic virus I	Adult T-cell leukemia/lymphoma
Human herpesvirus 8	Kaposi sarcoma

It's important to note that most people with these infections do *not* go on to develop cancer. Most people have been exposed to Epstein-Barr virus (EBV) by the time they reach adulthood, for example, and *H. pylori* infects about half the world's population. Many of these people not only remain cancer free but don't even develop symptoms of an infection. It's possible to go your whole life as a carrier of EW or human papilloma virus (HPV) and not even know it. Exposure to these infections does, however, increase the risk of cancer. Why do some people develop cancer while others do not? As you'd imagine, there is no single, definitive answer, and what we do know is both complex and multifaceted; many factors must come together simultaneously to create the conditions for cancer to develop. However, they all have a common denominator: chronic inflammation.

To begin with, if you combine any of these infections with one or more of the "traditional" risk factors for cancer, your risk rises significantly. For example, if you smoke; are overweight; face repeated exposure to cancer-causing toxins, pollutants, or UV radiation; eat a poor diet; or drink heavily, you're at far higher risk than the general population to develop cancer. (Having a chronic inflammatory illness also raises the risk, but we'll talk about that separately below.) Note that any of these individual risk factors triggers an inflammatory response, and if the issue persists—such as a long-term smoking habit or a habitually poor diet—so does the inflammation. Now combine the chronic inflammation associated with these unhealthy lifestyle habits or exposure to toxins with the natural inflammatory response that accompanies any kind of infection, and you've got the cancer "perfect storm" brewing and gathering force.

Still, even in the absence of traditional risk factors, infection can and does lead to cancer in some individuals. Very generally speaking, there are three reasons this can happen.

1. Some infections suppress the immune system. Without its normal defense system functioning at 100 percent, the body is less effective at fighting off precancerous or cancerous cells or infections that can lead to cancer.

2. Some infections can cause chronic inflammation in certain tissues and organs—for example, hepatitis causes chronic

inflammation of the liver. Over time, these inflamed areas may undergo genetic and chemical changes that lead to cancer.

3. Some viruses can insert their own genes inside cells, causing them to grow out of control and eventually form a tumor.[18]

On the other side of the equation, when the immune system is functioning properly, it does a very effective job protecting us against cancer. First, it eliminates pathogens that could induce cancer. Second, having eliminated those pathogens, it minimizes the chronic inflammation that makes for cancer-friendly conditions. And third, there is evidence that the healthy immune system routinely identifies and eliminates precancerous or cancerous cells before they can cause harm. This is a process known as *immune surveillance*. But obviously immune surveillance doesn't work all the time, and one reason could be that, much like viruses and bacteria and other pathogens, cancer cells can change and evolve over time—and in ways that enable them to sneak past the immune system's defenses. We've seen other cancer-causing pathogens use the same tactic.

A key DNA protein that's required for the Epstein-Barr virus to replicate, for instance, has evolved in such a way that the body doesn't recognize it as potentially harmful. It can thus escape immune system surveillance, leaving EBV free to proliferate, where it primarily infects certain white blood cells called B cells. EBV can send B cells into overdrive and make them divide rapidly—in other words, it can cause them to become cancerous.[19]

H. pylori is another cancer-causing pathogen that's displayed incredibly sophisticated ways to evade the immune system's defenses. Throughout the 30,000 years it's coexisted with people, *H. pylori*, the main cause of peptic ulcers and gastric cancer, has developed the ability to live *under* the stomach's protective mucosal lining, attach to the thin layer of cells that lines the digestive tract, and then hang out there, causing long-term infection. Macrophages can engulf *H. pylori* as they would any other pathogen, but *H. pylori* has even figured out a way to survive being eaten alive! These crafty critters cause macrophage apoptosis—a type of programmed cell death, or, put another way, cellular self-destruction.[20]

There are many other ways *H. pylori* can survive the inflammatory response, but the point is that it can readily outwit the immune system and colonize the stomach, causing long-term infection. And as we know, with persistent infection comes persistent inflammation. The longer it goes untreated, the worse the damage. *H. pylori* is responsible for up to 90 percent of stomach ulcers, and it's so closely associated with stomach cancer that the World Health Organization's International Agency for Research on Cancer has deemed it a Group 1 carcinogen,[21] sharing top billing with formaldehyde, tobacco products, and mustard gas.

Another extremely common and potentially cancerous pathogen is HPV. There are 150 types of HPV, but only about a dozen cause cancer. And of those, types 16 and 18 are responsible for 70 percent of cervical cancers.

HPV infection rates are very high—more than 90 percent of women will be infected with some type of HPV in their lifetimes—but most people will not develop cancer, and many never even have symptoms of HPV infection. The danger arrives when one of the cancer-causing forms of HPV causes an infection that becomes *chronic*. Whenever a pathogen is hanging around, the result is long-term activation of the immune system—in other words, chronic inflammation. However, chronic inflammation is only one of the factors that increase the risk of HPV developing into cancer. Others include smoking, having a weakened immune system, engaging in long-term oral contraceptive use, having many children, and practicing poor oral hygiene.[22] In addition to cervical cancer, HPV can cause cancers of the mouth, penis, anus, vulva, and vagina.

Fortunately, HPV-related cervical cancer prevention represents one of the great triumphs of modern medicine. We're talking about the HPV vaccine. Recent estimates project that the HPV vaccine has helped lower the prevalence of cancer-causing HPV by 64 percent in females ages 14 to 19 and by 34 percent in females ages 20 to 24.[23] The HPV vaccine also protects against genital warts, and it can be administered to males, as well.

The Inflammatory
Disease–Cancer Connection

So to recap, abundant evidence reveals that chronic inflammation is a factor in certain forms of cancer. However, it's important to keep things in perspective. As with cancers that arise from infections, most people with inflammatory conditions do *not* go on to develop cancer. And though their risk of these cancers is significantly higher than that of the general population's, for most people, the *overall* cancer risk still remains relatively low. For example, people with gastroesophageal reflux disease (GERD) have a higher risk of esophageal cancer, but most will never develop it. Of GERD sufferers, 10 to 15 percent will develop a more severe complication called Barrett's esophagus. This subset is at an even greater risk of esophageal cancer, but even so, only 1 out of every 860 Barrett's patients will go on to develop cancer.[24]

Large data collections have found that additional risk exists with other chronic infections. Prostatitis, for example, causes a roughly 14 percent increase in prostate cancer; ulcerative colitis increases the chance of colorectal cancer by about 25 percent, and pancreatitis increases the chance of pancreatic cancer by 10 to 20 times.[25] Where gastric cancer risk is concerned, estimates vary by country; Japan, Korea, and China, for instance, are known to have higher rates of gastric cancer along with a higher incidence of *H. pylori* infection. Results of one recent study conducted over 10 years found that in patients with *H. pylori* infection *and* gastritis, the risk of gastric cancer increased thirty-two-fold.[26]

One of the important things to understand about cancers that arise from inflammatory conditions is that they usually develop over decades. The longer the inflammatory condition persists, the higher the chance of cancer. And given what we know about chronic inflammation and how it heightens our cells' chance of DNA damage and accelerates the mutation process, this makes sense. Along the same lines, the severity of the inflammatory illness also plays a part in increasing the cancer risk. If ulcerative colitis affects a large part of the colon, for example, the risk of colorectal cancer is greater than if the disease is not extensive. Here are some of the most common types of inflammatory conditions that have been linked to cancer.

INFLAMMATORY CONDITION	LINKED WITH . . .
Inflammatory bowel disease (primarily ulcerative colitis and Crohn's disease)	Colorectal cancer Small bowel adenocarcinoma
Pancreatitis	Pancreatic cancer
Peptic ulcers Chronic gastritis	Stomach (gastric) cancer
Chronic gastroesophageal reflux disease Barrett's esophagus	Esophageal cancer
Prostatitis	Prostate cancer
Pelvic inflammatory disease	Cervical cancer Ovarian cancer
Hepatitis B Hepatitis C	Liver cancer Hepatitis C may also be linked with non-Hodgkin's lymphoma and T-cell leukemias
Chronic bronchitis Chronic asthma Other sources of chronic inflammation of the lungs (smoking, infections, asbestos or silica exposure)	Lung cancer
UV radiation–associated inflammation	Melanoma
Endometriosis	Endometrial cancer
Chronic cholecystitis (inflammation of the gallbladder)	Gallbladder cancer
Primary sclerosing cholangitis (a disease of the bile ducts)	Bile duct cancer
Recurrent cystitis (urinary tract infections)	Bladder cancer
Gingivitis	Oral squamous cell carcinoma
Sarcoidosis (a disease that causes abnormal collections of inflammatory cells)	Lung cancer Skin cancer Liver cancer
Sialadenitis (inflammation of the salivary glands)	Salivary gland carcinoma

Within this list, the connection between inflammatory bowel disease and colorectal cancer has been intensively studied. IBD takes two primary forms, Crohn's disease and ulcerative colitis (see Chapter 4 for more). The risk of colorectal cancer stemming from IBD increases with longer duration of IBD, extent of ulcerative colitis, a family history of colorectal cancer, the presence of a chronic inflammatory condition of the bile ducts known as sclerosing cholangitis, and the overall degree of inflammation present in the body.

Colorectal cancer accounts for one-sixth of ulcerative colitis–related deaths.[27] The other factor that increases the risk of colorectal cancer is a high BMI, as being overweight is a driver of chronic inflammation.

To decrease the risk of colorectal cancer, IBD patients should have regular screenings, keep their disease under control by staying on their medications, eat a healthy anti-inflammatory diet (see the next chapter for more), and exercise regularly. In addition, those with IBD can help keep inflammation in check with a few extra interventions. Regular aspirin, a readily available non-steroidal anti-inflammatory drug, has been shown to reduce the risk of colorectal cancer,[28] and many studies have shown that high vitamin D levels are associated with lower colorectal cancer risk, so talk with your doctor about these options if you've been diagnosed with IBD. To get maximum levels of vitamin D, go with a supplement. Food sources of vitamin D include fortified milks and juices, mushrooms, eggs, and fatty fish—but you should avoid anything that would trigger a food sensitivity or allergic reaction, however mild. Vitamin D is also absorbed through sunlight. For more on nutritional means to prevent colorectal cancer, be sure to read the Eating a Poor Diet section just ahead on page 206.

Of course, the same advice applies to anyone with any chronic inflammatory condition. If you know that your cancer risk is already higher than the general population's, it's more important than ever to get regular medical checkups, live an overall anti-inflammatory lifestyle, and avoid additional cancer risk factors. Read on for more anti-inflammatory, anticancer tips, and don't miss our full anti-inflammatory plan detailed in Part III.

Is Your Lifestyle Inflammalignant?

If inflammaging is the chronic inflammation associated with aging, we can coin another term, *inflammalignant,* to describe the chronic inflammation linked with cancer. Let's review some of the research on lifestyle factors that increase inflammation and raise cancer risk. If you recognize any of these inflammalignant habits in your own life, see what you can do to change them.

Smoking

Perhaps the number-one unhealthy lifestyle habit that raises inflammation and leads to cancer is smoking. (Though note that chewing tobacco causes cancers of the mouth and throat, too.) Smoking is a guaranteed way to keep your immune system operating in overdrive and to expose yourself and those around you to a bevy of carcinogens. It is the single largest *avoidable* cause of cancer in the world. Lung cancer remains the top killer of men and women worldwide. In 2012, it claimed 1.6 million lives.[29]

Science has established links between smoking and more than a dozen types of cancer, including cancers of the lung, larynx, esophagus, mouth, pharynx, bladder, pancreas, kidney, liver, stomach, bowel, cervix, ovary, nose, sinuses, and breast and some forms of leukemia. This is one inflammalignant habit you should do everything in your power to quit.

Being Overweight

A close runner-up to smoking is being overweight. Overweight and obesity are inflammatory illnesses. They're directly linked with several types of cancer, including breast, esophageal, colon, uterine, kidney, stomach, endometrial, gallbladder, prostate, liver, ovarian, pancreatic, and thyroid cancers. Being overweight also raises your risk of a type of brain tumor (meningioma) and a blood cancer (multiple myeloma). When your body is in a constant state of obesity-induced inflammation, premalignant cells are primed to become cancerous cells, and tumor growth is fueled by oxidative stress.[30]

The damage can begin very early. A recent study found that having both obesity and high inflammation during adolescence was associated with a higher risk of later developing colorectal cancer. The study was based on nearly 240,000 teens ages 16 to 20 who were followed an average of 35 years. The teens with a BMI of 27.5 to 29.9 (overweight) had more than twice the risk of developing colorectal cancer than those with a normal BMI. For teens whose BMI was 30 and above (obese), the risk climbed to 2.38 times higher.

And those with high systemic inflammation, as indicated by erythrocyte sedimentation rate, had a 63 percent greater risk of later developing colorectal cancer compared to those with low inflammation.[31]

The risk of cancer also climbs depending on how long the extra weight sticks around. Consider the results of one study that followed nearly 74,000 postmenopausal women for an average of 12.6 years. During that time, 6,301 of the women were diagnosed with an obesity-related cancer. Forty percent of the study pool were never overweight, while 60 percent were overweight for some time during adulthood, and of those, about half were obese at some point. Researchers found that the longer a person was overweight, the higher the risk of cancer. Being overweight for a longer duration during adulthood increased the overall incidence of obesity-related cancers by 7 percent, of postmenopausal breast cancer by 5 percent, and of endometrial cancer by 17 percent. Further investigation found that the higher the weight, the higher the risk: For every 10 years with a BMI of 10 units above normal, the risk of postmenopausal breast cancer was 8 percent higher, and it was 37 percent higher for endometrial cancer. The risk of colon and kidney cancers was higher, as well.[32]

On the other hand, as you might expect, losing weight directly reduces cancer risk. Another study divided 439 postmenopausal women into four groups and monitored them for 12 months: One group followed a reduced calorie diet, another engaged in regular aerobic exercise, the third adopted both a reduced calorie diet and exercise, and the last made no lifestyle changes whatsoever. Researchers compared the circulating biomarkers involved with angiogenesis, the growth of new blood vessels that support a tumor. The women in the diet plus exercise group lost the most weight, which was anywhere from 2 to 11 percent of total body weight. Consequently, the more weight the women lost, the greater their drop in angiogenic biomarkers. Interestingly, the women in the exercise-only group did not show lower levels of these biomarkers.[33] Ultimately, this study demonstrates that losing weight reduces the risk of any of the obesity-related cancers and lowers chronic inflammation, as well.

Joanne Nadovich

AGE: 55

- Reduced total cholesterol by 52 points
- Increased energy
- WEIGHT LOST: 12 pounds
- INCHES LOST: 4

When I heard how restrictive the first 2 weeks of the plan would be, I thought I'd never be able to do it. But I could and I did! I lost inches and pounds, and I gained a better feeling about myself.

I think one of the main benefits for me was how much I learned. The Whole Body Cure Plan isn't a diet—it's more of an education plan. I learned what I could do to improve my health and feel better. For example, I learned that it is best to eat my last meal at least 2 hours before bedtime. If I eat closer to bedtime, I get indigestion. I avoid processed foods entirely now. I'm also trying to avoid gluten because I notice a difference when I go without it. If I do occasionally have a piece of bread or a cracker, I don't always feel great after. That was one of the biggest lessons—to learn to connect how I feel with what I eat. It may be a food that's causing my bad feeling or bad reaction. Some of my food-related symptoms were a tingling on my tongue or inflammation in my joints. Once, I had cheese and crackers as a late-night snack, and I woke up the next morning with red, swollen eyes—almost like I had pinkeye. The symptoms were gone within a day. Could it have been due to something else? Possibly, but that wasn't an experiment I was willing to repeat!

The other main thing I learned was how delicious the high-quality food products tasted compared to what I'd been eating. I continue to use pasture-raised, grass-fed chicken and beef because the quality is so much better. The same goes for the organic vegetables. They're more expensive, but there's a clear difference in quality. More than once, I had people ask me where I got my produce because it tasted so good. I'm blessed to live near one of the oldest farmers' markets in town. It runs outdoors from March through November, and during the

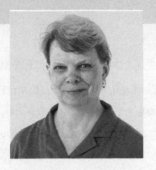

Joanne's Tips

Make a game of finding new ways to prepare food. Each time we introduced a new food, I'd google clean-eating recipes for that food. I love trying new recipes, so I'd gather new ones and make up my menu—it was a challenge I enjoyed. You do have to have the benefit of time to do that, as well as the dedication to stick with the plan. It is helpful to be in the right mind-set to dedicate yourself to this learning process. Go in with the mind-set that it *is* a process and that you're going to learn new things and find things you'll continue to do for good. I did, and I'm very glad I did it.

winter months, they have an indoor market. I can rely on my local farmers' market for high-quality food.

The food was one thing, but one of the most enjoyable parts for me was the qigong program. I was already practicing tai chi weekly. I'd studied tai chi for 2 years with Hilary, our instructor for the Whole Body Cure program, and 1 year before that with another instructor. Hilary is great. I've met students who've been with her for 17 years and longer. One has just turned 90, and many are healthy, vibrant people in their seventies and eighties. They firmly believe that tai chi has helped them age successfully, prevent falls because it improves balance, and recover from illnesses more quickly. It can take a full year to learn a short form of tai chi that's the basis for the next stage, which also takes a full year, and so on. Qigong is typically a shorter routine, and it's much easier to understand and follow, so it's much better suited to this program. The routine Hilary developed for the plan is good for the reduction of stress and inflammation, so it was a win-win. ■

Eating a Poor Diet

Central to the issues that surround overweight and obesity, of course, is diet. What you eat has an enormous impact on your cancer risk, not only because a poor diet can contribute to weight gain but also because many foods are highly inflammatory. Colorectal cancer, for example, has been linked to diets rich in animal proteins and fats, especially a high consumption of red meats and processed meats.

In 2015 the World Health Organization declared processed meats a Group 1 carcinogen. Processed meats are any meats that have been prepared by a process of smoking, curing, salting, or adding other chemical preservatives or flavor enhancers. Examples include bacon, sausage, ham, hot dogs, pastrami, and any cold cut that has gone through a chemical process. Meanwhile, red meat (beef, lamb, or pork products) was placed in Group 2A, which designates substances that are "probably" carcinogenic to humans. The evidence shows that regularly eating even small amounts of processed meat, such as one small hot dog, increases the chance of colorectal cancer by 18 percent compared to eating none. There was also a link observed between processed meat and an increased risk of stomach cancer. For red meat, eating 3.5 ounces daily was linked to an 18 percent increased risk of colorectal cancer as well as an increased risk of pancreatic and prostate cancer.[34]

Essentially, both processed and red meats are among the most inflammatory foods you can eat. They both have high amounts of sulfur-containing amino acids, saturated fats, and, in the case of processed meats, inorganic sulfur used as a preservative. Red meat is high in heme iron, which causes oxidative stress, and processed meats contain nitrates and nitrites from the preserving process. Meats cooked at high temperatures contain even more carcinogens.[35] If we may mix our metaphors, this is a veritable cocktail of inflammatory and carcinogenic substances! The typical Western diet, marked by a high consumption of processed and red meats, refined grains, soda, and sweets, has been shown many times to increase colorectal cancer risk.[36]

This brings us to the most important point when it comes to diet and cancer prevention. For the most effective means to reduce the risk of any type of cancer *and* lower inflammation, your best bet is to adopt an *overall healthy eating pattern*. So-called superfoods are no doubt healthy all on their own, but it's the *synergy* of all the vitamins, nutrients, fiber, antioxidants, healthy fats, and plant polyphenols that provides the most comprehensive cancer prevention and that keeps inflammation levels low. Evidence shows that fiber, calcium, vitamin D, folate (a B vitamin), and antioxidant nutrients (such as vitamins A, C, and E; lycopene; beta-carotene; and selenium) provide many protective effects against colorectal cancer, and these nutrients are best available through a varied diet. There are also many hundreds of cancer-protective polyphenolic compounds our bodies draw from plant foods—and remember this includes any food of plant origin, not just fruits and vegetables but also spices, nuts, and teas. Polyphenols' anticancer effects have been largely attributed to their antioxidant and anti-inflammatory activities.[37] We'll provide our own anti-inflammatory eating plan in the next chapter.

Consuming Too Much Alcohol

For years conventional scientific wisdom has assured us that "moderate drinking," which is up to one drink a day for women and up to two for men, is good for us. One drink is defined as 5 ounces of wine, 12 ounces of beer, 1.5 ounces of 80-proof spirits, or 1 ounce of 100-proof spirits. Overwhelming evidence has demonstrated that moderate drinking is associated with a lower incidence of heart disease and death, high blood pressure, gallstones, cognitive decline, and stroke. There's also evidence that it plays a role in preventing depression, type 2 diabetes, and even certain cancers.[38] It's important to remember, however, that most of these studies are looking at moderate *wine* consumption; much of the health benefits of alcohol comes from wine's polyphenolic content.

That said, an article published in the journal *Addiction* in mid-2016 grabbed headlines with the announcement that alcohol is a *direct* cause of seven different types of cancer and that even low to moderate drinking increases the risk. Based on a review of large sets of data from several studies, the author concluded that alcohol causes cancers of the pharynx, larynx, esophagus, liver, colon, rectum, and breast and that there is accumulating evidence for a causal relationship between alcohol and cancers of the pancreas, prostate, and skin (melanoma). As other researchers have noted, heavy drinking is associated with greater cancer risk, and smoking greatly compounds the risk.[39] Depending on the population studied, the combination of smoking and heavy drinking raises the risk by a factor of 50 or more.[40]

Other research has drawn somewhat different conclusions. Results of two large studies—based on data from over 88,000 women and over 47,800 men who were followed for over 30 years—found minimal overall cancer risk associated with light to moderate drinking. When results were broken down by gender, however, researchers found that women did have a higher risk of alcohol-related cancers, mainly in the form of breast cancer. The far stronger association, however, was between smoking and cancer risk, and that applies to both genders.[41] We'll add a final piece to this puzzle by taking a closer look at the results of two studies that examined alcohol's effects on inflammatory markers over several years. The first followed 8,209 adults (69 percent men) over a 10-year period. Researchers found that nondrinkers, former drinkers, and heavy drinkers had consistently elevated levels of three proinflammatory cytokines. But those who consistently consumed moderate levels of alcohol over a 10-year period had *lower* concentrations of inflammation compared to nondrinkers. Moderate drinkers had the best inflammatory profile, which is consistent with many other studies showing the heart-healthy benefits of moderate drinking.[42] Another study of 2,900 women over 8 years looked at different inflammatory biomarkers and found similar results. Researchers noted that the moderate wine drinkers (one glass per day) had significantly lower levels of inflammatory biomarkers, including CRP and fibrinogen, than women who drank less than one glass of wine per day or who didn't drink at all.[43] You could say, in other words, that results from these studies demonstrate the Goldilocks effect—not too much, not too little, but somewhere in the middle is just right.

What's abundantly clear is that heavy drinking is associated with the highest alcohol-related cancer risk and that smoking greatly elevates the risk. Liver cancer primarily occurs in people with cirrhosis resulting from heavy drinking. Without question, anything above moderate daily alcohol consumption, or binge drinking of any frequency, is detrimental to health and causes inflammation both systemically and at alcohol-related cancer sites, such as the liver, mouth, and esophagus. Women with any type of cancer risk should take extra care when it comes to drinking because of the link between alcohol and breast cancer.

Getting Poor Sleep

Maybe you wouldn't automatically associate sleeping difficulties with the other lifestyle issues we've already described as inflammalignant, but there is mounting evidence that poor sleep increases the risk of cancer. Until recently, most of the research on sleep and cancer risk has been conducted on breast cancer, and results were mixed.

Now results from a new study confirm the Goldilocks effect here, too—sleeping too much or too little is associated with increased cancer risk. Results were based on the sleep habits of 173,327 men and 123,858 women ages 51 to 72. The strongest link was found between male "short sleepers" (5 to 6 hours per night) and gastric cancer. Though the other associations didn't achieve clinical significance, researchers also noted links between male short sleepers and cancers of the head and neck, bladder, and thyroid and non-Hodgkin's lymphoma and myeloma. In women who slept more than 9 hours a night (long sleepers), there was an increased risk of non-Hodgkin's lymphoma but a *decreased* risk of ovarian cancer.[44]

As you saw from Chapter 2, insomnia is associated with chronic inflammation, and we also know that short sleepers (less than 6 hours a night) and people who sleep too much (9 or more hours a night) are at greater risk of obesity,[45] which on its own raises inflammation and cancer risk. Based on what we know about poor sleep's effect on weight, inflammatory markers, chronic stress, and mood disorders, it makes sense to follow the National Sleep Foundation's guidance: Adults ages 26 to 64 should get 7 to 9 hours of sleep per night, and adults 65 and over should get 7 to 8 hours.[46]

Immunotherapy

Some of the most exciting developments in the field of cancer treatment concern immunotherapy interventions, treatments that use your own immune system to help fight cancer. There are different types of immunotherapy, but all of them ultimately work to activate the immune system to fight cancer cells the same way it would fight bacteria or viruses. As we mentioned earlier, there is some evidence that immune surveillance—when the immune system identifies a precancerous or cancerous cell and eliminates it before it causes a problem—works in this way, but the system is far from perfect. Cancer cells evolve over time and can escape detection, ultimately tricking the immune system to work for their own ends. Immunotherapy drugs activate the immune system in different ways to harness its power and help shut down cancer.

There are three main types of immunotherapy (with more currently under investigation). *Checkpoint inhibitor* drugs are the most widely used type. To tell the difference between normal cells and threatening ones, the immune system uses "checkpoint" proteins, or molecules that need to be activated or inactivated to launch an immune response. Checkpoint proteins essentially keep the immune system from attacking normal cells. Under normal circumstances, cancer cells keep these checkpoint molecules inactivated and thus avoid receiving an immune system attack. Checkpoint inhibitors reverse this process and keep killer T-cells activated and free to attack. However, one of the hazards of checkpoint inhibitors is that when the immune system is unleashed, it attacks not just cancer cells but healthy ones, as well. Currently, checkpoint inhibitors have been used for lung, kidney, bladder, head and neck, and breast cancers, and in some cases, they have completely eliminated advanced melanomas.

Work is ongoing in another area of research, *cancer vaccines*. The HPV vaccine and vaccines for hepatitis have had tremendous success in preventing the infections that can lead to cancer, but cancer vaccines work differently. Instead of preventing a disease, they try to get the immune system to fight a disease that's already taken hold. Currently there is only one cancer vaccine approved for use in the United States, and it's used for advanced prostate cancer. Several different types of vaccines are currently undergoing research, and for many types of cancer, including brain, breast, cervical, colorectal, kidney, lung, pancreatic, and prostate cancers and lymphoma and melanoma, among others.

Lastly, *cell therapy* involves harvesting immune cells from a patient, genetically "reprogramming" them so they can fight cancer, and then administering them to the patient through IV drip. Cell therapy has been referred to as a "living drug," and it's created individually for each patient. This form of immunotherapy is still in the experimental phase, but early results have been extraordinarily promising, and a drug for blood cancers may reach the market by 2017. Around the world, many clinicians and people with cancer are hopeful about the potential for these new cell therapy treatments. Researchers at the Fred Hutchinson Cancer Research Center made headlines in early 2016 by announcing preliminary results of a new T-cell therapy for blood cancers. (Results have yet to be published in a peer-reviewed journal.) In one part of their study, 27 of 29 patients with acute lymphoblastic leukemia showed no trace of cancer after their infusions. Another group in the study, consisting of 19 of 30 non-Hodgkin's lymphoma patients, experienced partial or complete remission. In some patients, large tumors disappeared after a single dose of the engineered T cells within weeks of the infusion.[47] These results sound like science fiction, but they demonstrate just how revolutionary the field of immunotherapy can be—and they demonstrate the hidden power of our own immune systems, just waiting to be harnessed.

A Cancer-Free Future?

Extraordinary discoveries like these bring us back to where we began, with the results from the new immunotherapy intervention for pancreatic cancer, which gives us a sneak peek into the future of cancer treatment. If you'll remember, pancreatic cancer is one of the most lethal forms of the disease, with just 18 percent of patients alive a year after diagnosis and only 4 percent alive after 5 years. If pancreatic cancer has metastasized, the average survival rate from diagnosis is just 4.6 months. This new study compared a standard chemotherapy drug (gemcitabine) with gemcitabine plus an immunotherapy drug called IMM-101, which contains an inactive form of *Mycobacterium*. IMM-101, in effect, "wakes up" the immune system and causes it to attack pancreatic cancer cells while leaving healthy cells intact. Eighty-four percent of the study participants had metastatic pancreatic cancer. Those with metastasized disease who received gemcitabine alone survived for an average of 4.4 months, but those who also received IMM-101 survived for an average of 7 months. And as we mentioned at the beginning of the chapter, some lived for more than a year and one survived for nearly 3 years. What's more, IMM-101 produced zero side effects, which is unheard of for standard cancer drugs.[48] This was a small study, and the therapy worked better for patients with metastasized disease than for those whose cancer remained localized, so more research is clearly necessary.

But more research is exactly what's happening. Hundreds of clinical trials are currently under way throughout the world on many different immunotherapies for cancer, both on the types we've mentioned here as well as on new, emerging therapies. One class of drugs under investigation, for example, alters cancer cells' genetic programming and reteaches them to behave like healthy, normal cells. With such promising developments in cancer treatment already proving effective, might we indeed be moving toward a cancer-free future? Many experts believe such a future is within the realm of possibility. But treatment is only part of the equation, and to truly eradicate cancer, we need to prevent it from occurring in the first place. Fortunately, that's something we can start doing right now through healthy lifestyle choices, no special degree or additional research required.

PART III

The Whole Body Cure Wellness Plan

CHAPTER 11

Extinguishing the Fires

The Whole Body Cure Eating Plan

By now you're aware how a proinflammatory lifestyle impacts your overall health, so let's get right to the good news. The single most powerful change you can make to extinguish the fires of inflammation is to change the way you eat. You can prevent or reverse many major chronic illnesses simply by eating the right foods. What a joy to enjoy delicious, healthy foods as your medicine!

And that's exactly what this chapter is all about. The Whole Body Cure Eating Plan shows you how to leverage our most powerful tool—our diets—to lower inflammation and maintain whole-body health for the rest of your life. It's the most delicious medicine you'll ever taste. And if you're eating *this* kind of medicine, it's entirely possible you'll have less need for the kind that requires a prescription.

"Let Food Be Thy Medicine"

Hippocrates, the Greek physician known as the father of modern medicine, wrote these words more than 1,500 years ago—and they ring true today more than ever. The standard American diet is loaded with highly processed, lab-engineered "food" products that contain a long list of chemicals that few can pronounce, let alone grasp the cascade of negative effects they exert on our bodies.

When we consume such "foods," our bodies perceive these additives as foreign invaders and our immune system rightly launches the inflammatory response—and keeps it revved up if we eat this way regularly. Highly processed foods are among the main causes of inflammation and the chronic illnesses it spawns.

So the first principle of the Whole Body Cure Eating Plan is to eat *real* foods. The fuel our bodies truly need—whole, healthy, minimally processed foods—are fruits and vegetables that come from the garden, not from the lab, and proteins that come from sustainable sources rather than large industrial operations. We'll get into specifics for each food group later in this chapter, but the overall goal to remember is that the foods you eat should be nonprocessed or minimally processed and, if possible, organic so you can avoid harmful pesticides and other chemicals that can trigger inflammation. The foods we're talking about are by their very nature anti-inflammatory, and they also just happen to be the best food choices for keeping weight off for the long term. Though the Whole Body Cure Eating Plan is *not* a diet, most people who follow it lose weight, and weight loss can often be quite significant. (Some panelists, for instance, lost more than 20 pounds.) With what we know about unhealthy foods and inflammation-driven weight gain, this is just what we'd expect. If you're exchanging proinflammatory saturated fats and processed foods for organic, grass-fed meats and antioxidant-rich fruits and vegetables, you can expect to lose weight.

The Whole Body Cure Plan lasts just 12 weeks, but in order to reap the long-term rewards of lower inflammation, we hope you'll take what you learn and use it to create a new way of eating, for life. So let's get started by first discussing how you will neutralize the inflammation that's already present in your body and reset your system so you can discover what foods are best for your individual needs.

Reset Your Body and Eliminate Food Sensitivities—For Good

Throughout this book, you've read about the dangers of hidden food sensitivities, which are a common source of chronic inflammation as well as a variety of related symptoms, such as joint pain, headaches, gastrointestinal complaints, fatigue, and brain fog (a feeling of being spacey or out of it). Well now we're

THE CASE FOR ORGANICS

Organic foods may cost a little more than conventional foods, but you'll more than make up for the difference in health benefits. To earn the USDA Organic label, a food must be grown in soil that has had no prohibited substances—such as synthetic fertilizers and pesticides—applied for at least 3 years prior to harvest. As for organic meats, animals must be fed with 100 percent organic feed, must not be treated with antibiotics or hormones, and must be raised in conditions that allow their natural behaviors, such as grazing in a pasture. Additionally, organic foods must not contain any artificial colors, flavors, or preservatives, and they must not be genetically modified.[1]

What does all this mean for our health? It means less exposure to toxins routinely used in conventionally produced foods, and it means more nutritional value. A recent meta-analysis of 343 studies found that organic crops, on average, contain significantly higher concentrations of antioxidants than conventionally produced crops. Further, pesticide residues in conventionally produced crops were four times higher than in organic crops, while organic crops had 48 percent lower concentrations of the toxic heavy metal cadmium,[2] which has been linked to bone, kidney, and lung diseases. As for meats, a recent meta-analysis based on 67 studies found that organic meats (beef, chicken, lamb, and pork) were 47 percent higher in anti-inflammatory omega-3 fatty acids than conventionally produced meats.[3]

If you can't go all organic all the time, buy organic versions of the foods that consistently show the highest levels of pesticides. Each year the Environmental Working Group releases a "Dirty Dozen" list of the most pesticide-laden produce. You can see the full list at ewg.org. To help remove pesticides from conventional foods, always wash produce thoroughly, and for even more scrubbing power, try washing with a solution of four parts water and one part white vinegar. Rinse thoroughly with plain water afterward. Peeling fruits and vegetables after washing also helps, though you'll lose some of the fiber content.

going to show you how to deal with those food sensitivities head-on. The first step, of course, before you can identify exactly which foods are causing the problem, is to help your body free itself of as much inflammation as possible. Therefore, the Whole Body Cure Eating Plan begins with a 2-week reset phase that will detox your system and quickly neutralize any food sensitivities and systemic inflammation. This 2-week period calms your entire system and jump-starts the healing process. For those first 2 weeks, you'll be eating organic fruits and vegetables and tasty protein shakes and taking specially formulated supplements that support digestive health, lower inflammation, and ensure you're getting the nutrients you need. Here's an overview of what you'll eat during this time (we'll describe each component of the meals just ahead). Don't worry that you'll be hungry. Most people are surprisingly satisfied on this plan. But if you are hungry, eat more vegetables, fruit, and/or fat.

Breakfast

1 serving shake

1 serving fat

1 serving vegetables (if desired)

1 serving fruit (if desired)

Supplements

1 teaspoon CoCurcumin

1 tablespoon GI-Revive

Lunch

2 to 4 servings vegetables (half as raw veggies)

1 serving fat

1 serving fruit

Snack (Try to eat every 4 to 5 hours. Based on your schedule, a snack may be best in the afternoon or evening.)

½ serving shake

Supplements

1 teaspoon CoCurcumin

1 tablespoon GI-Revive

Dinner

2 to 4 servings vegetables (half as raw veggies)

1 serving fat

1 serving fruit

It's important to track your progress, Dr. Kirshner has found his patients start feeling better and forget they had some of the symptoms first listed on day one. So be sure to take the time to record your progress. It's also a great way to keep track of what you've eaten in case you start feeling poorly. You may be able to trace it back to something new or different you recently ate. You will find a sample log page and sample self-assessment worksheets in the Appendix beginning on page 365 so you can see how to record how you feel and keep track of your progress throughout the plan. The free journal you received with this book will make tracking your progress a breeze, so be sure to use it when starting the plan. You'll complete the first three self-assessment worksheets during this initial reset phase: at the very beginning of the plan (Day 1), at the end of the first week (Day 7), and at the end of the second week (Day 14). Though these first 2 weeks are the most restrictive of the program, many people report that it's during this time that they notice a dramatic uptick in energy and an improvement in general well-being. Comparing the self-assessments from Day 1 and Day 14 can be an eye-opening experience, as you'll see just how different your body looks and feels in just 2 weeks of living with less inflammation.

Once this 2-week reset phase is complete, you're ready for the next part of the plan, which shows you how to slowly and methodically reintroduce your body to specific foods so you can determine which, if any, trigger food sensitivities that lead to inflammation. Remember, everybody has a unique response to the foods he or she eats. And because we are omnivores and eat such a varied diet on any given day, without such a detailed, systematic approach, it's virtually impossible to pinpoint the exact food that may be causing your unique symptoms. This diagnostic eating strategy is commonly referred to as an elimination diet, and the beauty of this approach is it gives you the time and the tools to test out each type of food individually to see how your body responds. Here's how it works.

You'll test one food at a time, for 3 days each. Of course, if you have a known food allergy, or if you'd normally avoid a certain food, such as if you're a pescatarian or vegetarian, you will avoid that food and simply go on to the next food to test. But unless you develop a severe allergic reaction (widespread hives, trouble breathing, swelling), it's important to complete all 3 days of the test period, as it can take up to 3 days for the body's immune response to react to a food sensitivity or intolerance. So, for example, the first food you'll reintroduce is grass-fed beef. For 3 consecutive days, enjoy grass-fed beef alone or in any of the recipes starting on page 239 along with the breakfast shake and fruits and vegetables like you've been enjoying for the first 2 weeks, and you'll again complete a self-assessment worksheet to record how you feel. Make sure you record your body's reactions even if you don't think they're related to what you've eaten or if they seem to be a fluke, as food sensitivities can produce a wide range of symptoms. Whatever you experience, jot it down on the self-assessment—this is your chance to notice and record *your* body's feedback on individual foods. You can trust your body to tell you what's good for you and what isn't. One panelist, for example, found that her body spoke up loud and clear once she reintroduced eggs—in the form of extreme fatigue. If her fatigue had occurred on a single day, it would be easy to chalk it up to any number of causes, from an oncoming virus to poor sleep to stress. This is yet another reason you'll be testing foods for 3 days each. The panelist's fatigue only worsened on Days 2 and 3 of eating eggs, so then she had strong evidence to suspect that eggs were the culprit. Her final confirmation arrived when she eliminated eggs from her diet and her energy quickly returned.

Dr. Kirshner's Inflammation Insight

When Emma first came to see me, she had such extensive food intolerances her diet consisted of only five foods: tomatoes, cucumbers, coffee, rice, and turkey breast. Eating any other foods resulted in diarrhea and joint pain, and she never went out to eat. This was the most severe case of food intolerance I'd seen, and it took the longest to resolve. But through trial and error, an anti-inflammatory diet, and a gut-healing program, Emma found relief. It took about 2 months of detox and healing before she could even try any "new foods," but within 1 year, she could eat up to 45 different foods with no negative effects. Within 2 years, she could eat most foods and enjoy meals out at most restaurants with minimal complaints.

This panelist's experience gives you a snapshot of how our eating plan works. You'll be slowly reincorporating a variety of foods into your diet one at a time and then using self-assessments to monitor and record your reactions. Listen carefully to your body during this phase, and it will tell you which foods support your whole-body health and which ones don't. If a food causes no reactions, you're in the clear and free to enjoy it as you like. But if a food causes a negative symptom or prompts the return of symptoms you were happy to leave behind—and then eliminating that food relieves those symptoms—you'll know to avoid that food permanently.

If you're worried about the possibility of giving up a favorite treat, try looking at it from the perspective of how much better you'll feel after. As a matter of fact, one of the reactions we heard most consistently from our panelists was they didn't miss foods that caused negative symptoms because they loved the way they felt without them. And the only foods you will be eliminating from this point on will be those that cause negative reactions like fatigue, digestive issues, joint pain, and headaches. Eliminating a food that's making you sick is a small price to pay for the reward of whole-body health and wellness. By the end of the program, you'll have your own customized eating practice, one that will serve you well for life.

Here's an example of how you'll eat each day during the 3-day test period. Remember if you are hungry, add more vegetables, fruit, and/or fat.

Breakfast

1 serving shake

1 serving fat

1 serving vegetables (if desired)

1 serving fruit (if desired)

Supplements

1 teaspoon CoCurcumin

1 tablespoon GI-Revive

Lunch

1 serving of the food you are testing (such as grass-fed beef, eggs, shellfish)

2 to 4 servings vegetables (half as raw veggies)

1 serving fat

1 serving fruit

Snack (Try to eat every 4 to 5 hours. Based on your schedule, a snack may be best in the afternoon or evening.)

1 serving fruit or

1 serving vegetables or

½ shake

Supplements

1 teaspoon CoCurcumin

1 tablespoon GI-Revive

Dinner

1 serving of the food you are testing (such as grass-fed beef, eggs, shellfish)

2 to 4 servings vegetables (half as raw veggies)

1 serving fat

1 serving fruit

There is an order in which you should reintroduce the foods you've eliminated from your diet, although it is not necessarily specific. Because beef and eggs are perfect proteins, the Whole Body Cure Plan has you try these foods first (one at a time, of course). Below is a Dr. Kirshner's suggested order; however, if you need to proceed in a different order, it's fine to do so. Just be sure to reintroduce the foods in 3-day increments. And remember, if there is a food on the list that you would never eat, simply skip it and go on to the next one on the list.

- Grass-fed beef

- Organic eggs

- Organic chicken

- Organic turkey

- Wild fish like salmon, cod, tuna, etc.

- Grass-fed lamb

- Raw nuts

- Organic beans and legumes

- Organic dairy products

- Organic soy products like edamame, tempeh, tofu (avoid highly processed soy products like soy protein bars or textured vegetable protein)

Once you've tested all the foods, you're free to enjoy the ones that didn't cause a negative reaction, and you'll also know which, if any, to avoid. If you need to lose weight, pay attention to portion sizes, but remember that the Whole Body Cure Plan is *not* a diet. When you're hungry, feel free to eat any of the acceptable foods. Rather than counting calories or adhering to strict portion sizes, this program encourages you to learn how to follow your body's cues.

So after you complete all the test periods, here's an overview of how you'll eat from then on (these serving sizes are suggestions).

Breakfast

1 serving protein or shake

1 serving fat

1 serving vegetables (if desired)

1 serving fruit (if desired)

Lunch

1 serving protein

2 to 4 servings vegetables (half as raw veggies)

1 serving fat

1 serving fruit

Snack (Try to eat every 4 to 5 hours. Based on your schedule, a snack may be best in the afternoon or evening.)

1 serving fruit or

1 serving vegetables or

1 serving raw nuts or

½ shake

Enjoy 1 ounce of dark chocolate (70 percent or higher), if desired, daily.

Dinner

1 serving protein

2 to 4 servings vegetables (half as raw veggies)

1 serving fat

1 serving fruit

Okay, So What Do I Eat?

Great question! By now you're sure to be curious about what you'll be eating for the 12 weeks of the Whole Body Cure Plan. And here's where things get fun. The plan is built around whole, real, anti-inflammatory foods—and Mother Nature provides these foods in abundance. You may just eat a more varied, exciting diet with this anti-inflammatory style of eating than you ever have in your life!

Pop into your local farmers' market any time of year, and you'll catch a glimpse of the vast array of delicious foods available, from fruits and vegetables to grass-fed meats to nearly any kind of nut and seed, not to mention healthy sources of fat such as olive oil and coconut oil. Of course, all these foods are typically available at your local grocery store, as well, but take care to stick to nonprocessed or minimally processed options. Let's take a quick look at each type of food on the plan, followed by a list of all the foods you can enjoy. At the end of this chapter, we'll give you lots of scrumptious recipes using these all-natural healing foods.

Heal Yourself by Eating Plenty
of These Foods

The mainstays of the plan are organic fruits and vegetables, protein shakes, healthy fats, and beverages that keep you fully hydrated and do not promote inflammation. As the weeks continue, you'll incorporate organic, free-range meats, poultry, organic eggs, wild-caught fish and shellfish, and nuts and seeds. Eventually, barring a food sensitivity, you'll be able to add in beans, legumes, and even certain dairy products, as well. So you see, there will be plenty to eat, drink, and enjoy as you launch your very own health transformation.

Let's take a closer look at what's on the menu.

Vegetables

With just a few exceptions, the types of vegetables and the amount you can eat on the Whole Body Cure Plan are *unlimited*. The three vegetables that do not make the cut are white potatoes, corn, and iceberg lettuce. These foods have limited nutritional value, and corn constitutes a double whammy because it's one of the top causes of food sensitivities. You should also eat no more than half a yam or sweet potato per day because of their relatively high carbohydrate content and because they tend to be quite large anyway. Other than these exceptions, however, we encourage you to eat as many vegetables as you can and to look for new opportunities to get more vegetables into your meals, such as featuring them as a main dish, sautéing some veggies along with your scrambled eggs, or using greens like baby spinach or baby kale in your shakes. With their high antioxidant, vitamin, mineral, and fiber content and zero saturated fat, vegetables are anti-inflammatory powerhouses, and you can hardly eat too many of them. Try to eat about twice as many vegetables per day as fruits.

If you don't see your favorite veggie on the list opposite, feel free to add it. And on the other hand, if you find an unfamiliar vegetable on the list, just give it a try! "Eating the rainbow," from dark leafy greens to bright yellow bell peppers to multihued heirloom tomatoes and beyond, gives you the full complement of health-promoting phenolic compounds found in plant foods.

You're also encouraged to try new combinations of vegetables or new ways of preparing them. Use as many fresh herbs and spices as you like, and don't forget that turmeric, garlic, and ginger are especially effective at lowering inflammation. In addition to new flavors, many of our panelists were delighted to find how much they loved roasted vegetables and how easy they are to prepare. You can also prepare vegetables by steaming them for around 4 minutes or by stir-frying them for approximately 5 minutes using olive oil, coconut oil, or grape-seed oil. Steaming and stir-frying will allow veggies to retain more nutrients.

On the opposite end of the spectrum, try and eat half of your vegetables raw. Certain vitamins, minerals, and enzymes that aid in digestion are lost when veggies are exposed to heat, especially vitamins A and C and folate. Raw vegetables also have a higher water content, which helps you feel full faster and thus can promote weight loss. And speaking of water content, you're free to drink delicious fresh juices made from blended vegetables, so dust off that juicer or blender and come up with your own creations.

Do use organic vegetables whenever possible. Frozen vegetables are okay, but avoid all dried or canned vegetables. If you get stuck at any point and must use canned veggies, make sure the cans are BPA-free.

Vegetables List

Any vegetable, except white potatoes, corn, and iceberg lettuce, is allowed.

- Artichokes
- Asparagus
- Bamboo shoots
- Bean sprouts
- Beets, red*
- Bok choy
- Broccoflower
- Broccoli
- Broccoli rabe
- Brussels sprouts
- Cabbage (all types)
- Carrots
- Cauliflower
- Celery
- Chives
- Cucumbers
- Eggplant
- Fennel
- Garlic
- Ginger
- Green beans
- Herbs (basil, cilantro, cumin, dill, oregano, parsley, sage, thyme, etc.)
- Jicama
- Kohlrabi
- Leeks
- Mushrooms
- Okra
- Olives

*Remember, consuming beets may change the color of urine and bowel movements, but this is of no concern.

- Onions
- Parsnips
- Peppers (any type, any color)
- Pimientos
- Radishes
- Rutabaga
- Scallions

- Sea vegetables (arame, dulse, hijiki, kombu, nori, etc.)
- Summer squash (zucchini, yellow squash)
- Sweet potatoes (½ per day)
- Tomatillos
- Tomatoes
- Turmeric

- Turnips
- Water chestnuts
- Wax beans
- Winter squash (spaghetti, butternut, acorn)
- Yams (½ per day)
- Zucchini

Lettuces and Greens List

- Arugula
- Beet greens
- Collard greens
- Dandelion greens
- Endive
- Escarole

- Kale
- Mustard greens
- Radicchio
- Red and green leaf lettuce
- Romaine

- Spinach
- Swiss chard
- Watercress

Fruits

With the exception of bananas, which are calorie-dense and high on the glycemic index, any fresh fruit is allowed on the plan. That said, the stars of the show when it comes to anti-inflammatory power are berries, so get in the habit of eating these antioxidant-rich superfruits. Frozen fruits are okay to use, especially in the cold months when fresh fruits aren't as available. Fresh or frozen, organic is always best.

As with vegetables, you're encouraged to "eat the rainbow" to benefit from a variety of different phenolic compounds—and you just may find some new favorites on our list! Fruits have a naturally higher sugar content than vegetables, so overall, eat half as much fruit as vegetables. Also bypass canned fruits, especially ones which are often packed in sugary syrups. Within these parameters, you can enjoy delicious fruits throughout all 12 weeks of the plan.

Fruits List

- Apples
- Apricots
- Aronia berries (chokeberries)
- Avocado
- Blackberries
- Blueberries
- Cantaloupe
- Cherries
- Cranberries
- Figs
- Grapefruit

- Grapes
- Guava
- Honeydew melon
- Kiwifruit
- Kumquats
- Lemons
- Limes
- Loganberries
- Mango
- Mulberries
- Nectarines

- Oranges
- Papaya
- Peaches
- Pears
- Pineapple
- Plums
- Pomegranates
- Raspberries
- Strawberries
- Tangerines
- Watermelon

WHOLE-BODY TIPS FOR WHOLE-YEAR EATING

If you're wondering how to stick to the plan during the winter months, when fresh fruits and vegetables aren't as abundant, rest assured that many people have successfully completed the plan throughout all four seasons. While many of the favorite summer vegetables, such as tomatoes and cucumbers, are less abundant in the colder months, there is still plenty to eat during the winter, and during these months, you'll likely be cooking more of your vegetables. Organic greens are available year-round for salads, but instead of adding summer veggies to the bowl, add shredded beets, carrots, or kohlrabi; sautéed onion and mushrooms; or roasted vegetables. Roasting vegetables is a simple and delicious way to prepare winter vegetables. Chop a variety—onion, garlic, broccoli, cauliflower, winter squash, bell peppers, parsnips, or even radishes—and toss with some oil, herbs (if desired), and a sprinkle of sea salt and pepper, then roast together until tender and you'll have a meal or a snack waiting for you in the fridge. Finally, don't forget about soups, always a cold-weather favorite. Vegetables can become creamy, rich soups without the addition of inflammatory ingredients. Check out all the delicious recipes starting on page 239.

Healthy Fats

Fats are healing foods when you're choosing the right ones. We know the dangers of hydrogenated oils, and we also want to avoid oils that are high in proinflammatory omega-6 fatty acids, such as canola oil, corn oil, soybean oil, or vegetable oil. Furthermore, the healthy fats you'll find listed below boast anti-inflammatory benefits all on their own, and there's ample evidence that combining a healthy fat with other ingredients increases the absorption of nutrients. One well-known example is turmeric. Turmeric has incredible anti-inflammatory properties, but eaten alone, its nutrients are hard for the body to absorb. Adding a healthy fat, such as extra-virgin olive oil or coconut oil, however, prevents the active compounds in turmeric from being broken down by the liver or stomach acids before they can make it into the bloodstream.[4]

As always, organic is best, but whether you opt for organic or not, make sure to look for the least-processed oils you can find—depending on the type, you'll see them labeled as cold-pressed, expeller-pressed, unprocessed, or unrefined. You're aiming for high-quality oils that have not been exposed to heat or chemicals during production.

Here are the fats you can use for cooking, for salad dressings, or for drizzling over vegetables, all of them just as healthy as they are tasty.

Healthy Fats List

Standard serving size is ½ to 1 tablespoon, 4 to 7 servings per day.

- Avocado oil
- Coconut oil
- Extra-virgin olive oil
- Fish oil
- Flaxseed oil (keep refrigerated and do not heat; use for salad dressings)
- Grape-seed oil
- Pumpkin seed oil
- Walnut oil

Protein Shakes

As stated earlier, during the reset phase of the plan, you will rid your body of sensitivities and inflammation to prepare for the elimination diet. Protein shakes provide protein in the most digestible form possible, making the shakes easier than meat and eggs for the body to digest. This allows the body to focus its energy on reducing inflammation instead of digesting protein.

Since protein shakes are so popular these days, it's important that you read ingredient lists to be sure you are not getting a sugary treat. Look for ones that have at least 20 grams of protein and less than 5 grams of sugar per serving. See the Resources section on page 369 for our guide to the best brand selections. Enjoy one shake for breakfast and half a shake for a snack for the elimination part of the plan. After that, you may continue having quick and delicious shakes for breakfast, along with any proteins that don't cause sensitivities.

Supplements

Two supplements are an important part of the program. The first is a dry powder you mix into beverages or add to foods called CoCurcumin, which is a blend of curcumin (the active compound in turmeric), coenzyme Q10, and coconut oil. We know that curcumin is an anti-inflammatory powerhouse, and studies show that added fat (such as the coconut oil) helps enhance the absorption of curcumin. The anti-inflammatory benefits are even greater with the addition of coenzyme Q10, an antioxidant that helps convert food into energy. CoCurcumin may be added to shakes or to warm coconut milk or almond milk, or it may be stirred into boiling water to make tea. You can also stir it into soups or stews just before serving. Use 2 teaspoons of CoCurcumin for the first 6 weeks of the plan, and 1 teaspoon thereafter.

The other suggested supplement you'll use is called GI-Revive. Most people with chronic inflammation have some gastrointestinal issues, including intestinal permeability, also known as leaky gut syndrome. When the gut is too permeable (leaky), toxins, bacteria, and other harmful substances can pass through the intestinal wall and into the bloodstream, increasing inflammation. GI-Revive helps to heal the gastrointestinal wall and assists in regularity. Take 2 tablespoons daily for the first two phases by adding it to your shake or stirring it into water.

Meat, Poultry, Fish, and Eggs

You'll incorporate these proteins back into your diet one at a time, beginning in Week 3 with beef. If you are a pescatarian or vegetarian, you'll simply ignore the recommendations to eat foods you normally avoid and skip ahead to the first food that you eat. For example, skip the week that tests for beef and go on to eggs. The same goes for any known food allergy. If you know you have an allergy to eggs, for instance, skip that week and go on to the first food that you do eat. You should use organic protein foods wherever possible. Organic eggs and meats ensure that you're getting antibiotic- and hormone-free foods, and, where applicable, opt for animals that are grass-fed. All fish should be wild, not farm-raised, as farm-raised fish are routinely treated with antibiotics and they tend to have a lower anti-inflammatory omega-3 content than wild fish.

To keep down the cost of organic, free-range meats and other proteins, try buying from local providers or consider joining a CSA, a community-supported agriculture group, in your area. Food co-ops as well as CSAs often allow several consumers to go in together to buy products in bulk, thus reducing the cost for all.

After the first 2 weeks of the Whole Body Cure Plan, which will detox your body and lower inflammation quickly, you'll add proteins back into your meals, one new one every 3 days, in this suggested order: beef, eggs, chicken, turkey, pork, shellfish, fish, and lamb. The standard serving size for meats and fish is about 3 ounces cooked, which equates to 4 ounces when raw (roughly palm-size). If you're still hungry after your meal, don't feel guilty about going back for a little more. Portion control is great, but listen to *your* body and follow its cues.

Prepare meats and fish by broiling, baking, roasting, grilling, or poaching. Avoid any sort of processed meat products, such as cured or smoked meat or lunchmeat, as they've been exposed to chemical processing and are highly proinflammatory. Here are the proteins to enjoy.

Meat List
- Grass-fed beef
- Grass-fed lamb
- Grass-fed pork
- Organic chicken
- Organic eggs
- Organic turkey

Shellfish List

- Clams
- Crab
- Crawfish
- Lobster

- Mussels
- Octopus
- Oysters
- Scallops

- Shrimp
- Squid

Fish List

All fish should be wild-caught, not farm-raised.

- Arctic char
- Atlantic mackerel
- Barramundi
- Bass
- Black sea bass
- Catfish
- Cod
- Haddock

- Halibut
- Lionfish
- Mahi mahi
- Monkfish
- Pollock
- Pompano
- Rainbow trout
- Rockfish

- Salmon
- Sardines
- Striped mullet
- Trout
- Tuna
- Wahoo
- Wreckfish

Nuts and Seeds

Nuts and seeds are excellent sources of protein, fiber, minerals, and antioxidants, and you only need a handful to enjoy their great health benefits. A single Brazil nut, for example, contains your entire Recommended Dietary Allowance (RDA) of cancer-fighting selenium, almonds contain an impressive 75 milligrams of calcium per ounce, and an ounce of chia seeds contains nearly half of your RDA of fiber. And though nuts and seeds are naturally high in fat, this is healthy, monounsaturated fat we're talking about, and research has shown time and again that eating nuts and seeds does *not* promote weight gain. In fact, people who eat nuts regularly actually tend to weigh less than those who don't. Their risk of type 2 diabetes is lower, as well.[5]

Nuts and seeds are excellent options for snacks between meals, and you can add them to salads, too. You'll be able to eat nuts and seeds once you determine you don't have any sensitivity to them. If you have diverticulitis, you may want to avoid seeds; check with your doctor to make sure. Finally, raw, unsalted nuts and seeds are best for lowering inflammation, but it's fine to toast them occasionally for an entirely new flavor (see recipe on page 290).

Nuts List

Standard serving size is about 1 ounce or a handful.

- Almonds
- Brazil nuts
- Cashews
- Hazelnuts
- Macadamias
- Pecans
- Pistachios
- Walnuts

Seeds List

If you have diverticulitis, check with your doctor before eating seeds.

- Chia seeds
- Flaxseeds
- Hemp seeds
- Pine nuts
- Pumpkin seeds
- Sesame seeds
- Sunflower seeds

Beverages

You will be eliminating alcohol and dairy milks while you're on the program. Once the 12 weeks are complete, it's up to you if you'd like to reincorporate alcohol and/or dairy, but remember that both promote inflammation, especially if consumed in large quantities, and you should test out these items just as you did with every other food. If you discover that you have a sensitivity to dairy, eliminate it permanently.

Otherwise, keep yourself well hydrated with any of the beverages listed below. Enjoy unlimited amounts of spring or filtered water, green tea, and herbal tea. For coffee and black tea, aim for no more than 2 cups per day. If you get bored with plain water, spritz it up with fresh lime, lemon, or orange or drop in fresh cucumber or mint for an easy, delicious thirst quencher. Adequate hydration helps to flush out toxins, and it keeps your digestive system functioning regularly.

Beverages List

- Spring water or filtered water
- Green tea*
- Herbal tea* (examples include chamomile, ginger, lemon balm, mint, rooibos, etc.)
- Black tea*
- Coffee*

*Avoid using half-and-half, milk, or creamer during the first 12 weeks, but you may add 1 tablespoon of coconut oil, if desired.

TIPS FOR STICKING TO THE PROGRAM WHEN EATING OUT

Here are some tips you can use to stay on track when eating away from home.

- When choosing a restaurant, select one that serves foods that are on the approved list. Look up menus online to decide what you'll be eating before leaving the house; this will prevent ordering something not on the plan and reduce stress.

- When traveling, pack a cooler of foods, including fresh fruit and sliced raw vegetables. Don't forget the water bottles!

- When attending a social gathering, bring a dish to share that's on the plan, like a fruit/veggie tray or chicken kabobs.

Sea Salt

Sea salt is the least processed salt available—it's made by simply evaporating water from ocean water or saltwater lakes. Table salt is usually sourced from underground mines, and very often, chemicals are added to prevent salt crystals from clumping. Though sea salt and table salt taste the same, sea salt is the most minimally processed; contains trace minerals, such as potassium, iron, and zinc; and contains no additives.

With salt, a little goes a long way—and you may find this to be especially so after completing the detox portion of the eating plan. Each recipe we've included needs no more than ½ teaspoon sea salt.

Heal Yourself by Temporarily Avoiding These Foods

You will be eliminating soy products, beans, legumes, and all dairy products during the beginning weeks of the Whole Body Cure. But once you've tested all the other foods on the plan and have identified any food sensitivities, you can test these food groups in the same way you did the others and see how your body reacts. If there are no problems, you may reincorporate these foods. We've provided a list of examples starting on the next page.

Take special care with dairy, however, as many people are lactose intolerant, and you should continue to avoid dairy products that are high in saturated fat, such as butter, cheese, ice cream, whipped cream, and full-fat sour cream. Also opt for organic dairy products to avoid exposure to antibiotics, hormones, preservatives, flavor enhancers, or other chemicals. Many of our panelists, even some of the diehard ice cream fans, felt so much better without dairy that they opted to go dairy-free for life. Plant and nut milks are easy, healthier substitutions if you have a need for milk, such as to use in coffee. Other panelists elected to eat dairy only as an occasional treat, such as a fine cheese. Still others reincorporated dairy in the form of yogurt and kefir. These fermented dairy products are among the healthiest options as they are easier to digest and offer health benefits from their probiotic content. Even if you are able to reincorporate dairy back into your diet, don't overdo it. If you really enjoy it in your coffee, add it back. If yogurt makes a great lunch or snack for you, occasionally add organic sugar-free yogurt back to your meals. Just remember that dairy can still have an inflammatory effect, so keep it to a minimum.

Soy Products

Soy is a very common food allergen, and most of the soybeans grown in this country are genetically modified organisms (GMO), which in animal studies have been linked with allergic reactions, autoimmune disorders, infertility, and accelerated aging. So if you do decide to test out soy products, use an abundance of caution. This is one case where you shouldn't compromise on organic, which will rule out GMO soy. Further, continue to avoid processed soy products like textured vegetable protein (TVP) and soy protein isolate. Make sure soy sauce is gluten-free as the gluten found in soy sauce may cause inflammation. Further, use only small amounts of wheat-free soy sauce since it can cause water retention.

Soy Products List
Make sure to choose organic products.

- Edamame
- Miso
- Natto
- Soy sauce
- Tempeh
- Tofu

Beans and Legumes

Note that peanuts, which are a legume, are not on the eating plan at any time since they're the source of so many allergic reactions. But if you're a peanut fan, you can test them after the 12-week period to see if you can consume them. If you can add peanut butter back, be sure it's an organic, natural variety with no added fats or sugar.

Beans and Legumes List

- Beans of all types (adzuki, black, navy, kidney, red, cannellini, great northern, lima, pinto, fava, mung, etc.)
- Chickpeas
- Lentils
- Peas (green, crowder, black-eyed, sugar snap, snow, yellow)

Dairy

Continue to avoid dairy products that are high in saturated fat, such as butter, ice cream, whipped cream, half-and-half, creamer, full-fat sour cream, whole milk, and cheese. If you do decide to reincorporate dairy, stick with organic products.

Dairy List

- Buttermilk
- Cheese
- Kefir
- Milk
- Sour cream
- Yogurt

Heal Yourself by Avoiding These Foods

Now that we've gone over the anti-inflammatory foods you can indulge in to stay healthy, let's talk about what you should avoid, and why. You may find a few of the items on this list surprising, as some of them *do* offer some health benefits.

An occasional glass of red wine, for example, is well known to promote heart health and to boost mood. But if your primary goal is to lower inflammation, avoiding these foods and beverages is the best way to maintain the *maximum* anti-inflammatory benefit. If you find some of these foods difficult to avoid, focus instead on how good you feel without them.

Alcohol

As we mentioned earlier, you'll be avoiding alcohol during the 12 weeks of the Whole Body Cure Plan because alcohol increases inflammation, and different types can cause food sensitivities in a number of people. (Not to mention that wine and beer contain quite a bit of added sugar, which is proinflammatory all on its own.) If you wish to reincorporate alcohol once the 12 weeks are up, you can test individual types (white wine, red wine, beer) for sensitivity just like you did with the other foods. If the beverage you're testing produces no negative symptoms, you may resume drinking alcohol in moderation. Moderation is defined as no more than one alcoholic beverage per day for women, and no more than two for men.

Grains and Flours

The Whole Body Cure Eating Plan encourages you to eliminate all grains and grain products, including rice, barley, oats, millet, wheat, and items made from flour, such as bread, pasta, cereal, and baked goods. Again, it's not that whole grains are without nutritional value, but grains and flours are known

---

THE SKINNY ON FERMENTED FOODS

Fermented foods have gained a great deal of attention in recent years because of their fantastic health benefits. They are a wonderful source of probiotics and great healing foods for an unhealthy gut.

If you want to reincorporate fermented foods into your diet after the Whole Body Cure Plan concludes, treat each food as you did the rest by testing it individually for 3 days. Start with sauerkraut and kimchi, and if you like, move on to miso to see if you can tolerate soy. Save your final tests for yogurt and kefir as dairy tends to give people more trouble. If you have no problems with any of these foods, feel free to enjoy them all, including the fermented soy products natto and tempeh and the fermented tea drink kombucha.

to raise inflammation levels. Grains and grain-based flour products can increase intestinal permeability (leaky gut), as well, which further drives up inflammation. Finally, eliminating grains automatically avoids any sensitivity to gluten, which increases inflammation.

Sugar and Sugar Substitutes

Sugar and sugar substitutes (artificial sweeteners) are notorious inflammation promoters, not to mention that highly processed sugar substitutes are synthetic products with zero nutritional value. So you'll be eliminating sugar, raw and organic included, as well as synthetic sugar substitutes while following the program. Though don't forget that dark chocolate (70 percent cacao or greater) is allowed once you complete the elimination-diet phase.

In the meantime, if you find that you just can't live without a bit of sweetness in your coffee or tea, you may use small amounts of local honey or stevia. Raw, local honey may improve allergy symptoms, so a teaspoon in your tea is fine. And stevia, unlike some of the other sugar substitutes that are purely synthetic, is made from an herb. This South American plant has been used for thousands of years as a sweetener. The plant's leaves are 200 to 300 times sweeter than sugar but contain no carbohydrates or calories. Do, however, proceed with caution: Too much pure stevia can be bitter, so many companies cut it with less healthful sweeteners or with cellulose powder. Avoid brands that list dextrose or cellulose on the package. Instead, reach for pure stevia powder or liquid. A pinch is all you'll need, and if you continue with an anti-inflammatory manner of eating, you may find that your taste buds change and you no longer need any sweetener.

Highly Processed Foods

Your body will love you if you eliminate prepackaged, highly processed foods not just during the eating plan but permanently. Certainly some packaged foods are better than others—just to cite one example, compare a box of organic vegetable broth with canned broth. In the former you'll find whole, real foods straight out of the garden, such as organic celery, onion, carrots, mushrooms, garlic, and herbs. Meanwhile, canned vegetable broth will serve up hydrolyzed vegetable protein (soy, corn, wheat), monosodium glutamate (MSG), hydrolyzed whey protein, wheat bran protein, dextrose, autolyzed yeast protein, hydrochloride, disodium inosinate, and disodium guanylate, not to mention the harmful BPA found on the inner lining of the can. So while you're following the plan (and, we hope, forever after!), stick with fresh, whole foods. This is the most reliable way to get the biggest inflammation-lowering impact, and you're sure to treat yourself to a wider range of those healthy phenolic compounds that come from fruits and vegetables. Eliminating highly processed packaged foods automatically eliminates all or most of our last category, too.

MSG and All Chemicals

Simply put, this plan encourages you to eliminate all chemical additives. MSG, aspartame, food colorings, preservatives, taste enhancers, thickeners, and any other additives are not allowed on the Whole Body Cure Plan. Fortunately, if you're eating whole, real foods, you've automatically eliminated these lab-engineered "ingredients" that not only drive up inflammation but also have the potential to cause a wide range of unwanted symptoms and reactions.

Remember—You Are What You Eat

You now have the basic blueprint for how you should eat for the rest of your life! One of the beauties of the Whole Body Cure Eating Plan is that it empowers each person to determine the optimal way of eating and staying healthy based on *individual* needs. Food sensitivities vary widely from person to person, as do their symptoms. Taking the time to eat according to *your* body's needs will transform the way you feel, and it will give you the very best chance of staying healthy and energetic for the long term—all while treating yourself to foods that are as healthy as they are delicious.

Recipes

Strawberry Shake

PREP TIME: 5 MINUTES ● TOTAL TIME: 5 MINUTES

1½ cups frozen strawberries

1 cup red chard (optional)

1 cup water

2 scoops vanilla protein powder

¼ avocado, cubed

In a blender, combine the strawberries, greens, water, protein powder, and avocado. Blend until smooth.

SERVES: 1

Very Berry Shake

PREP TIME: 5 MINUTES ● TOTAL TIME: 5 MINUTES

½ cup frozen strawberries

½ cup frozen raspberries

¼ cup frozen blueberries

1 cup beet greens or red chard (optional)

1 cup almond milk or water

2 scoops vanilla protein powder

1 tablespoon almond butter

In a blender, combine the berries, greens, milk or water, protein powder, and almond butter. Blend until smooth.

SERVES: 1

Peach-Raspberry Shake

PREP TIME: 5 MINUTES • TOTAL TIME: 5 MINUTES

½ cup frozen peaches

½ cup frozen raspberries

1 cup beet greens or chard (optional)

1 cup water

¼ avocado, cubed

2 scoops vanilla protein powder

In a blender, combine the peaches, raspberries, greens, water, avocado, and protein powder. Blend until smooth.

SERVES: 1

Chocolate-Cherry Shake

PREP TIME: 5 MINUTES • TOTAL TIME: 5 MINUTES

1 cup ice water

½ cup frozen cherries

2 scoops chocolate protein powder

In a blender, combine the water, cherries, and protein powder. Blend until smooth.

SERVES: 1

Tropical Shake

- 1 cup ice water
- ½ cup fresh or frozen pineapple
- ½ cup fresh or frozen mango
- ¼ cup fresh or frozen peaches
- ¼ avocado, cubed
- 2 scoops vanilla protein powder

In a blender, combine the ice, pineapple, mango, peaches, avocado, and protein powder. Blend until smooth.

SERVES: 1

Neapolitan Shake

- 1½ cups frozen strawberries
- 1 cup water
- 1 scoop vanilla protein powder
- 1 scoop chocolate protein powder
- ¼ avocado, cubed

In a blender, combine the strawberries, water, protein powders, and avocado. Blend until smooth.

SERVES: 1

Mocha Shake

  1 cup ice water

  ¼ avocado, cubed

  2 scoops chocolate protein powder

  ⅛ teaspoon coffee granules

   Pinch of cinnamon (optional)

In a blender, combine the ice, avocado, protein powder, coffee, and cinnamon, if desired. Blend until smooth.

SERVES: 1

Spring Salad with Asparagus and Radishes

PREP TIME: 10 MINUTES • TOTAL TIME: 10 MINUTES

¼ cup extra-virgin olive oil

2 tablespoons sherry vinegar or wine vinegar

¼ teaspoon sea salt

8 cups mixed greens

1 pound asparagus, trimmed and cut into 2" pieces

5 radishes, sliced

1 tablespoon chopped fresh mint (optional)

In a large bowl, whisk together the oil, vinegar, and salt. Add the greens, asparagus, and radishes and toss to combine. Sprinkle with the mint, if desired, just before serving.

SERVES: 8

Spinach and Fennel Salad

PREP TIME: 15 MINUTES ● TOTAL TIME: 15 MINUTES

2 tablespoons extra-virgin olive oil

2 tablespoons white or red wine vinegar

2 teaspoons Dijon mustard

1 bulb fennel

1 small red onion

1 bag (5–6 ounces) baby spinach

1. In a large bowl, whisk together the oil, vinegar, and mustard.

2. In a food processor with the slicing blade or with a mandoline, thinly slice the fennel and onion. (If you'd prefer, use a knife and cut into very thin slices.) Add to the vinaigrette and toss to coat well.

3. Divide the spinach among 4 plates. Top with the fennel mixture.

SERVES: 4

Fennel and Beet Salad

PREP TIME: 15 MINUTES ● TOTAL TIME: 15 MINUTES

    2 tablespoons extra-virgin olive oil
    2 tablespoons balsamic vinegar
    ½ teaspoon Dijon mustard
    1 bulb fennel
    1 beet, peeled
    2 bags (5–6 ounces each) mixed greens
    2 oranges, sectioned

1. In a medium bowl, whisk together the oil, vinegar, and mustard.

2. In a food processor with the slicing blade or with a mandoline, thinly slice the fennel. (If you'd prefer, use a knife and cut into very thin slices.) Change the blade of the food processor to a shredding blade. Shred the beet. Add the fennel slices and shredded beet to the vinaigrette and toss to coat well.

3. Divide the greens among 4 plates. Top with the fennel and beet mixture and orange sections.

SERVES: 4

Anti-Inflammation Slaw

PREP TIME: 10 MINUTES • TOTAL TIME: 10 MINUTES

2 large stalks broccoli, shredded
(reserve the florets for another use)

½ small red cabbage, shredded

2 carrots, shredded

1 recipe Avocado Salad Dressing (page 249)
or Roasted Garlic Dressing (page 250)

In a large bowl, toss together the broccoli, cabbage, carrots, and half the dressing. Toss to coat well, adding more dressing if needed.

Note: To save time, look for preshredded broccoli among the bagged salads in your grocer's produce section.

SERVES: 4

Creamy Caesar Dip

PREP TIME: 10 MINUTES ● TOTAL TIME: 10 MINUTES

5 cups cauliflower florets

1 tablespoon anchovy paste or fish sauce

1 tablespoon fresh lemon juice

1 clove garlic

½ teaspoon Dijon mustard

1 teaspoon extra-virgin olive oil

Carrot, celery, and cucumber spears

1. Place a steamer basket in a medium saucepan with 1" of water. Bring to a boil over high heat. Steam the cauliflower in the basket for 15 minutes, covered, or until very tender. Remove from the heat and let cool.

2. In a food processor, combine the cauliflower, anchovy paste or fish sauce, lemon juice, garlic, and mustard. Process until smooth. Transfer the mixture to a small serving bowl and drizzle with the oil. Serve with the carrot, celery, and cucumber spears.

SERVES: 8

Balsamic Vinaigrette

PREP TIME: 10 MINUTES • TOTAL TIME: 10 MINUTES

 2 tablespoons balsamic vinegar

¼ to ½ teaspoon Dijon mustard

 ½ teaspoon dried herb such as basil, tarragon, or dill

 ½ teaspoon sea salt

 ¼ teaspoon ground black pepper

 2 tablespoons extra-virgin olive oil

 2 tablespoons flaxseed oil

In a jar with a lid, combine the vinegar, mustard, herb, salt, and pepper. Seal and shake to blend. Add the oils, seal, and shake until well-blended.

Note: This can be made with ¼ cup (4 tablespoons) olive oil if desired. Using fresh herbs instead of dried is a delicious option—use ½ to 1 tablespoon minced fresh herbs of your choice.

SERVES: 8

Avocado Salad Dressing

PREP TIME: 5 MINUTES • TOTAL TIME: 5 MINUTES

 1 avocado, chopped

 ½ teaspoon sea salt

 ¼ teaspoon cracked black pepper

 3 tablespoons apple cider vinegar

 2 tablespoons lemon fish oil, or 2 tablespoons
   olive oil and 1 tablespoon lemon juice

1. In a medium bowl, mash the avocado, salt, and pepper with a fork until completely smooth. Add the vinegar and oil and stir until completely blended.

2. Store in an airtight container for up to 5 days.

Note: This can be prepared in a food processor for a very smooth consistency.

SERVES: 4

Roasted Garlic Dressing

PREP TIME: 10 MINUTES ● TOTAL TIME: 1 HOUR 15 MINUTES

1 large bulb garlic

1 tablespoon + ¼ cup extra-virgin olive oil

2 tablespoons apple cider vinegar

½ teaspoon sea salt

¼ teaspoon ground black pepper

1. Preheat the oven to 400°F.

2. Cut the top ½" of the garlic skin from the top of the bulb. Place in the center of a piece of foil and drizzle with 1 tablespoon of the oil. Wrap the foil around the garlic and seal. Bake for 55 minutes, or until browned and very soft. Let cool for 10 minutes.

3. Squeeze the garlic cloves from the skins into a blender or small food processor. Add the vinegar, salt, and pepper and pulse until smooth. With the machine running, gradually add the remaining ¼ cup oil until a creamy dressing develops.

SERVES: 4–6

Creamy Broccoli Soup

PREP TIME: 5 MINUTES ● TOTAL TIME: 50 MINUTES

2 bunches broccoli

1 tablespoon olive oil

1 large onion, chopped

3 ribs celery, chopped

2 cloves garlic, smashed

2 cups vegetable broth

½ can (13.5 ounces) coconut milk

   Sea salt and pepper to taste (optional)

1. Trim the broccoli stalks just to the lowest woody section and discard. Cut florets off the top of the stems and reserve. Chop the remaining stalks.

2. Heat the oil in a large saucepan over medium-high heat. Cook the onion, celery, garlic, and chopped broccoli stalks for 10 minutes, stirring occasionally, or until browned. Add the broth and bring to a simmer.

3. Reduce the heat to low, cover, and simmer for 30 minutes or until the vegetables are very tender. Remove to a blender or food processor, working in batches if necessary, and puree until smooth. (Or, you may use an immersion blender to puree the soup.)

4. Return the soup to the pan along with the coconut milk and reserved broccoli florets. Simmer for 5 minutes, stirring occasionally, or until broccoli is tender.

Note: For a change of pace, you may make this with a large bunch of asparagus. Cut off and reserve the tip and chop the stems.

SERVES: 4

Butternut Squash Soup

PREP TIME: 5 MINUTES • TOTAL TIME: 50 MINUTES

1 butternut squash

2 tablespoons olive oil

1 large onion, chopped

2 ribs celery, chopped

2 carrots, chopped

1 box (32 ounces) vegetable broth

1. Preheat the oven to 350°F. Pierce the squash several times and place on a baking sheet. Bake for 50 minutes or until very tender when pierced with a fork. Remove to a cutting board. Let cool 10 minutes. Cut in half, and remove and discard the seeds.

2. Meanwhile, heat the oil in a large saucepan over medium-high heat. Cook the onion, celery, and carrots, stirring, for 10 minutes or until lightly browned. Add the broth and bring to a simmer.

3. Reduce the heat to low, cover, and simmer for 30 minutes or until the vegetables are very tender. Scoop the butternut squash from the shell and add to the vegetable mixture.

4. Remove to a blender or food processor, working in batches if necessary, and puree until smooth. (Or, you may use an immersion blender to puree the soup.) Return to the pan and cook for 3 minutes or until heated through.

SERVES: 4

Spring Artichoke Sauté

PREP TIME: 15 MINUTES • TOTAL TIME: 30 MINUTES

2 tablespoons extra-virgin olive oil

1 large red onion, cut into thin wedges

½ teaspoon dried thyme

2 cups baby carrots, halved lengthwise

1 bunch asparagus, cut into 2" pieces

1 package (9–12 ounces) frozen artichoke hearts, thawed

3 tablespoons water

½ teaspoon sea salt

Juice of 1 lemon (optional)

In a large skillet, heat the oil over medium heat. Cook the onion and thyme, stirring, for 5 minutes, or until softened. Add the carrots and asparagus and cook for 2 minutes. Add the artichokes, water, and salt. Simmer, stirring occasionally, for 5 minutes, or until the vegetables are crisp-tender. Sprinkle with the lemon juice, if desired.

SERVES: 4–6

Garlicky Asparagus

PREP TIME: 10 MINUTES • TOTAL TIME: 15 MINUTES

1 tablespoon extra-virgin olive oil

5 cloves garlic, minced

1 pound asparagus, trimmed

½ teaspoon sea salt

¼ teaspoon ground black pepper

In a large skillet, heat the oil over medium-high heat. Cook the garlic for 1 minute, or until lightly browned. Add the asparagus and cook for 5 minutes, or until crisp-tender. Sprinkle with the salt and pepper.

SERVES: 4

Roasted Green Beans

PREP TIME: 5 MINUTES • TOTAL TIME: 30 MINUTES

1 pound green beans

1 large red onion, cut into wedges

2 cloves garlic, minced (optional)

2 tablespoons olive oil

½ teaspoon sea salt

½ teaspoon dried oregano

1. Preheat the oven to 450°F.

2. Place the beans and onion on a rimmed baking sheet. Sprinkle with the garlic (if desired), oil, salt, and oregano and toss to coat.

3. Bake for 25 minutes, turning occasionally, or until browned.

SERVES: 4

Roasted Vegetables

PREP TIME: 10 MINUTES ● TOTAL TIME: 1 HOUR

2 cups Brussels sprouts, halved

2 cups baby carrots

2 cups peeled, sliced parsnips

2 tablespoons extra-virgin olive oil

2 cloves garlic, minced

1 teaspoon dried Italian seasoning

½ teaspoon sea salt

1. Preheat the oven to 400°F.

2. Place the Brussels sprouts, carrots, and parsnips on a rimmed baking sheet. Sprinkle with the oil, garlic, seasoning, and salt and toss to coat.

3. Bake for 45 to 50 minutes, turning occasionally, or until the vegetables are browned.

SERVES: 4

Roasted Cauliflower in Red Wine Vinaigrette

PREP TIME: 10 MINUTES ● TOTAL TIME: 35 MINUTES

2½ tablespoons extra-virgin olive oil, divided

5 cups cauliflower florets

1½ tablespoons sherry vinegar or red wine vinegar

1 teaspoon minced garlic

½ teaspoon Dijon mustard

3 tablespoons chopped fresh parsley

1. Preheat the oven to 450°F.

2. Place the florets in a single layer on a rimmed baking sheet. Toss the florets with 1 tablespoon oil. Roast, stirring once, for 25 minutes, or until golden brown.

3. In a small bowl, whisk together the vinegar, garlic, mustard, and the remaining 1½ tablespoons of the oil. Stir in the parsley and toss with the florets before serving.

SERVES: 4

Curried Vegetable Sauté

PREP TIME: 15 MINUTES ● TOTAL TIME: 40 MINUTES

2 tablespoons extra-virgin olive oil

1 onion, chopped

1 tablespoon grated fresh ginger

2 teaspoons mild curry powder

1 zucchini, chopped

2 carrots, chopped

1 red bell pepper, chopped

½ teaspoon sea salt

1. In a large skillet, heat the oil over medium heat. Cook the onion, stirring occasionally, for 5 minutes, or until softened. Add the ginger and curry powder. Cook, stirring frequently, for 5 minutes, or until the onion is golden.

2. Add the zucchini, carrots, pepper, and salt. Cover and reduce the heat to medium-low. Cook for 15 minutes, or until the vegetables are tender.

SERVES: 4

Spaghetti Squash
with Basil Pesto

PREP TIME: 10 MINUTES ● **TOTAL TIME: 50 MINUTES**

　1　spaghetti squash, halved and seeded

　1　teaspoon + 2 tablespoons extra-virgin olive oil

1¼　cups packed fresh basil

　1　clove garlic

　¼　teaspoon sea salt

1. Preheat the oven to 450°F. Coat a baking sheet with cooking spray.

2. Brush the spaghetti squash with 1 teaspoon of the oil and place cut side down on the baking sheet. Roast for 40 minutes, or until fork-tender. Let stand for 15 minutes, or until cool enough to handle.

3. Meanwhile, in a food processor, combine the basil, garlic, salt, and the remaining 2 tablespoons oil. Process, stopping the machine once or twice to scrape down the sides, until pureed. (Stir in 2 or 3 tablespoons of warm water if a creamier texture is desired.)

4. Use a fork to scrape the strands of squash crosswise from the inside of the skin. Place in a large bowl and toss with the pesto.

Note: Any leftovers will make a delicious lunch served cold or at room temperature.

SERVES: 4

Moroccan Veggie "Noodles"

PREP TIME: 10 MINUTES ● **TOTAL TIME:** 45 MINUTES

1 spaghetti squash, halved and seeded

1 teaspoon + 2 tablespoons extra-virgin olive oil, divided

¼ cup fresh lemon juice

1 clove garlic, minced

1 teaspoon ground cumin

3 large carrots, shredded

½ cup chopped fresh cilantro

1. Preheat the oven to 450°F. Coat a baking sheet with cooking spray.

2. Brush the spaghetti squash with 1 teaspoon of the oil and place cut side down on the baking sheet. Roast for 40 minutes, or until fork-tender. Let stand for 15 minutes, or until cool enough to handle.

3. Meanwhile, in a large bowl, whisk together the lemon juice, remaining 2 table-spoons of oil, garlic, and cumin until well blended. Use a fork to scrape the spaghetti squash into the bowl. Add the carrots and cilantro. Toss to coat well. Serve immediately or chill to serve later.

SERVES: 4

Spaghetti Squash with Salsa

PREP TIME: 20 MINUTES • TOTAL TIME: 1 HOUR 10 MINUTES

1 spaghetti squash, halved lengthwise

3 teaspoons olive oil, divided

10 plum tomatoes, chopped

¼ cup chopped fresh basil

¼ cup chopped fresh parsley

3 cloves garlic, minced

1 tablespoon lime juice

1 teaspoon + 1 tablespoon olive oil

¼ teaspoon sea salt

¼ teaspoon ground black pepper

1. Preheat the oven to 450°F. Coat a baking sheet with cooking spray.

2. Brush the spaghetti squash with 1 teaspoon of the oil and place cut side down on the baking sheet. Roast for 40 minutes, or until fork-tender. Let stand for 15 minutes, or until cool enough to handle.

3. Using a fork, separate the squash into strands and transfer to a large bowl.

4. Meanwhile in a food processor, combine the tomatoes, basil, parsley, garlic, lime juice, remaining 1 tablespoon of oil, salt, and pepper. Process until combined but slightly chunky. Pour over the squash and toss to coat.

Note: Feel free to substitute prepared salsa if desired.

SERVES: 4

Zucchini Noodles with Pesto

PREP TIME: 15 MINUTES ● TOTAL TIME: 15 MINUTES

2 cups packed fresh basil leaves

2 tablespoons almonds

1 clove garlic

1 teaspoon fresh lemon juice

¼ cup olive oil

2 zucchini, spiralized
  (or 6 cups precut zucchini noodles)

1. In a food processor or blender, combine the basil, almonds, garlic, and lemon juice. Pulse to finely chop. With the machine running, slowly drizzle in the oil until a thick paste forms.

2. Transfer the mixture to a large bowl (add more lemon juice if desired). Add the zucchini noodles and toss to coat.

SERVES: 4

Vegetable Chips

2 large vegetables such as zucchini,
beets, parsnips, or carrots

1 tablespoon olive oil

¼ teaspoon sea salt

¼ teaspoon ground black pepper

1. Preheat the oven to 400°F. Coat 2 baking sheets with cooking spray.

2. Thinly slice the vegetables on the diagonal, about ⅛" thick (or use a mandoline). In a large bowl, toss the slices with the oil, salt, and pepper. Arrange in a single layer on the baking sheets.

3. Bake, turning once, for 25 minutes. Reduce the oven temperature to 300°F and bake for 10 to 15 minutes, or until lightly brown and crisp. Remove to paper towels and cool.

SERVES: 4

Creamy Mashed Cauliflower

PREP TIME: 5 MINUTES • TOTAL TIME: 30 MINUTES

1 head cauliflower, cut into florets

1 tablespoon olive oil

½ teaspoon sea salt

¼ teaspoon ground black pepper

1. Place a steamer basket in a large saucepan with 2" of water. Place the cauliflower in the basket. Cover and bring to a boil over high heat. Reduce the heat to medium-low and simmer for 25 minutes, or until tender. Place the cauliflower in a medium serving bowl.

2. Add the oil, salt, and pepper. With a potato masher, mash until well blended and of desired consistency.

Note: A large steamer or pasta pot works well for cooking the cauliflower instead of a saucepan. For a creamier mash, use an immersion blender or food processor to mash.

SERVES: 4

Italian-Style Spinach

PREP TIME: 5 MINUTES • TOTAL TIME: 10 MINUTES

¼ cup extra-virgin olive oil

4 cloves garlic, thinly sliced

⅛ teaspoon red-pepper flakes

3 bags (5–6 ounces each) spinach

¼ teaspoon sea salt

1. In a large skillet, heat the oil over medium-high heat. Cook the garlic and red-pepper flakes, stirring occasionally, for 1 minute, or until the garlic is lightly browned.

2. Add half the spinach and cook, tossing, for 1 minute until wilted. Add the remaining spinach, sprinkle with the salt, and cook, turning, for 2 minutes, or until wilted and hot.

SERVES: 4

Zucchini, Tomato, and Basil Toss

PREP TIME: 5 MINUTES • TOTAL TIME: 15 MINUTES

- 1 tablespoon extra-virgin olive oil
- 1 zucchini, halved lengthwise and cut into ½" slices
- 4 scallions, chopped
- 2 cups grape tomatoes, halved
- ¼ teaspoon sea salt
- 2 tablespoons chopped fresh basil

1. In a large skillet, heat the oil over medium heat. Cook the zucchini and scallions for 5 minutes, or until they begin to soften.

2. Add the tomatoes and salt. Cook, partially covered, for 3 minutes, or until the vegetables are lightly browned. Stir in the basil just before serving.

SERVES: 2–4

Zucchini and Squash with Fresh Mint

PREP TIME: 5 MINUTES • TOTAL TIME: 10 MINUTES

- 1 tablespoon extra-virgin olive oil
- 1½ pounds small zucchini and yellow squash, chopped
- ½ teaspoon sea salt
- 1 tablespoon fresh lime juice
- ¼ cup chopped fresh mint (optional)

In a large skillet, heat the oil over medium-high heat. Cook the zucchini and squash for 5 minutes, or until lightly browned. Sprinkle with the salt and lime juice. Toss with the mint, if desired, just before serving.

SERVES: 4

Grilled Steak with Avocado

PREP TIME: 10 MINUTES ● TOTAL TIME: 40 MINUTES

1 tablespoon ground cumin

½ teaspoon + ⅛ teaspoon sea salt

½ teaspoon ground red pepper

1 lime, halved

1 pound flank steak

2 cloves garlic, crushed

1 ripe avocado, cubed

½ cup salsa verde

1 scallion, sliced

2 tablespoons chopped fresh cilantro

1. In a small bowl, combine the cumin, ½ teaspoon of the salt, and the pepper.

2. Squeeze half of the lime over one side of the steak and rub with half the garlic. Sprinkle half of the spice mixture over the steak. Turn the steak and repeat with the remaining lime half, garlic, and spice mixture. Let stand 15 minutes at room temperature.

3. Preheat the grill to medium-high or heat a grill pan over medium-high heat.

4. Grill the steak for 8 minutes for medium-rare, turning once, or until a meat thermometer inserted in the center reaches 145°F. Transfer to a cutting board and let stand for 5 minutes.

5. In a medium bowl, combine the avocado, salsa verde, scallion, cilantro, and the remaining ⅛ teaspoon salt. Cut the steak into thin strips. Serve topped with the avocado mixture.

SERVES: 4

Mediterranean Beef Stew

PREP TIME: 15 MINUTES ● TOTAL TIME: 1 HOUR 5 MINUTES

2 teaspoons extra-virgin olive oil

1½ pounds beef top round steak, cut into ¾" strips

4 cloves garlic, minced

3 onions, cut into thin wedges

2 green bell peppers, chopped

1 pound cremini or button mushrooms, sliced

1 teaspoon ground allspice

¼ teaspoon ground black pepper

3 cups beef broth

1 can (6 ounces) tomato paste

4 tablespoons red wine vinegar

1. In a large stock pot or Dutch oven over medium-high heat, heat the oil. Cook the beef and garlic, turning the beef occasionally, for 10 minutes, or until browned.

2. Add the onions, bell peppers, mushrooms, allspice, and black pepper and cook for 10 minutes, stirring occasionally, or until the vegetables soften. Stir in the broth, tomato paste, and vinegar. Bring to a boil, reduce the heat to low, cover, and simmer for 30 minutes, or until the meat is fork-tender.

SERVES: 8

Beef and Vegetable Roast

PREP TIME: 10 MINUTES   ●   TOTAL TIME: 1 HOUR 40 MINUTES

4 pounds beef rib-eye roast

3 tablespoons extra-virgin olive oil, divided

4 cloves garlic, finely chopped, divided

3 teaspoons dried or 1½ tablespoons minced
  fresh rosemary, divided

1 teaspoon sea salt, divided

½ teaspoon ground black pepper

1 pound turnips, chopped into 1" pieces

1 bag (1 pound) baby carrots

1 head cauliflower, cut into florets

1. Preheat the oven to 350°F. Coat a large shallow roasting pan with cooking spray.

2. Place the beef in the pan and rub with 1 tablespoon of the oil, half of the garlic, and 2 teaspoons of the rosemary. Sprinkle with ½ teaspoon of the salt and the pepper.

3. In a large bowl, combine the turnips, carrots, and cauliflower with the remaining 2 tablespoons oil, garlic, 1 teaspoon rosemary, and ½ teaspoon salt. Spread the vegetables in a single layer around the roast.

4. Roast the beef and vegetables for 1 hour to 1 hour and 30 minutes, or until a thermometer inserted in the center of the roast registers 145°F for medium-rare/160°F for medium/165°F for well-done. Let the roast stand for 10 minutes before slicing.

SERVES: 8

Burgers with Caramelized Onion

PREP TIME: 20 MINUTES • TOTAL TIME: 45 MINUTES

1 pound lean ground beef

½ teaspoon smoked paprika

½ teaspoon sea salt

½ teaspoon ground black pepper

2 tablespoons olive oil

1 large red onion, sliced

2 tablespoons balsamic or apple cider vinegar

8 leaves butter lettuce

1. In a medium bowl, combine the beef, paprika, salt, and pepper. Shape into 4 burgers. Place on a plate, cover, and chill while preparing the remaining ingredients.

2. In a large skillet, heat the oil over medium heat. Cook the onion, stirring, for 5 minutes, or until browned. Reduce the heat to low, cover, and cook for 10 minutes, or until very soft. Increase the heat to medium-high and stir in the vinegar. Cook for 2 minutes.

3. Preheat the grill to medium-high or heat a grill pan over medium-high heat.

4. Grill the burgers for 5 minutes, turning once, or until a thermometer inserted in the center registers 145°F for medium-rare/160°F for medium/165°F for well-done. Place 1 lettuce leaf each on 4 plates. Top each with a burger and the onion mixture. Place the remaining lettuce leaves on top to use as a roll.

SERVES: 4

Thai Beef Lettuce Wraps

PREP TIME: 10 MINUTES • TOTAL TIME: 25 MINUTES

12 ounces flank, skirt, or sirloin steak

¼ teaspoon sea salt

2 limes

2 tablespoons fish sauce

1 tablespoon sriracha sauce

1 head Bibb lettuce, leaves separated

1 carrot, grated

½ red onion, thinly sliced

½ cup chopped fresh cilantro

1 jalapeño pepper, thinly sliced
    (wear plastic gloves when handling)

1. Preheat grill to medium-high or heat a grill pan over medium-high heat. Season the steak on both sides with the salt. Cook for 8 minutes, turning once, or until a thermometer inserted in the center registers 145°F for medium-rare/160°F for medium/165°F for well-done. Remove from the heat and let stand for 5 minutes.

2. In a small saucepan over low heat, cook the juice of 1 lime, fish sauce, and sriracha for 1 minute or until heated through. Slice the steak thinly against the grain and drizzle half of the warm sauce over it.

3. Arrange the beef, lettuce leaves, carrot, onion, cilantro, pepper, the remaining lime cut into wedges, and the remaining sauce on a serving platter. Use the leaves like tortillas, wrap up the steak slices and top with the vegetables as desired.

SERVES: 3

Grilled Beef and Arugula Salad

2 tablespoons + 1 teaspoon extra-virgin olive oil

2 tablespoons raspberry vinegar

1 scallion, thinly sliced

½ teaspoon sea salt, divided

¼ teaspoon ground black pepper, divided

4 ripe apricots, halved

4 2¾"-thick filet mignons (4 ounces each)

1 bag (5 ounces) baby arugula or spinach

1. Preheat the grill to medium-high or heat a grill pan over medium heat.

2. In a large bowl, whisk 2 tablespoons of the oil, the vinegar, scallion, ¼ teaspoon of the salt, and ⅛ teaspoon of the pepper and set aside.

3. Brush the cut surface of the apricots with the remaining 1 teaspoon oil. Season the beef with the remaining ¼ teaspoon salt and ⅛ teaspoon pepper. Grill the beef and apricots, cut side down. Cook the apricots for 6 minutes, or until soft. Cook the beef for 8 minutes or until a thermometer inserted in the center registers 145°F for medium-rare/160°F for medium/165°F for well-done, turning once.

4. Let stand for 5 minutes. Cut the apricots into slices. Thinly slice the beef against the grain.

5. Add the arugula or spinach to the reserved dressing and toss to coat. Transfer to 4 serving plates. Top with the beef and apricot slices.

SERVES: 4

Roasted Squash Salad with Poached Eggs

PREP TIME: 20 MINUTES ● TOTAL TIME: 1 HOUR 30 MINUTES

2 tablespoons olive oil

1 delicata squash, halved, seeded, and thinly sliced

½ teaspoon sea salt

4 ounces mixed greens

4 tablespoons Balsamic Vinaigrette (page 249)

4 eggs

4 tablespoons hazelnuts, toasted and chopped

1. Preheat the oven to 425°F. Coat a baking sheet with cooking spray and drizzle with the oil.

2. Place the squash in a single layer on the baking sheet. Sprinkle with the salt, toss to combine, and roast, turning once, for 25 minutes, or until browned and tender.

3. Divide the greens and squash between 2 plates and drizzle each with 2 table-spoons of the vinaigrette.

4. Bring a large skillet with 1½" of water to a bare simmer over medium-high heat. Working quickly, crack the eggs into a saucer, one at a time, and slide into the barely simmering water. Cook for 4 minutes, or until the egg white is opaque. Remove the eggs with a slotted spoon and pat dry with a paper towel. Place 2 eggs on the greens of each plate. Sprinkle with the hazelnuts before serving.

SERVES: 2

Egg Salad "Sandwich"

PREP TIME: 10 MINUTES ● **TOTAL TIME:** 10 MINUTES

4 peeled hard-cooked eggs

2 ribs celery, finely chopped

2 small carrots, finely chopped

¼ small red onion, minced (optional)

3 tablespoons Roasted Garlic Dressing (page 250)

4 leaves Bibb or romaine lettuce

1. In a medium bowl, mash the eggs with a fork. Add the celery, carrots, onion, and dressing and stir to blend.

2. Divide the lettuce between 2 plates and place one-quarter of the egg salad into each lettuce leaf. Roll to eat.

SERVES: 2

Grilled Jerk Chicken with Pineapple and Red Pepper

PREP TIME: 10 MINUTES • TOTAL TIME: 20 MINUTES

- 2 tablespoons extra-virgin olive oil, divided
- 1 red bell pepper, quartered
- 4 thick, fresh pineapple slices
- ¼ teaspoon sea salt
- 1 tablespoon jerk seasoning
- 4 boneless, skinless chicken thighs

1. Preheat the grill to medium-high or heat a grill pan over medium-high heat.

2. In a large bowl, combine 1 tablespoon of the oil, the pepper, and the pineapple. Sprinkle with the salt and toss to coat. Transfer to a platter.

3. In the same bowl, combine the jerk seasoning and the remaining 1 tablespoon oil. Add the chicken and toss to coat. Grill the chicken, pepper, and pineapple for 10 minutes, turning once, or until a thermometer inserted in the thickest section of the chicken registers 165°F.

SERVES: 4

Roasted Spiced Chicken and Vegetables

PREP TIME: 15 MINUTES • TOTAL TIME: 35 MINUTES

1 clove garlic, minced

1 teaspoon ground cumin

1 teaspoon grated fresh ginger

1 teaspoon sea salt, divided

4 boneless, skinless chicken breast halves

1 red onion, sliced

1 small eggplant, cut into ¼"-thick slices

1 zucchini, cut lengthwise into ¼"-thick slices

¾ pound mini sweet peppers

1 tablespoon olive oil

1. Preheat the oven to 400°F. Coat a large rimmed baking sheet with cooking spray.

2. In a small bowl, combine the garlic, cumin, ginger, and ½ teaspoon of the salt. Rub the spice mixture all over the chicken. Place on one side of the baking sheet. Bake for 10 minutes.

3. Meanwhile, in a large bowl, combine the onion, eggplant, zucchini, peppers, oil, and the remaining ½ teaspoon salt. Toss to coat. After 10 minutes of cooking the chicken, add the vegetables to the other side of the baking sheet. Bake for 10 minutes, or until the vegetables are browned and a thermometer inserted in the thickest portion of the chicken registers 165°F.

SERVES: 4

Grilled Chicken with Garlic-Parsley Sauce

PREP TIME: 15 MINUTES ● TOTAL TIME: 30 MINUTES

1 cup loosely packed flat-leaf parsley

3 tablespoons lemon juice

2 tablespoons extra-virgin olive oil

2 tablespoons water

1 tablespoon fresh oregano

1 clove garlic

½ teaspoon sea salt

Pinch of ground red pepper (optional)

4 small boneless, skinless chicken breast halves

1. In a food processor or blender, combine the parsley, lemon juice, oil, water, oregano, garlic, salt, and red pepper, if using. Process until nearly smooth, stopping the machine once or twice to scrape down the sides.

2. Place the chicken in a plate and spoon 3 tablespoons of the garlic-parsley sauce over the chicken. Turn to coat, and let stand while preheating the grill or heating a grill pan over medium-high heat.

3. Grill the chicken, covered, turning once, for 8 minutes, or until lightly browned and a thermometer inserted in the thickest portion registers 165°F and the juices run clear. Serve the remaining sauce with the chicken.

SERVES: 4

Chicken Breasts Stuffed with Spinach and Sun-Dried Tomatoes

PREP TIME: 15 MINUTES ● TOTAL TIME: 30 MINUTES

4 cups boiling water

2 cups spinach, coarsely chopped

4 small boneless, skinless chicken breast halves
   (about 1¼ pounds total)

½ teaspoon sea salt

½ cup chopped oil-packed sun-dried tomatoes

2 tablespoons extra-virgin olive oil

1 tablespoon red wine vinegar

1. In a colander in the sink, pour the boiling water over the spinach to wilt. Drain well.

2. Place the chicken breasts between 2 sheets of parchment or wax paper and use the bottom of a heavy skillet to pound to ¼" thickness. Sprinkle with the salt.

3. Divide the spinach and tomatoes evenly over the breasts to within ½" of the edges. Roll up each breast from one short end. Fasten with a wooden pick.

4. In a large skillet, heat the oil over medium heat. Cook the chicken, turning occasionally, for 6 minutes, or until browned on all sides. Cover and cook for 6 minutes, or until a thermometer inserted into the center of a breast registers 165°F and the juices run clear.

5. Transfer the chicken to a platter and cover to keep warm. Add the vinegar to the skillet and cook for 1 minute, scraping up any brown bits from the bottom of the pan. Drizzle over the chicken.

SERVES: 4

Tarragon Chicken Salad

PREP TIME: 15 MINUTES ● TOTAL TIME: 30 MINUTES

1 pound boneless, skinless chicken breasts

2 cups reduced-sodium chicken broth

3 tablespoons Dijon mustard

2 tablespoons white wine vinegar

2 tablespoons extra-virgin olive oil

2 teaspoons dried tarragon

¼ teaspoon sea salt

⅛ teaspoon ground black pepper

1 cup seedless red grapes, halved

½ cup toasted pecans, coarsely chopped

4 leaves lettuce or radicchio

1. In a large saucepan, place the chicken and add the broth to cover. Bring to a boil over high heat. Reduce the heat to low, cover, and simmer for 10 minutes, turning halfway through, or until a thermometer inserted into the center of a breast registers 165°F. Set the chicken aside until cool enough to handle.

2. Meanwhile, in a large bowl, whisk together the mustard, vinegar, oil, tarragon, salt, and pepper.

3. Cut the chicken into 1" cubes and add to the bowl. Then add the grapes and pecans. Toss to mix. Serve on the lettuce or radicchio.

SERVES: 4

Southwestern Chicken Salad

PREP TIME: 15 MINUTES ● TOTAL TIME: 30 MINUTES

2 tablespoons salsa

2 tablespoons olive oil, divided

1 lime, halved and divided

¾ pound boneless, skinless chicken breast,
    cut into ½" pieces

2 teaspoons fajita seasoning

8 cups torn romaine lettuce

1 large tomato, chopped

1 avocado, chopped

2 tablespoons chopped fresh cilantro (optional)

1. In a small bowl, combine the salsa, 1 tablespoon of the oil, and the juice from half a lime. Whisk and set aside.

2. In a large skillet, heat the remaining 1 tablespoon oil over medium heat. Cook the chicken, stirring frequently, for 10 minutes, or until the chicken is no longer pink in the thickest part. Sprinkle with the fajita seasoning and squeeze the juice from the remaining lime half over the chicken. Cook for 1 minute.

3. In a large bowl, toss the warm chicken mixture with the lettuce, tomato, and avocado. Add the reserved salsa dressing and toss to coat. Sprinkle with the cilantro, if desired.

SERVES: 4

Easy Chicken Chili

PREP TIME: 10 MINUTES • TOTAL TIME: 35 MINUTES

1 tablespoon extra-virgin olive oil

2 scallions, thinly sliced, white and green
   parts separated

1 clove garlic, finely chopped

1 teaspoon chili powder

½ teaspoon ground cumin

1 can (14.5 ounces) diced tomatoes, drained

1 cup chicken broth

2 cups shredded cooked chicken breast

1. In a medium saucepan, heat the oil over medium-high heat. Cook the scallions and garlic, stirring, for 1 minute or until golden. Add the chili powder and cumin and cook, stirring, for 1 minute.

2. Add the tomatoes and broth. Simmer for 15 minutes, or until the liquid is slightly reduced. Stir in the chicken and simmer for 5 minutes.

SERVES: 4

Barbecued Chicken and Sweet Potatoes

PREP TIME: 15 MINUTES ● TOTAL TIME: 1 HOUR 10 MINUTES + MARINATING TIME

1 small onion, finely chopped

1 can (8 ounces) tomato sauce

¾ cup water

2 tablespoons red wine vinegar

2 tablespoons Worcestershire sauce

1 tablespoon chili powder

4 small bone-in chicken breast halves, skinned

2 small sweet potatoes

2 tablespoons extra-virgin olive oil

½ teaspoon sea salt

1. In a medium saucepan, bring the onion, tomato sauce, water, vinegar, Worcestershire sauce, and chili powder to a boil over high heat. Reduce the heat to low and simmer, uncovered, for 15 minutes, or until thickened. Remove from the heat and let cool for 20 minutes.

2. Place the chicken in a resealable plastic bag with ⅔ cup of the sauce. Seal and shake to coat. Refrigerate for 1 to 8 hours along with the remaining sauce.

3. Just before grilling or broiling, halve the potatoes lengthwise. Cut each half into 3 wedges. In a large bowl, place the potato wedges and drizzle with the oil and salt. Toss to coat.

4. Preheat the grill or broiler.

5. Remove the chicken from the marinade and place on the grill rack or broiler pan. Discard the marinade. Grill or broil for 20 minutes, or until a thermometer inserted in the thickest portion registers 165°F and the juices run clear. Place the potatoes on the edges of the grill or roasting pan during the last 15 minutes of cooking the chicken, turning once.

SERVES: 4

Lemon Turkey

PREP TIME: 5 MINUTES • TOTAL TIME: 20 MINUTES

8 ounces turkey cutlet

2 tablespoons fresh lemon juice

1 tablespoon extra-virgin olive oil

$\frac{1}{2}$ teaspoon dried oregano

$\frac{1}{4}$ teaspoon sea salt

1. Preheat the oven to 375°F. Coat a small baking dish with cooking spray.

2. Place the turkey in a single layer in the dish. Drizzle with the lemon juice and oil. Sprinkle with the oregano and salt.

3. Bake for 15 minutes, or until no longer pink.

SERVES: 2

Tuna-Stuffed Endive

PREP TIME: 10 MINUTES • TOTAL TIME: 10 MINUTES

  2 cans (6 ounces each) water-packed
     wild light tuna, drained and flaked

  1 rib celery, finely chopped

¼ cup chopped red onion

¼ cup chopped fresh cilantro

  2 tablespoons fresh lime juice

¼ teaspoon ground black pepper

  2 tablespoons extra-virgin olive oil

15 Belgian endive leaves (about 2 heads)

In a medium bowl, combine the tuna, celery, onion, cilantro, lime juice, and pepper. Stir in the oil. Divide the tuna mixture evenly among the endive leaves.

SERVES: 3

Herb-Crusted Salmon

PREP TIME: 5 MINUTES • TOTAL TIME: 25 MINUTES

¼ cup chopped herb, such as parsley,
   basil, or cilantro

3 cloves garlic, minced

1 tablespoon olive oil

½ teaspoon sea salt

1 wild salmon fillet

1. Preheat the oven to 425°F. Line a baking sheet with foil or parchment paper.

2. In a small bowl, combine the herb, garlic, oil, and salt.

3. Place the fillet on the baking sheet and spread the herb mixture over the fillet.
Bake for 15 minutes, or until opaque.

SERVES: 4–6

Mustard Cod with Roasted Vegetables

PREP TIME: 20 MINUTES ● TOTAL TIME: 1 HOUR

2 cups baby carrots

2 cups broccoli florets

1 package (8 ounces) sliced mushrooms

1 large onion, cut into wedges

2 tablespoons extra-virgin olive oil

½ teaspoon sea salt

½ teaspoon ground black pepper

1 pound cod fillets, fresh or frozen and thawed

2 teaspoons Dijon mustard

1. Preheat the oven to 425°F. Coat 2 rimmed baking sheets with cooking spray.

2. Combine the carrots, broccoli, mushrooms, and onion on 1 baking sheet. Toss with the oil, and sprinkle with the salt and pepper. Bake for 20 minutes.

3. Place the cod on the remaining baking sheet. Spread the mustard evenly over the fish. Add to the oven with the vegetables and bake for 10 minutes, or until the fish flakes easily and the vegetables are browned and tender.

SERVES: 4

Warm Shrimp Salad

PREP TIME: 5 MINUTES • TOTAL TIME: 10 MINUTES

2 tablespoons olive oil

1 clove garlic, minced

1 pound peeled and deveined shrimp

1 cup grape tomatoes, halved

1 tablespoon white wine vinegar

1 teaspoon grated orange peel

½ teaspoon sea salt

1 bag (5 ounces) baby arugula, spinach, or mixed greens

1. In a large skillet, heat the oil over medium heat. Cook the garlic and shrimp for 2 minutes, stirring. Add the tomatoes, vinegar, orange peel, and salt and cook for 2 minutes, or until the shrimp is opaque.

2. In a large bowl, place the arugula, spinach, or greens. Top with the shrimp mixture, and toss to coat.

SERVES: 4

Seared Scallops

2 tablespoons olive oil

1 pound wild sea scallops

$\frac{1}{4}$ teaspoon sea salt

$\frac{1}{4}$ teaspoon cracked black pepper

1 tablespoon lemon juice

1 tablespoon chopped fresh flat-leaf parsley (optional)

1. In a large skillet, heat the oil over medium-high heat. On a plate, toss the scallops with the salt and pepper. Cook the scallops for 5 minutes, turning once, or until opaque. Remove the scallops to a plate.

2. Add the lemon juice and parsley, if using, to the skillet and cook for 1 minute, stirring to break up the brown bits. Pour the sauce over the scallops.

SERVES: 4

Lamb Kabobs with Mushrooms and Tomatoes

PREP TIME: 15 MINUTES • TOTAL TIME: 25 MINUTES
+ MARINATING TIME

- 2 tablespoons gluten-free soy sauce
  (Bragg Liquid Aminos is a good option)
- 1 teaspoon sesame oil
- 1 clove garlic, minced
- 1 teaspoon grated fresh or $\frac{1}{2}$ teaspoon
  ground ginger
- $1\frac{1}{2}$ pounds lamb cubes
- 16 cherry tomatoes
- 16 small mushrooms

1. In a large bowl, combine the soy sauce, oil, garlic, and ginger. Add the lamb, tomatoes, and mushrooms, tossing to coat. Cover and refrigerate for up to 12 hours, tossing once or twice.

2. Preheat the grill to medium-high or heat a grill pan over medium-high heat.

3. Thread the lamb, tomatoes, and mushrooms onto metal skewers. Grill for 10 minutes, turning to brown all sides, or until the meat is pink.

SERVES: 4

Lamb Burgers with Tomato

PREP TIME: 10 MINUTES • TOTAL TIME: 25 MINUTES

1½ pounds ground lamb

2 cloves garlic, minced

1 teaspoon dried thyme

½ teaspoon sea salt

½ teaspoon ground black pepper

1 cup canned crushed tomatoes

1. In a large bowl, combine the lamb, garlic, thyme, salt, and pepper. Shape into 6 burgers.

2. Heat a large, heavy skillet over medium-high heat until hot. Cook the burgers for 5 minutes, turning once, or until browned. Pour off any fat, reduce the heat to low, and pour the tomatoes around the patties (the tomatoes will boil briefly).

3. Cook for 10 minutes, turning the burgers once, or until a thermometer inserted in the center registers 160°F.

SERVES: 6

Grilled Lamb Chops with Orange Relish

PREP TIME: 15 MINUTES ● TOTAL TIME: 25 MINUTES

3 navel oranges, peeled and coarsely chopped

3 tablespoons finely chopped red onion

2 tablespoons chopped fresh basil

½ teaspoon sea salt, divided

8 bone-in loin lamb chops (4 ounces each)

¼ teaspoon ground black pepper

1. Preheat the grill to medium-high or heat a grill pan over medium-high heat.

2. In a large bowl, combine the oranges, onion, basil, and ¼ teaspoon of the salt. Set aside.

3. Sprinkle the lamb chops with the pepper and remaining ¼ teaspoon salt. Grill the chops for 8 minutes, turning once, or until browned and a thermometer inserted in the center registers 145°F for medium-rare. Serve with the orange relish.

SERVES: 4

NUT RECIPES

Enjoy nutritious nuts in many ways, including:

- Eat out of hand for snack.
- Toss in salads.
- Sprinkle over stir-fries.
- Finely chop and press into chicken or turkey breasts before baking.
- Add raw cashew butter (no sugar) to shakes.
- Add to curries or chili.

Toasted Nuts

PREP TIME: 5 MINUTES • TOTAL TIME: 15 MINUTES

1 pound raw organic nuts such as almonds, cashews, or walnuts

1. Preheat the oven to 300°F.

2. Spread the nuts on a rimmed baking sheet. Bake for 5 minutes. Remove and shake the baking sheet to turn the nuts. Continue baking the nuts, checking every 2 minutes, until browned.

Note: Don't walk away from the nuts—they can go from not browned to burnt very quickly.

SERVES: 16

Curried Cashews

PREP TIME: 15 MINUTES • TOTAL TIME: 15 MINUTES

1 tablespoon olive oil

1 teaspoon curry powder

1 cup raw cashews, almonds, walnuts, or pecans

Pinch of sea salt

1. Preheat the oven to 400°F.

2. In a small saucepan, cook the oil and curry powder over medium-low heat, for 1 minute. Stir in the cashews and cook for 1 minute. Spread on a rimmed baking sheet. Sprinkle with the salt.

3. Bake for 5 minutes. Remove and shake the baking sheet to turn the nuts. Continue baking the nuts, checking every 2 minutes, until browned.

SERVES: 4

Citrus Ice

PREP TIME: 15 MINUTES ● TOTAL TIME: 15 MINUTES + FREEZING TIME

Juice of 8 oranges

Juice of ½ lime

Pinch of sea salt

3 tablespoons honey

1. In a large measuring cup, combine the orange and lime juices. Add enough water to equal 4 cups. Stir in the salt and honey until the honey dissolves.

2. Pour into a 9" x 9" metal pan (not nonstick). Cover with plastic wrap and freeze for 1 hour. Stir with a fork, breaking up the chunks. Cover and return to the freezer. Stir every 30 minutes for 2 hours or until the mixture is evenly icy and granular. Spoon into dessert bowls.

SERVES: 4

Baked Peaches with Blueberries

PREP TIME: 15 MINUTES • TOTAL TIME: 15 MINUTES + FREEZING TIME

2 firm peaches, halved and pitted

1 tablespoon lemon juice

4 teaspoons maple sugar or brown sugar

1 tablespoon grass-fed butter, cut into 4 cubes

2 cups fresh blueberries

Juice of ½ lime

⅛ teaspoon ground cinnamon

¼ cup plain 2% Greek yogurt

1. Preheat the oven to 350°F.

2. Place the peaches in an 8" x 8" baking dish and sprinkle with the lemon juice. Top each half with 1 teaspoon of maple syrup and 1 cube of the butter. Bake for 1 hour or until tender and browned. Let cool.

3. Meanwhile, in a medium saucepan over medium heat, cook the blueberries, lime juice, and cinnamon for 5 minutes or until the berries release their juices and begin to soften. Let cool.

4. Divide the blueberries among 4 dessert plates and set 1 peach half on top of each. Top with 1 tablespoon of yogurt.

SERVES: 4

Chocolate Pistachio Bark

PREP TIME: 10 MINUTES ● TOTAL TIME: 10 MINUTES + COOLING TIME

16 ounces dark chocolate (60 percent cacao or higher), coarsely chopped

½ cup toasted pistachios (see page 290), chopped

½ teaspoon fine sea salt (optional)

1. Line a large rimmed baking sheet with parchment paper.

2. Place the chocolate in a microwave-safe glass bowl. Microwave on medium power for 5 minutes, stirring every 30 seconds, or just until melted and smooth. Stir in the pistachios.

3. Spread the mixture about ¼" thick on the baking sheet. Sprinkle with the salt, if using. Let the chocolate cool for 1 to 1½ hours or until very firm. Break into 16 pieces.

SERVES: 16

Chocolate Fondue

PREP TIME: 5 MINUTES ● TOTAL TIME: 10 MINUTES

4 ounces dark chocolate

¼ teaspoon almond extract

2 apples, sliced

2 oranges, sectioned

1. Place the chocolate in a microwave-safe glass bowl. Microwave on medium power for 3 minutes, stirring every 30 seconds, until smooth. Stir in the almond extract.

2. Serve the fruit with the chocolate.

SERVES: 4

CHAPTER 12

A Healthy Way to Tame the Flame

Exercising to Break the Cycle of Chronic Inflammation

When it comes to exercise and inflammation, the best strategy is to avoid the extremes. On one end of the spectrum, imagine the person who is always pounding the pavement, pumping iron, chanting the phrase "no pain, no gain" through gritted teeth, and spending her free time engaged in extreme sports. At the other end is the proverbial couch potato who can't remember the last time he's broken a sweat.

What we want to achieve is the happy medium between those two examples. Most doctors recommend that adults get 150 minutes of moderate-intensity aerobic activity per week, which translates to half an hour 5 days a week. Moderate-intensity activity has been defined by public health experts as any activity that burns 3.5 to 7 calories per minute. The classic example is walking a mile at a 15- to 20-minute pace. Other examples are bicycling on level ground, water aerobics, using a rowing machine, or ballroom dancing.

Whatever form of exercise you choose, finding a good middle ground is the key when it comes to keeping inflammation in check. It is normal to have some postexercise muscle soreness and mild inflammation; in fact, these are signs that you're achieving a sufficient level of muscle fatigue, but numerous studies have observed that extreme exercise can be incredibly taxing on the body. In one study, researchers compared the incidence of upper respiratory infections in three different groups: elite athletes, recreationally competitive athletes, and sedentary controls. The highest rates of infection over a 5-month period occurred in the elite athletes, followed by the sedentary folks.[1] Athletes also face a higher risk of developing osteoarthritis than the general population because they put more wear and tear on their joints and face greater susceptibility to injury—it's estimated that up to 50 percent of people who suffer ligament injuries or meniscus tears will have painful, debilitating osteoarthritis 10 to 20 years later.[2] And of course, overexertion causes inflammation—locally at the sites of joints, muscles, and any injuries, as well as systemically. Overtraining syndrome is a recognized clinical diagnosis that occurs when a person exercises excessively without adequate rest in between workouts. Symptoms can include fatigue, depression, slow heart rate, lack of appetite, disruptions to sleep, and, ironically, decreased athletic performance. What's at the root of all of these symptoms? Chronic inflammation.[3]

Now all this said, the other extreme—a sedentary lifestyle—is even more harmful in the long run. A sedentary lifestyle puts you at greater risk for a huge array of health problems, including some of our nation's top killers—diabetes, heart disease, stroke, and Alzheimer's among them. Further, if you

Dr. Kirshner's Inflammation Insight

For overall brain and body health, try exercises that challenge your balance, such as ones that require a wobble board or fitness ball, or other exercises that use resistance bands, which makes for more complex movements. When you're using muscles required to stay upright on an unbalanced surface, or when you're using complex, nonlinear movements, you're not only strengthening muscle but also activating your cerebellum, which coordinates muscular activity. Exercises that use repetitive motions, such as weight lifting, do not activate the cerebellum to the same degree, and therefore they have less impact on total health.

don't exercise, you're missing out on one of the most effective and all-natural means to beat stress, depression, anxiety, and insomnia—all of which are both causes *and* effects of chronic inflammation. We now also know the many health concerns associated with prolonged periods of sitting, such as a greater risk of being overweight or developing high blood pressure, blood clots, cardiovascular disease, and even cancer. You really do lose all around if you're not engaged in some sort of regular physical activity.

So here's where exercising in moderation comes in. In addition to directly reducing inflammation, regular exercise helps maintain a healthy BMI, lowers LDL cholesterol, boosts HDL cholesterol, lowers blood pressure, alleviates depression, assuages anxiety, and promotes sufficient sleep. Great low-impact exercise options include walking, yoga, Pilates, tai chi, qigong, swimming, and cycling. If you want to up the ante part of the time, there's running, tennis, hiking, dancing, inline skating, higher-intensity workouts such as jumping rope or group fitness classes, and team sports such as volleyball, softball, or basketball.

Yoga is usually the first thing that comes to mind for gentle, low-impact exercise, and for good reason. But because most people are already familiar with yoga, in this chapter we've decided to shift the spotlight to the ancient Chinese practice known as *qigong* (pronounced "chee-gung"), which boasts many well-documented health benefits and is quickly gaining popularity in the West. Our test panel of volunteers practiced qigong throughout the 12 weeks of the anti-inflammatory eating plan. Our qigong expert, Hilary Smith, will show you, step by step, the exact routine that our test panel practiced. But first, some qigong basics.

Qigong: Cultivating Energy through Practice

Qigong was developed nearly 5,000 years ago in China. The word itself is made up of two Chinese words, *qi* + *gong*. *Qi*, which is a variant of the more familiar spelling *chi*, means "life force or energy." Qi, or vital energy, is said to circulate throughout the body as well as everything in the universe. *Gong* is translated as "an accomplishment attained through steady practice." Qigong, then, is a practice for enhancing life force and vitality. One of its literal translations is "life-energy cultivation," and qigong has been described as "meditative movement" and "mindful exercise."

There are many different styles of qigong with different emphases, but we'll be focusing on medical qigong, whose main intent is to restore health and keep the body and mind in a state of wellness. According to traditional Chinese medicine, sickness, pain, and discomfort result when the flow of qi through the body's meridians, or energy channels, is blocked or becomes stagnant. What can block the flow of qi? The answers are legion, but the main culprits involve extremes and irregularities—for example, being too hot or too cold, eating too much or too little, engaging in too much or too little physical activity, and sleeping too much or too little. Other things that can cause qi stagnation are poor posture, injury, illness, toxins, and unresolved extremes in emotion—for example, grief, fear, anger, or resentment.

In the context of Chinese medicine, when qi isn't flowing freely, we may feel stuck, tired, stressed, and sick. Qigong unblocks and increases the flow of qi, our vital energy.

> *Tension is what you think you should be; relaxation is who you are.*
> —Chinese proverb

Along with *tai chi*, another ancient form of meditative movement, qigong is practiced by millions of people around the world. Tai chi may be more familiar to Americans than qigong, and people often wonder about the differences between the two. Some schools of thought consider tai chi to be a form of qigong, but unlike tai chi, qigong is not based in the martial arts. Both tai chi and qigong involve engaging in gentle, flowing movements and deep, diaphragmatic breathing and cultivating a state of calm, focused awareness. Some forms of qigong, including the one featured here, also incorporate visualization, body alignment, and massage.

Qigong's simplicity is one of the main reasons we're including it as part of our whole-body wellness plan. It's much easier to learn than traditional tai chi, which can take many years to master and involves more complex movements. No special equipment or attire is needed—just comfortable clothing that allows you to move freely. It may also be the most adaptable form of exercise around. Qigong can be done standing, sitting, or even lying down, so people of any fitness level and any age can practice it, even those who are ill or are recovering from injury or illness. For instance, a form of qigong that requires less complex movements and balance poses has been used by those with mild traumatic brain injury,[4] and qigong can be adapted for practice by wheelchair users.[5] People with chronic illnesses—including muscular dystrophy, fibromyalgia, heart disease, kidney disease, diabetes, neurological disorders, chronic obstructive pulmonary disease, and cancer—have also successfully practiced qigong and experienced health improvements. On the other end of the spectrum, if you're in good health and already have a dedicated aerobic exercise practice, qigong can be an excellent add-on to increase flexibility and help protect joints from injury.

Hilary Smith is a registered nurse, certified fitness trainer, and a third-degree black belt. She's been studying tai chi and qigong since 1989, and she now teaches tai chi and qigong several times a week to people of widely varying ages and fitness levels. Smith lent her expert guidance to our test panel of volunteers during their qigong practice, which emphasized conscious breathing, holding poses, mental focus, and setting a healthy intention.

"The body is very good at self-healing if you give it the proper environment," Smith points out. "Qigong provides the environment for gentle movement; deep, relaxing breathing; a quiet mind; and focused intention," which supports health "from the inside out by increasing the flow of qi to the organs, muscles, bones, nervous and lymphatic systems, mind, and spirit—to everything that makes you uniquely you."

Eastern medicine asserts that body and mind are not separate, but instead work synergistically, each exerting effects on the other. Therefore, emotional stress has a direct negative effect on physical health, for example. But the converse is true as well: Any positive intervention will have a holistic beneficial effect. "Rather than focusing on, say, the heart or the joints or the brain, qigong is about the universal flow of energy and vitality coursing through the entire body," Smith says. "What benefits strength benefits flexibility benefits stress reduction, and what benefits the immune response benefits mental calmness and clarity, and so on."

The Science behind Qigong

Perhaps it is exactly this holistic, synergistic effect that's responsible for qigong's astonishing diversity of health benefits. Clinical trials and observational studies have demonstrated qigong's ability to reduce stress, lower blood pressure, reduce heart rate, improve heart rate variability, lower lipid levels, reduce BMI, improve respiratory function, promote better balance, increase flexibility, improve immune function, reduce inflammation, decrease chronic pain, decrease anxiety, improve depression, prevent bone loss, improve overall quality of life in healthy and chronically ill people, and even prolong survival in cancer patients.[6] Let's look at some of the latest research, beginning with a condition related to many of the doctor visits in America: stress.

Many studies consistently demonstrate that qigong has a powerful stress-reducing effect. Some people experience relief from anxiety even after one session of qigong, but not surprisingly, the stress-relieving effect is greatest in those who engage in a regular practice. Considering that as many as half of the illnesses in the United States are stress-related,[7] a regular practice of qigong can be an effective means to prevent illness and maintain overall well-being for most people. EEG (electroencephalogram) scans of qigong practitioners have shown increased levels of alpha, beta, and theta brain wave activity, suggesting greater relaxation and attentiveness. Blood tests have shown increased levels of endorphins (neurotransmitters that can induce feelings of euphoria and reduce pain) and reduced inflammatory biomarkers, including CRP, the stress hormone cortisol, and adrenocorticotropic hormone (which regulates cortisol).[8] Qigong has also been shown to be effective in reducing the severity of depressive symptoms.[9]

Qigong has also been proven effective as a method of pain control. In three separate clinical trials, people with osteoarthritis of the knee who practiced qigong experienced reduced pain and improved ease of movement.[10] Other studies have pointed out that qigong can reduce arthritis pain by promoting relaxation and increasing bloodflow to the affected areas. Because improved bloodflow leads to more efficient delivery of oxygen, nutrients, and natural painkillers such as endorphins, pain in the affected area is lessened; improved bloodflow also helps remove metabolic waste products that can contribute to pain.[11] In another study of office workers who use computers most of the day, a half-hour of daily qigong relieved neck pain and disability;[12] a separate study of similar office workers demonstrated qigong's ability to relieve lower-back pain and reduce stress.[13]

Qigong can also be helpful to people living with fibromyalgia, a chronic condition with symptoms that include fatigue, widespread pain, gastrointestinal issues, and sleep disruption. Fibromyalgia can be very difficult to treat, but recent studies have found that a regular qigong practice (daily for 6 to 8 weeks) improved pain, sleep, and overall physical and mental function. Those who continued their practice beyond 8 weeks experienced even greater benefits.[14] For people living with chronic fatigue or chronic fatigue syndrome, a 4-month qigong program was shown to significantly improve fatigue symptoms as well as mental functioning compared to controls. Blood tests also revealed significant improvement in telomerase activity.[15] As you'll recall from our earlier discussion about aging, telomeres are DNA sequences found at the ends of chromosomes; without sufficient telomerase activity, cells prematurely age and die.

Aside from lessening pain, anxiety, and fatigue, there's also strong evidence that qigong can help improve metabolic disorders. Adults with type 2 diabetes who practiced qigong for 12 weeks (60 minutes per week with an instructor plus two 30-minute sessions at home) experienced significant reductions in fasting blood glucose levels. Improved insulin resistance, while not clinically significant, was observed, as well.[16] In another study, 16 weeks of qigong practice was even found to increase flexibility and decrease "subcutaneous adipose accumulation" in healthy adults. Translation? Less belly fat! The 110 subjects in this study ranged in age from 20 to 59, and they practiced qigong three times a week for 30 to 60 minutes.[17] Fat that accumulates at the abdomen is known to be one of the most dangerous forms of fat because it produces proinflammatory cytokines as well as hormones that contribute to insulin resistance.

Qigong has also been shown to lower systolic and diastolic blood pressure,[18] both immediately after a single session[19] and for the long term. In a trial of 88 patients with mild hypertension, half practiced qigong for 16 weeks while half followed a conventional exercise program. *Both* groups experienced significant decreases in blood pressure; heart rate, weight, BMI, waist circumference, and total cholesterol decreased, as well.[20]

Qigong has also been studied extensively as a complementary therapy for cancer patients, where it's been shown to improve fatigue, immune function, and cortisol levels.[21] One study compared 162 people with cancer (predominantly breast and colorectal) to a control group. Those who practiced medical qigong for 10 weeks exhibited significant reductions in fatigue, anxiety, and depression, and they scored an average of 8.23 points higher than the control group on a quality of life test that evaluated physical, social, emotional, and functional well-being. The other notable outcome? The qigong group had significantly lower CRP levels. Exactly why and how qigong had a positive influence on inflammation isn't known, but the researchers of this study point out that one possible explanation is that qigong exerted an overall improvement to the immune system.[22]

There are actually many studies that have examined qigong's effect on inflammation. One study looked at the effects of 12 weeks (3 days per week) of qigong on bone density and a well-known inflammatory cytokine, IL-6, in middle-aged women. Not only did the qigong group experience less bone mineral density loss *and* a substantial decrease (−27 percent) in IL-6 by the close of the study, the control group, who did not practice qigong, experienced an *increase* (+23 percent) in IL-6. Why such a big difference between the experimental and control groups? Researchers speculate that the style of qigong subjects practiced was extremely relaxing and soothing, which decreased inflammation, and that it elevated estrogen, which has an inhibitory effect on IL-6.[23] Another study examined the effect of qigong practiced twice a week for 10 weeks on measures of stress and biomarkers of immunity. After 10 weeks, qigong practitioners showed a significant improvement in scores of anxiety, stress, and depression, as well as an increase in the secretion rate of salivary immunoglobulin A, an immune system antibody. They also exhibited a decrease in salivary cortisol concentrations,[24] indicating a reduction in psychological stress. Once again, we see qigong's synergistic effect at work: Qigong reduces stress, which reduces inflammation, which improves the immune system, which prevents a wide range of illnesses and improves overall health.

Your Qigong Practice

The accompanying DVD is all you'll need to start a qigong practice. However, if you'd like to expand beyond these moves, here's how to get started. One of the first things to do is find an instructor in your area. A good way to start is identifying your goals with qigong and searching for a teacher whose focus aligns with yours. For instance, some teachers emphasize the spiritual component of qigong, while others emphasize its stress-reducing outcomes, while others offer qigong strictly as a form of exercise. Try a few different classes and see which one best addresses your needs.

Also, consider the teacher's experience, not just the number of years she's practiced and taught qigong but also the kind of students with whom she works. Classes at a martial arts school may not be the best fit for older adults, for instance, or for those looking for more of a meditative experience. If you're recovering from an illness or injury, you'll want an instructor who has experience with a variety of medical conditions and who is readily able to adapt positions and movements to your individual needs.

But qigong instructor Hilary Smith points out that finding a teacher with whom you resonate is just as important as the teacher's experience. "Maybe you find someone whose technique isn't so perfect, but they can teach well," she says. "Style is not as important as someone you can learn from." Smith advises that you trust your instincts. You'll know when you find that person who just "clicks."

Once you find a teacher and a class, all you need to do is wear comfortable clothing that allows you to move, and leave your anxieties behind. "Any person can do qigong," Smith says. "Any body size, any level of fitness, any age, people who've suffered recent injuries or undergone recent surgeries. If you get tired, you can sit down—follow your own body's cues. Qigong is highly adaptable, and in general, you'll find that other students are very supportive and compassionate because they remember what it was like to be a beginner. It's also important to remember that everyone is still learning. If they knew how to do everything, they wouldn't have come to class."

How often should you practice? Ideally, every day! "Qigong is a very powerful practice that works its magic only by doing it," Smith says. "In a perfect world, we'd all practice every day and at the times when certain meridians are most active—the transition times of dawn and dusk are classic times to practice, for instance. But what I tell people is that whenever you can do it is the right time to practice—whatever works into your world with the least amount of stress. Practice without feeling like it's troublesome; otherwise it's defeating the purpose. It should feel like a respite from your to-do list, not another thing on it."

Smith recommends aiming for 20 minutes of practice on most days. "A consistent practice can cause changes that some practitioners consider miraculous," she says. "Others feel subtler changes, but beneficial ones nonetheless. I've found that a well-rounded practice can keep the body strong but relaxed and the mind sharp but calm."

Now, what if there are no qigong classes in your area? Plenty of books and online resources explain the philosophy of qigong and provide some basic instructions. Luckily for you, the DVD that accompanies this book gives you Smith teaching the qigong sequence she designed for our test panel. Starting on page 305, you'll find photographs and her step-by-step instructions for each move on the DVD.

From the Expert: Qigong Instructor Hilary Smith

To practice on your own at home, first find a quiet space where you won't be distracted or interrupted. Some people relax more readily with music; others prefer silence.

A very important consideration is to bring your mind into your body and listen closely to what you feel. Is your body saying "yes" to a certain technique, or is it saying "no way"? Follow your body's cues, and modify movements so you stay comfortable. For example, you might need a smaller range of motion or fewer repetitions.

Then, check your alignment. The feet are generally parallel, with the weight evenly distributed across the front and back and the inside and outside of the foot. The toes are spread, and the arches of the feet drawn up. Feel that you are standing *in* the ground, not on the ground. The knees are always softly bent—never locked. The pelvis is level, the ribs are drawn in and up, and the shoulders are wide and down. The head is floating upward, with the chin kept level. The tailbone feels heavy, and the head, light. The upper arm bone is rooted into the shoulder girdle. All the joints feel spacious—and if they don't, visualize them that way. This posture is called "natural stance."

Now bring your attention to your breath. Allow it to be deep and rhythmical, filling your lungs from the bottom to the top, and emptying them from the top to the bottom. Deepen each breath and be certain the exhalation is complete. As you exhale, think *let go*. Let go of what? Listen to your body! Perhaps you can let go of tension in your shoulders or in your jaw or forehead. Maybe there is some gripping in your hips or thighs that can be released. How about your mind? Are there thoughts, worries, or regrets you can exhale out? As you let go with each exhalation, you'll feel a little lighter, a little softer, and you'll give the qi an opportunity to flow with more ease. If you notice body parts that are uncomfortable or tight, use your mind to encourage the flow of breath and qi to them. Visualize them softening, melting, releasing.

Now we're ready to begin. Practice slowly and mindfully, and visualize that you are moving through water so the movements are not tense or limp, but alive. Each movement is the length of a slow breath.

Dawn Awakening

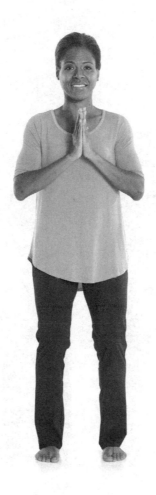

Start in a natural stance, with feet hip distance apart and knees slightly bent, toes pointing forward; ribs back and up, shoulders down, eyes gazing forward open or lightly closed. With hands in prayer position by your heart. Hands press together lightly, elbows droop, weight roots down. Breathe slowly and deeply, allowing the body to soften and the mind to become clear.

Awash In Sunshine

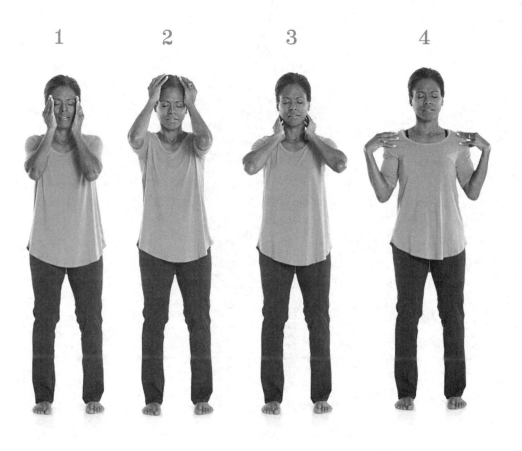

1   2   3   4

1 Rub the hands together, generating warmth and energy.
2 Place your hands to your face, as if gently washing, visualizing a cleansing, fresh start. 3 Continue by combing your fingertips over your scalp, 4 then gently drawing the hands

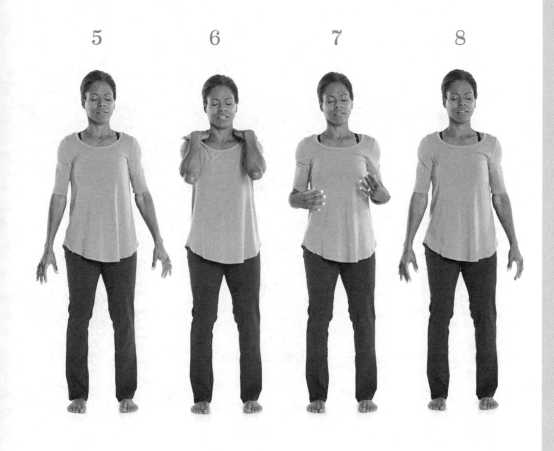

down the side of the neck, **5** visualizing pulling tension out of
the neck and shoulders and **6** releasing it, letting the arm drop.
7 **8** Bring fingertips behind shoulders and draw forward,
pulling tension out of the shoulders and release arms down.

Bringing in the Light

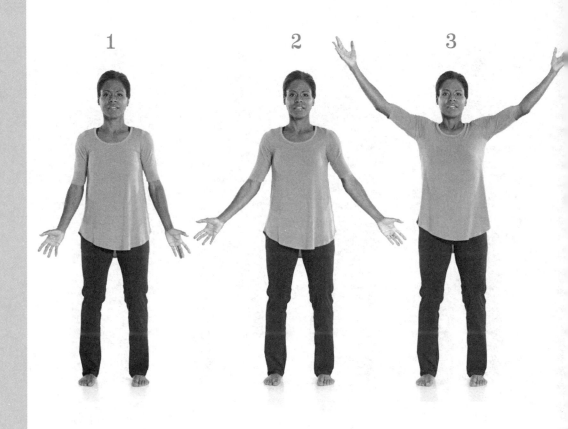

1   2   3

① Come back to natural stance with knees bent, arms by your sides. ② Roll the arms palms out. ③ Then open them out to the sides, ④ lift them overhead. ⑤ Bring the palms together overhead and ⑥ while knees drop bring the arms down in front of the body to prayer hands in front of the heart.

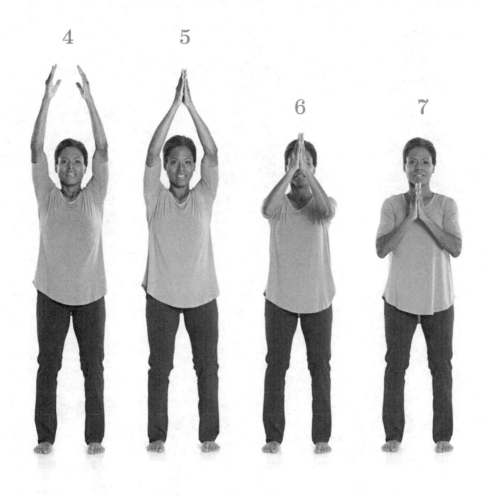

4   5

6   7

7 Bend and straighten the knees as much as comfortable—or
go from more deeply bent to slightly bent. Inhale as the arms
rise; knees bend and exhale as the arms descend to prayer
hands. (Complete 6 times.)

Gathering Earth's Bounty and Heaven's Magic

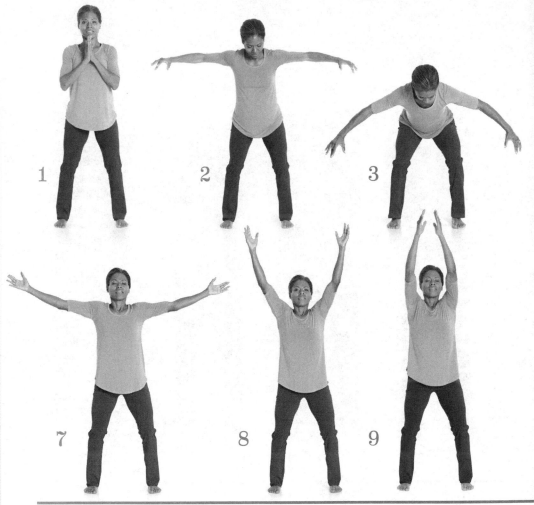

1 Start in natural stance. **2** Bend forward at hips and knees, arms spread wide, and **3** **4** gather energy from the earth. **5** Standing up, return to prayer hands. **6** Arms then reach open out to sides; looking up slightly, **7** **8** bring your arms overhead, **9** gathering energy from the heavens and **10** **11**

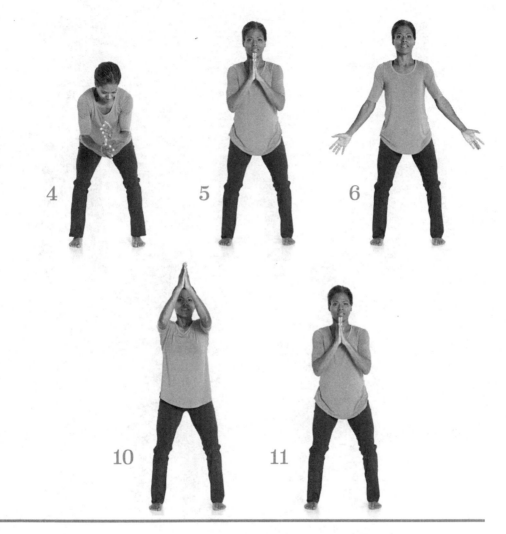

bringing it into the heart in prayer hands. Knees rise and inhale while gathering; lower and exhale while coming to prayer hands. Only bend forward as far as is comfortable. (Complete 3 to 6 times.)

Note: If you've been told by your doctor to avoid your head going lower than your heart, only go down to an appropriate level.

Moving into Openness

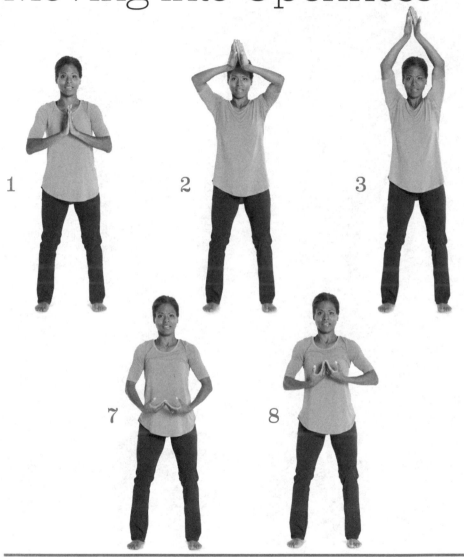

1 4 From prayer hands, 2 the arms start to rise up the midline of the body. 3 Arms roll so palms face out and the backs of the hands touch. 4 5 From overhead, 6 fingertips and elbows curve down to the sides, palms down, and then coil palms up and fingertips touch in front of the lower abdomen.

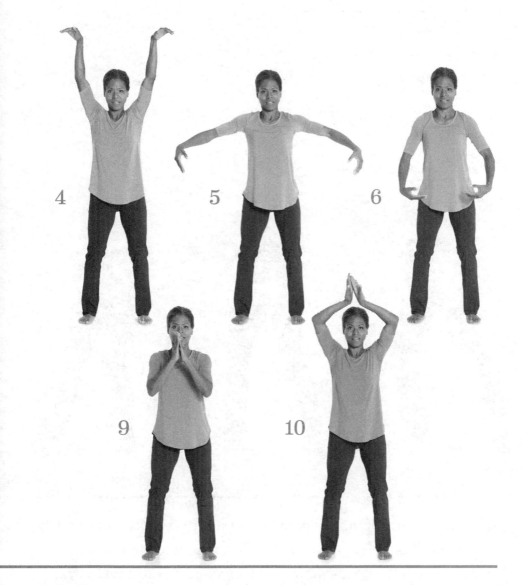

7 8 The hands rise up the midline with the backs of the hands touching, and 9 then roll to palms touching in prayer hands in front of the heart. 10 Knees rise and inhale while arms come up; knees bend and exhale while the arms descend. (Complete 6 times.)

Embracing Qi

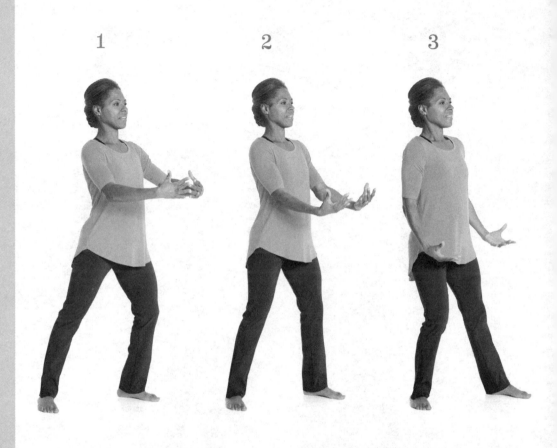

1   2   3

1 From natural stance, step one foot back about 12 inches and turn it out about 30 to 45 degrees. The arms are rounded in front, about waist height, as if hugging your favorite person. **2** Shift your weight back to the rear leg, the hands turn fingertips up and drop back along the sides of the body. **3** The arms open widely to the sides and come forward as the weight comes forward, rotating the hands to return to the hugging position. Point your fingertips up and as you shift your weight to the rear

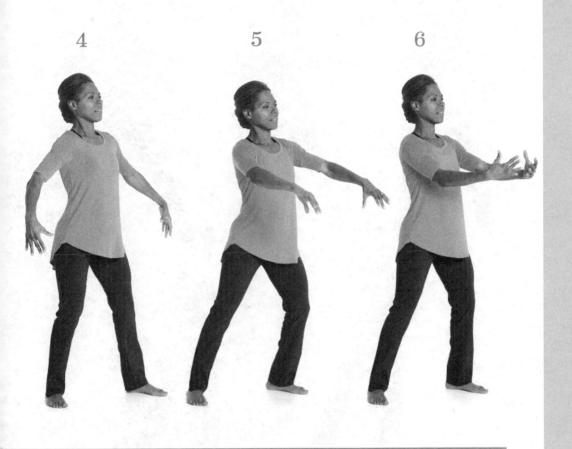

4   5   6

leg slowly ④ drop your hands back along the sides of the body.
The arms open widely to the sides and ⑤ come forward as the
weight comes forward, ⑥ rotating the hands to starting position with thumbs up. Inhale as the weight shifts back; and arms
move back; exhale as the weight comes forward. Be mindful
that the knee stays over the toe. Change legs and repeat. (Complete 3 to 6 times each side.)

Wind in the Willows

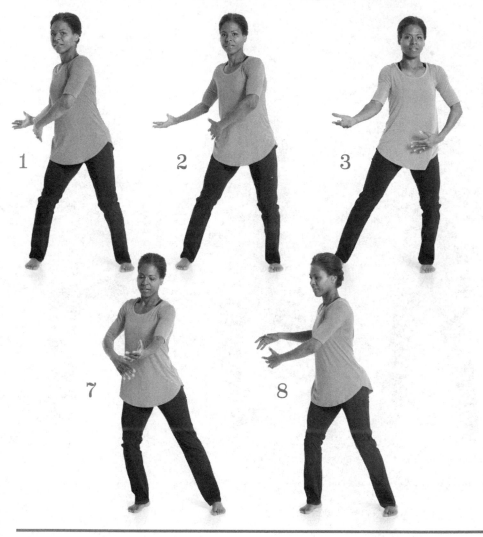

1   2   3

7   8

1 Starting in the natural stance, shift your weight to the right leg. Bring your right arm waist height, palm up, behind you. Keep your left palm facing inwards in front of the lower abdomen. 2 3 Weight shifts to the left with the arms following the body. 4 5 Switch arms so the left hand is behind, palm up, and the right hand in front, palm in, and shift

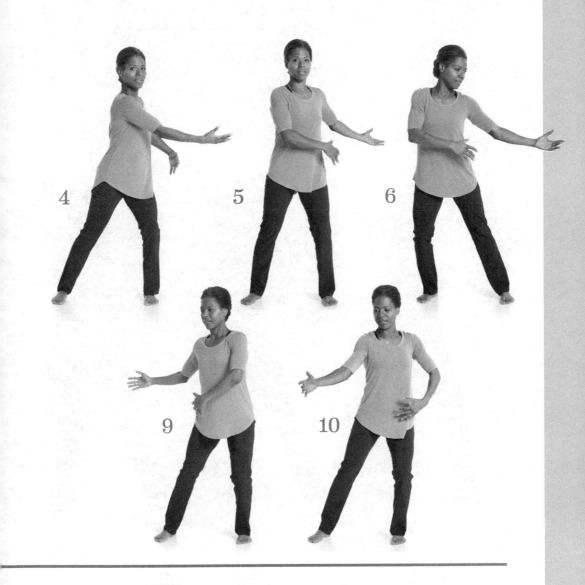

4   5   6

9   10

to the right. (6-10) Shift weight side to side, arms following similar to the feeling of moving through water as the arms change position. Inhale as the arm reaches in front; exhale while it returns. Feel as if the hip helps move the arms. (Complete 6 times.)

Rocking for Tranquility

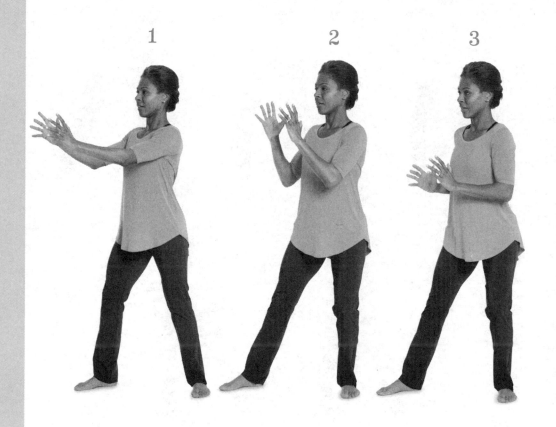

1   2   3

① From the natural stance, step one foot forward and turn it out at an angle. Bring the weight to the forward leg. The hands are in front of the abdomen, fingertips up, palms facing each other about 6" apart. **②** **③** Shifting the weight to the rear leg, draw hands in toward the heart. **④** Shift the weight to the

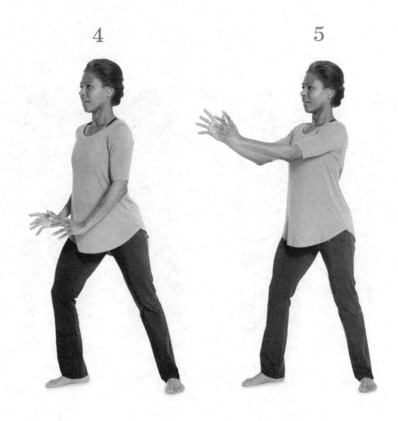

4   5

front leg and return to the starting position ⑤. Palms stay facing each other the whole time. Inhale as the weight shifts back; exhale as the weight comes forward. Keep the movements slow and enjoy the feeling of rocking! (Complete 3 to 6 times each side.)

Flowing Like Water

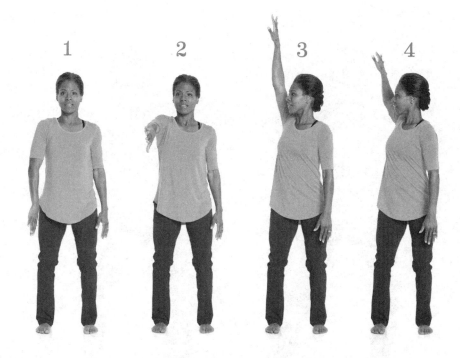

1   2   3   4

1 From natural stance with knees bent, rotate the right arm so the pinkie side of the hand is facing upward and the palm, away from the body. **2** Bring the arm forward, overhead, behind and down, and then forward. Rotate the arm as needed so the pinkie is always leading. **3** Keeping your shoulder down, **4** follow the arm with your eyes, bringing a

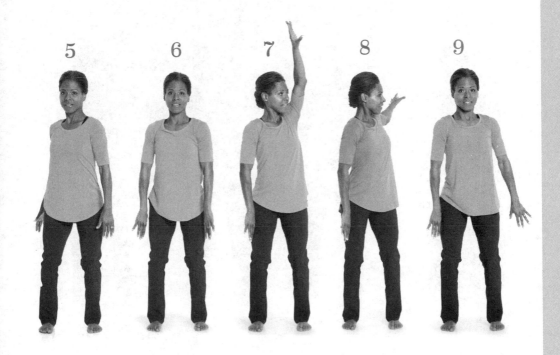

5   6   7   8   9

gentle twist into the body. As the arm comes up and back the knees rise and inhale; as it comes down and forward, the knees bend and exhale. ⑤ Bringing the palm around the back facing the body. ⑥ Twist the arm to face the palm back. (Complete 3 to 6 times right side. Repeat on left side.)

Taking Flight

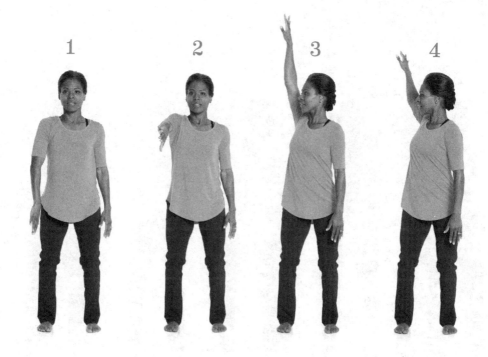

This move is the same as Flowing Like Water, but instead of completing the right arm before moving to the left, you will be alternating arms. ❶ From natural stance with knees bent, rotate the right arm so the pinkie side is forward. ❷ Bring the arm forward, overhead, behind and down. ❸ Rotate the arm as needed so the pinkie is always leading.

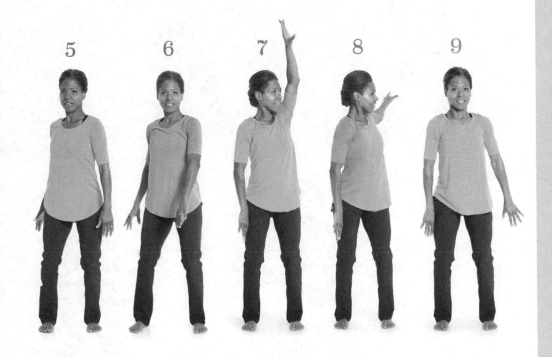

4 **5** Keeping your shoulder down, follow the arm with your eyes, bringing a gentle twist into the body. As the arm comes up and back the knees rise and inhale; as it comes down and forward, the knees bend and exhale. **6-9** Repeat on left side. (Complete 3 to 6 times each side.)

Reaching for the Stars

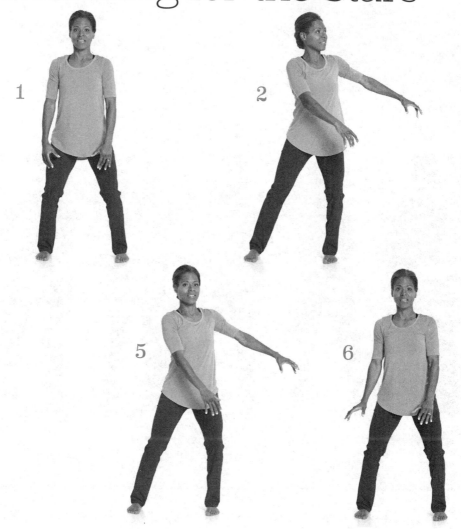

1 From natural stance, 2 shift weight to the left and keeping your shoulders back and down, 3 4 reach both arms up to the left. 5 6 As you shift your weight toward the right and draw both hands down to the middle of the lower abdomen.

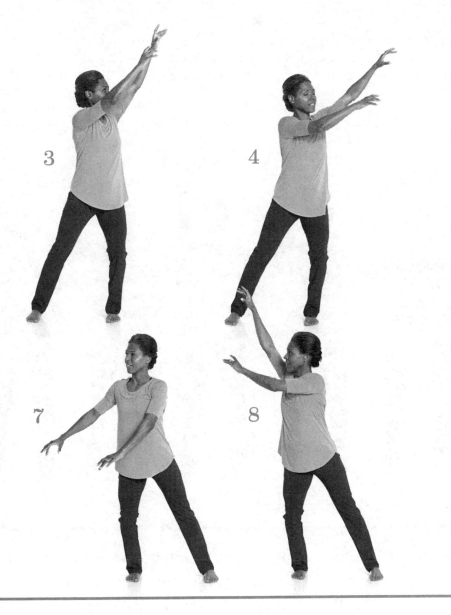

7 Shift your weight to the right and **8** reach hands up to the right (remembering to keep your shoulders back and down). Repeat moving side to side. Inhale as arms rise; exhale as they draw down. (Complete 6 times.)

Rooted and Rising

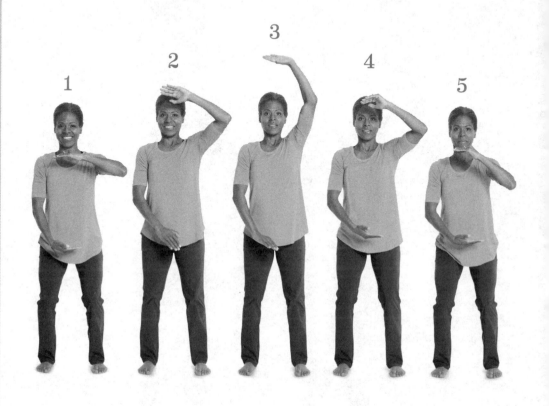

1 2 3 4 5

From natural stance, **1** keeping your elbows soft, move your left arm in front of your chest, palm down, and your right arm in front of the lower abdomen, palm up. Feel as if you're holding a large ball. **2** Turn the palms away from each other. **3** Press the left hand palm up and reach it overhead pressing the right hand palm down toward the earth, keeping the shoulders down. **4** Bring the hands back to the starting

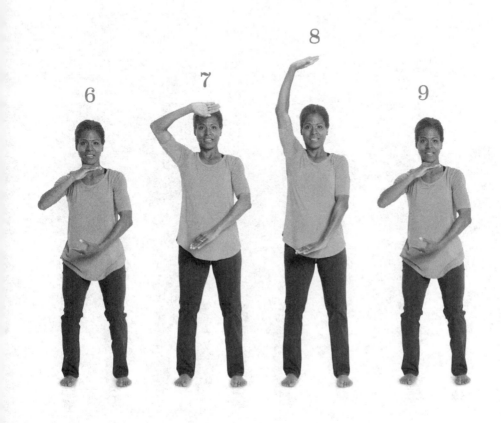

position, ⑤ palms facing each other as if holding a ball. As the hands separate, the knees rise and inhale; as they return to the ball, knees bend and exhale. ⑥ Change to the right palm facing down and the left palm facing up. ⑦ ⑧ Return to starting position ⑨. Be mindful of the arm rising but not the shoulder. You will feel a stretch in the side. (Complete 3 times each side.)

Opening the Pathways

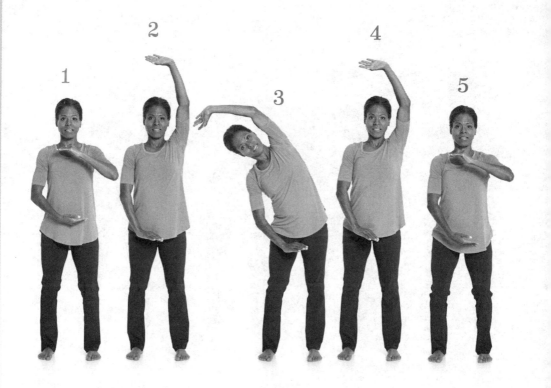

1   2   3   4   5

1 From the Rooted and Rising position (previous pose) with the left hand on top, **2** separate the arms up and down. **3** Bend the right knee and bend the body gently toward the right. **4** Straighten the right knee to return to the upright position, and then bring **5** hands back to the starting position. **6** Start with the right hand on top and **7** separate the

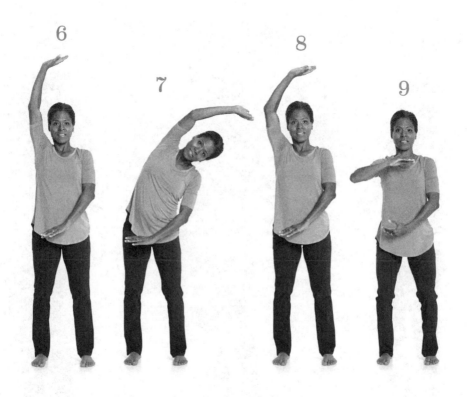

arms up and down. Bend the left knee and bend the body gently toward the left. **8** Straighten the left knee to return to upright, then bring hands **9** back to the starting postion. Inhale as arms separate; exhale as the body bends; inhale as the body straightens; exhale to starting position. Change sides. (Complete 3 times each side.)

Movement in Stillness

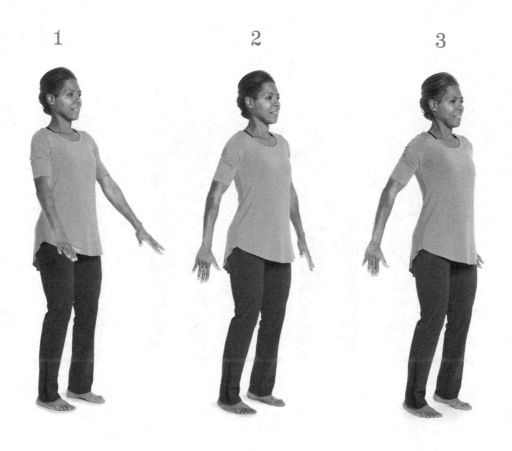

1   2   3

1 From the natural stance, with arms by your sides, **2** **3** shift the weight forward toward the balls of the feet as the palms press back. **4** Shift the weight back toward the heels as the **5** arms rotate and palms press forward. Inhale while

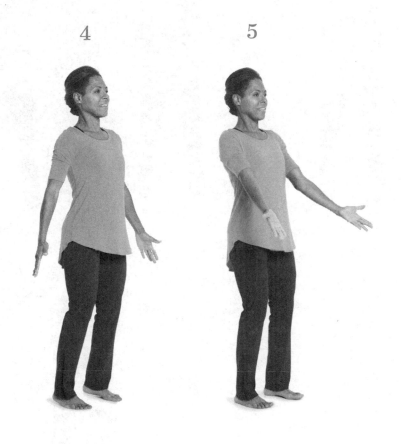

4

5

the weight shifts back; exhale as the weight comes forward
and lift the toes when the weight is back. Knees stay slightly
bent the entire time. (Complete 6 times.)

Cleansing the Organs

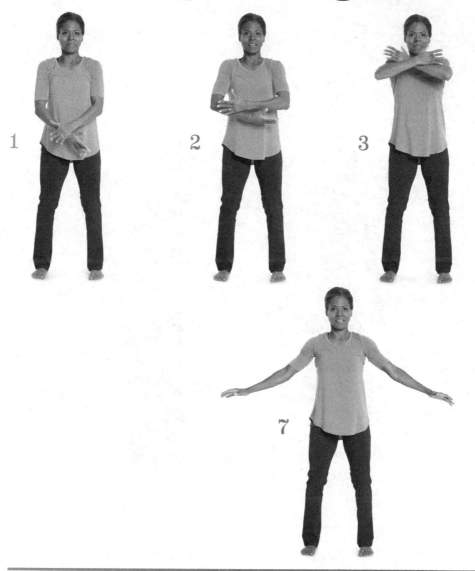

1 From natural stance with the knees bent, the arms cross in front of the lower abdomen 2 3 then rise up the front of the body to overhead, 4 turning the palms up toward the heavens. 5-8 Bring the arms down to the sides,

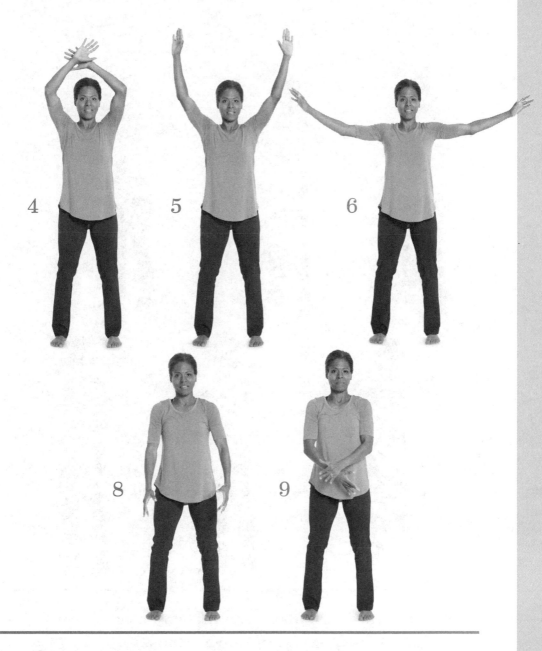

4

5

6

8

9

⑨ returning to the crossed position over the lower abdomen. Knees rise and inhale as the arms rise up the midline; knees bend and exhale as arms come down by the sides. (Complete 6 times.)

Clearing the Space

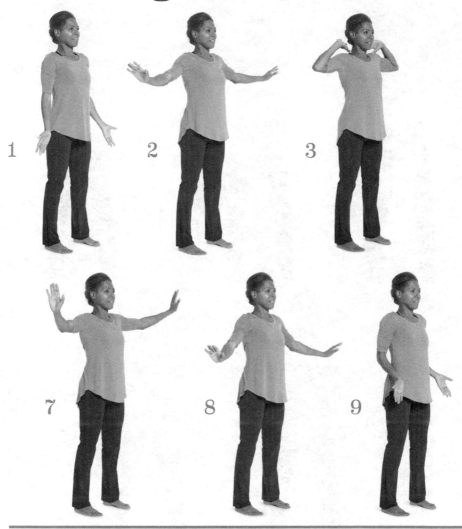

1. From natural stance with your arms by your sides, knees rise and inhale as 2. the arms rise out to the sides then 3. bring the backs of the hands to the tops of the shoulders with the palms up. 4. 5. Slowly exhale, bend the knees, draw the abdomen in, and press the palms upward with tension. 6-8. Inhale, knees rise, hands circle down the sides to the

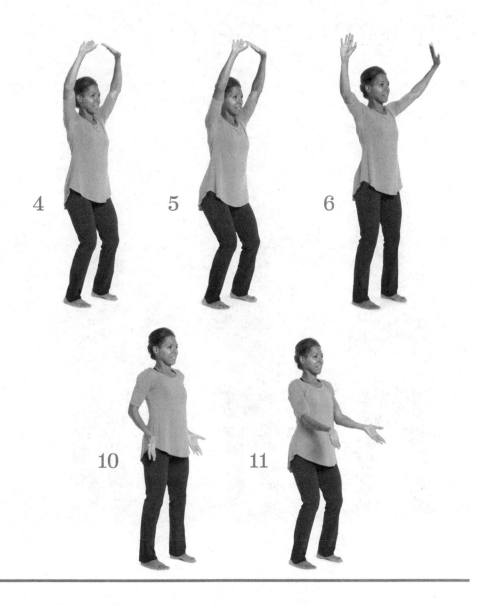

hips. **9** Press the palms forward; slowly exhale, knees bend, abdomen draws in, and **10** **11** push the palms forward with tension. Visualize pushing out pain, sorrow, anger, or regret, or visualize keeping negative influences pushed away. (Complete 3 times.)

Widening the Field

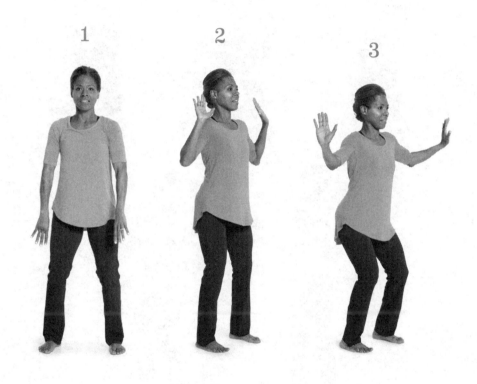

1   2   3

1 From natural stance with the arms by the sides, knees rise and inhale as the arms rise out to the sides and **2** come to the outside of the shoulders, palms facing out to the sides. **3** Slowly exhale, bend the knees, draw the abdomen in, and press the palms out to the sides with tension.

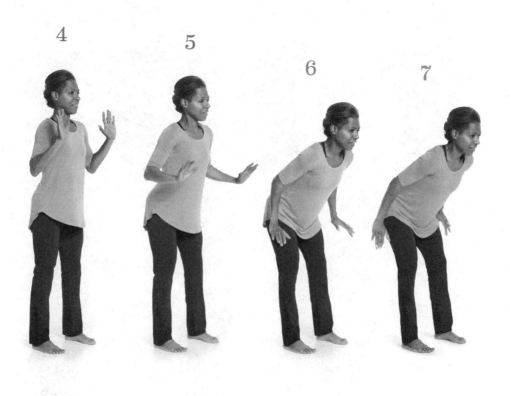

④ Inhale, knees rise, and arms come in front of the body; exhale, ⑤ bend forward slightly at the hip, and ⑥ ⑦ push the palms back with tension. Rise and repeat. Use the same visualization as Clearing the Space. (Complete 3 times.)

Moving the Qi

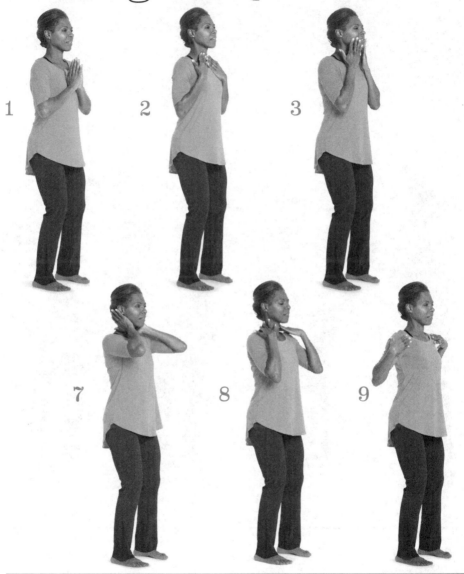

1

2

3

7

8

9

① From natural stance, bring the hands to prayer hands in front of the heart. Take a few deep breaths, rub the hands together to warm them, and ② place them on the chest. Feeling your body with your hands and your hands with your

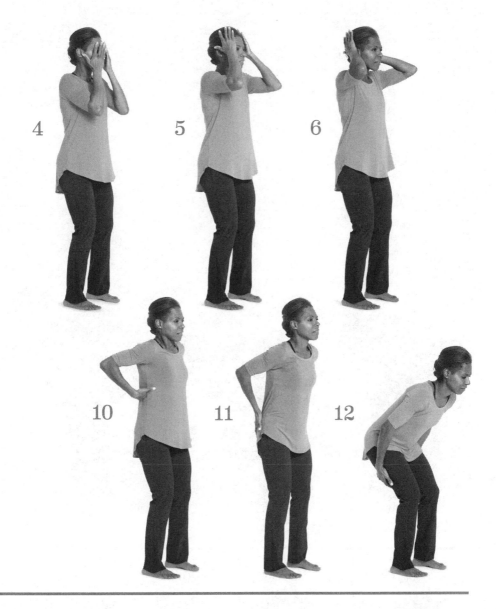

body, ③ ④ gently massage up the neck and face, 5-7
massage over the top of the head. ⑧ ⑨ Massage the neck
and shoulders then ⑩ down the back, ⑪ past the kidneys
and the sacrum. ⑫ The hands fan out so the fingers come

(continued)

Moving the Qi *(cont.)*

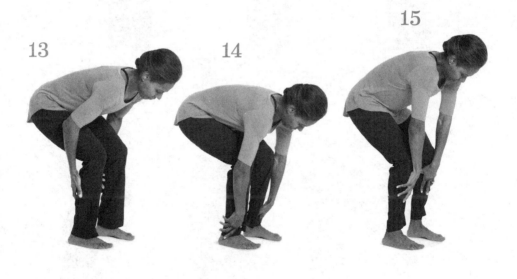

down the back of the legs, **13** thumbs down the outside of the legs. **14** Hands come forward at the ankles and **15** travel up the front and **16** inside of the legs, **17** through the groin creases, **18** over the abdomen, and **19** back to the chest.

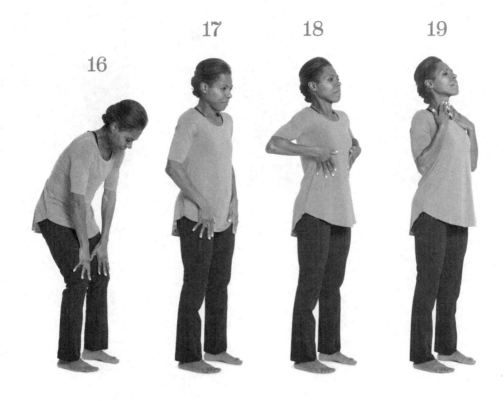

16   17   18   19

Breathing is slow and rhythmical. Visualize encouraging the flow of qi down the back of the body and up the front. Try a light or firm touch to your liking and allow the hands to conform to the contours of the body. (Complete 3 to 6 times.)

Awash in Qi

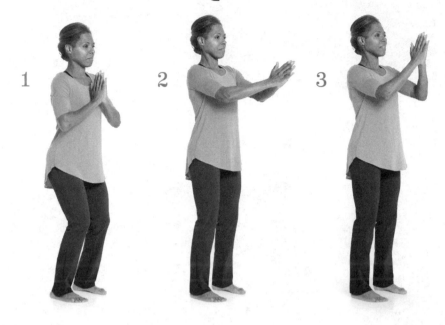

1   2   3

1 From natural stance with knees bent and hands in prayer hands by the heart, 2 extend the hands forward, up a few inches (inhale, knees rise), in toward the body, and 3 4 then down to the heart (exhale, knees bend).

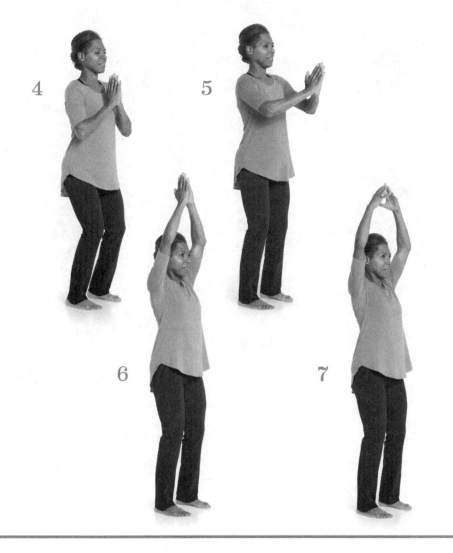

5 **6** Reach prayer hands up overhead (inhale, knees rise), and then descend hands toward the top of the head and **7** separate the palms, letting the middle fingers be the last to separate (exhale, knees bend).

(continued)

Awash in Qi *(cont.)*

8   9   10

8 The arms rise up overhead and 9 open to the sides, palms up at shoulder height (inhale, knees rise) and 10 the elbows draw in slightly (exhale, knees bend).

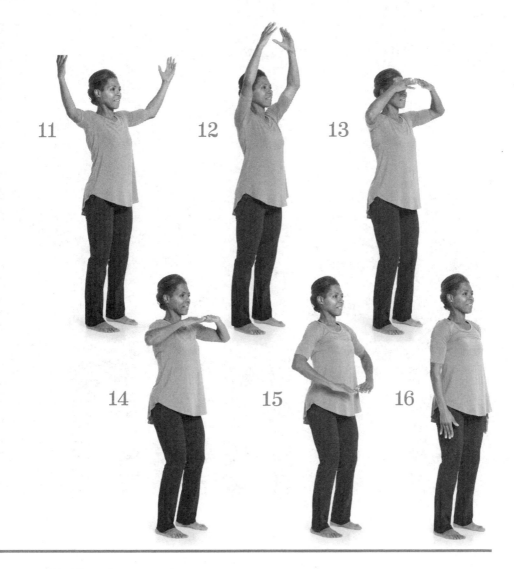

11 12 Extend the arms back out and up (inhale, knees rise), 13 turn palms toward the earth, and 14 15 slowly press arms down in front of the body (exhale, knees bend), 16 arms by the sides. (Complete 3 times.)

Coming Home

This move is a repeat of Bringing in the Light.

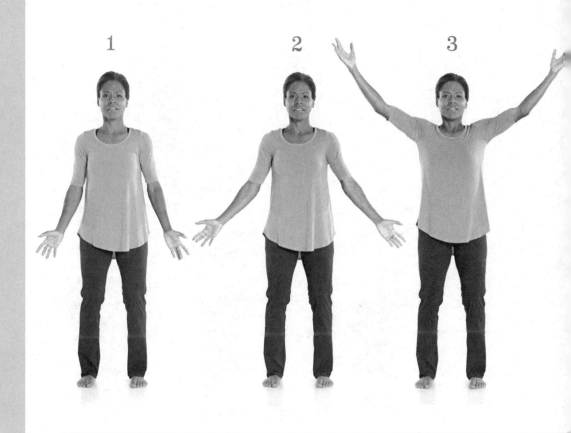

1   2   3

1 Come back to natural stance with knees bent, arms by your sides. 2 3 Roll the arms palm out, then open them out to the sides, 4 lift them overhead. 5 Bring the palms together overhead and 6 while knees drop bring the arms down in front of the body to 7 prayer hands in

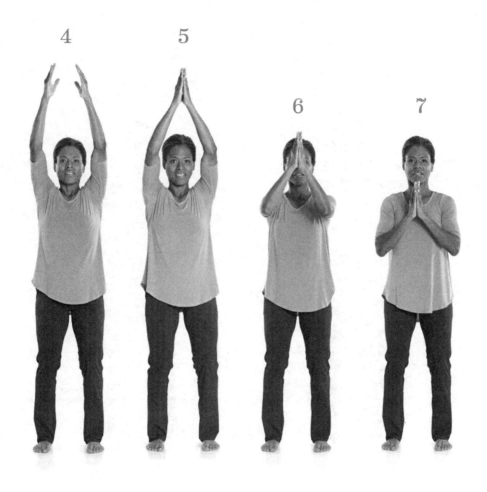

front of the heart. Bend and straighten the knees as much as comfortable–or go from more deeply bent to slightly bent. Inhale as the arms come up; knees bend and exhale as the arms descend to prayer hands. (Complete 6 times.)

Sealing the Qi

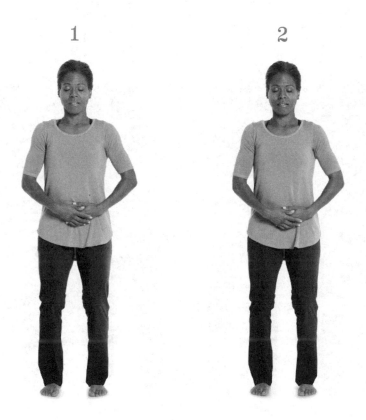

In natural stance, **1** cross the hands are placed crossed over the lower abdomen. Together as a unit, one on top of the other, **2** the hands circle first one direction, then the other,

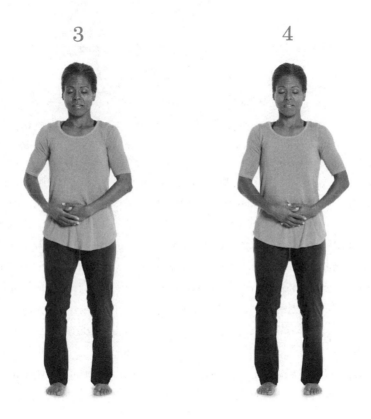

3

4

and then **3** come to stillness. **4** Repeat with other hand on top. Close your eyes, and rest quietly while breathing deeply for as long as you wish.

Healing Waters

Holistic Interventions for Chronic Inflammation

There's no question that the body and the mind are intimately and inextricably connected—they work together in a beautiful, powerful, and complex dance that we'll never fully understand. But we don't need a raft of research studies to know that the mind affects the body. Thoughts and emotions trigger physiological effects. If you've ever experienced sweaty palms, a dry mouth, a racing heart, or butterflies in your stomach from nervousness or anxiety; ever had a stress-induced headache; or ever experienced muscles that ache from tension, you've experienced the mind-body connection. Of course, the effects aren't just confined to negative experiences! If you've ever experienced arousal from a sexual fantasy, used visualization to bolster your confidence, or enjoyed the stress-busting effects of meditation, you've experienced the positive aspects of the mind-body connection, as well.

In this final chapter, we're going to look at some ways you can harness the power of the mind over the body. These practices are powerful, they're completely nonpharmacological, and they're available to us for little or even no money. All that's required is a little time and an open mind. So let's look at holistic, all-natural ways to reduce stress, stay healthy in body and mind, and, yes, quench the fires of chronic inflammation.

Mindfulness and Mindfulness Meditation

Mindfulness is simply the quality or state of being aware. It can describe a mental stance or attitude, but it's also an entire way of life.

Practicing mindfulness entails bringing attention to the present moment and calmly acknowledging it, without judgment. Mindfulness keeps us grounded in the here and now, fully conscious of the present moment. It's an antidote to coasting through our days on autopilot, barely aware of the inner workings driving our outer reactions. Many of us don't stop to examine our inner motivations or our interior landscape until something happens to demand our attention. If you've ever had the experience of losing your temper "over nothing" or bursting into tears "for no apparent reason," you know what we're talking about. Or perhaps our lack of awareness comes in the form of blowing through the day with such distraction that we barely register what's occurring. Before we know it, half a day has vanished while we dashed from one meeting to the next or surfed the Internet or ruminated on an old hurt or multitasked ourselves into exhaustion. Mindfulness puts a halt to living in this state of oblivion. The goal is to live mindfully, with moment-to-moment awareness, in all of life.

How do we get there? Through mindfulness meditation. If you've never meditated, don't be intimidated by the prospect. Think of mindfulness meditation as practice sessions for learning to live with greater awareness, a time set aside to make room for mindfulness. Even a few minutes a day of quiet awareness is an excellent start and can make a big difference in terms of stress reduction and learning to live consciously. Mindfulness meditation can take the form of a traditional sitting meditation, a walking meditation, or a breath-awareness practice, or it can be used as part of a qigong or yoga practice. One of the most well-known mindfulness practices is mindfulness-based stress reduction (MBSR), an 8-week program that combines mindfulness training and yoga. MBSR is widely taught and practiced in hospital and other health-care settings. While there are many ways to learn and practice mindfulness, you basically just need to be willing to become quiet for a period of time each day and try to cultivate awareness.

This brings us to an important point. Many people think about meditation as "zoning out" or achieving a state of "empty mind" in which thoughts no longer intrude. There are such meditation practices, but mindfulness meditation is not one of them. Mindfulness meditation is about zoning *in*. Rather than overcoming or eradicating thoughts, mindfulness meditation is about a truthful, focused awareness of thoughts, feelings, and experiences. If we become aware of negative thoughts or experiences—anything from anxiety to physical pain—rather than try and deny them or become upset over them, which will only worsen the situation, we calmly acknowledge what we find in the present moment.

If you're wondering how becoming aware of the present moment can help—especially if what you find there is negative—part of the answer lies in mindfulness's ability to drastically reduce stress and anxiety. Stress and anxiety worsen any physical and mental discomfort, and they're powerful inflammation triggers. Research demonstrates an extensive array of benefits from a mindfulness practice. It can enhance immune function, increase telomerase activity, and preserve cognitive function and memory. Mindfulness can improve symptoms of irritable bowel syndrome, anxiety, chronic stress, chronic fatigue syndrome, inflammatory skin conditions, chronic pain, fibromyalgia, ADHD, menopause, and insomnia, and it can even reduce stress-related overeating. It's been used to enhance overall quality of life in those with HIV, diabetes, rheumatoid arthritis, and cancer, and it has been used to help overcome eating disorders, substance abuse, and trauma and to speed recovery from illness, injury, and surgery.[1]

Now, how about inflammation specifically? With so many benefits, especially in the realm of stress reduction, perhaps you can already begin to see how mindfulness reduces inflammation. Here are some specifics from the research.

A review of 20 randomized controlled trials on mindfulness meditation found positive effects on four different parameters: a reduction in the activity of proinflammatory tumor necrosis factor-beta (TNF-ß), a reduction in levels of the proinflammatory cytokine CRP, immune system improvements in patients with HIV in the form of an increase in CD4+ T-cell count, and an increase in telomerase activity, which guards against aging.[2]

In a study of young women with depression, 31 were assigned to a 4-week mindfulness-based intervention while 33 served as controls. By the end of the study, those in the mindfulness group had lower levels of IL-6 and TNF-α, proinflammatory cytokines that have been associated with depression. And their IL-6 levels remained low at a 3-month follow-up. Both groups experienced an improvement in depression, but those with more severe depression showed more benefit with mindfulness training.[3]

Forty-nine adults (average age 66.3 years) who were having trouble sleeping were assigned either to a mindfulness awareness intervention or a sleep program that met for 2-hour sessions for 6 weeks. After the training, participants practiced their techniques for 1 year. They were assessed before and after the intervention, as well as at 10-week intervals. While both groups experienced better sleep and a decline in the proinflammatory cytokine NF-κB, the mindfulness group experienced better sleep quality and better secondary outcomes for insomnia symptoms, depression symptoms, fatigue interference, and fatigue severity.[4]

Fifty women with a history of trauma enrolled in an 8-week MBSR program; they were assessed on psychological functioning and inflammatory markers. They experienced significant decreases in perceived stress, depression, anxiety, emotional dysregulation, and post-traumatic stress symptoms and reported an increase in mindfulness. They also experienced significant decreases in IL-6 levels.[5]

Noting that previous studies found that lonely older adults have a higher risk of cardiovascular disease, Alzheimer's disease, and death from any cause, researchers set out to see if MBSR could assuage loneliness *and* lower the proinflammatory profile. They found that compared to controls, an 8-week MBSR program decreased self-reported loneliness and downregulated proinflammatory NF-κB-related gene expression in circulating white blood cells. Researchers also observed a trend toward lower CRP levels in the MBSR group.[6]

In another fascinating study, researchers decided to investigate the power of mindfulness on stress and symptoms of the inflammatory response on skin. First they gave a group of participants 8 weeks of MBSR training, while a control group received 8 weeks of training in a well-matched stress reduction program with no emphasis on mindfulness. Then, in the lab, they induced psychological stress through the Trier Social Stress Test, which required volunteers to deliver a 5-minute impromptu speech and complete 5 minutes of mental math. Afterward, the researchers applied a capsaicin cream to volunteers' forearms to assess their inflammatory response. Researchers measured immune and endocrine levels before and after the training. The results? While both types of training lowered overall stress, the people in the MBSR group displayed less inflammatory reaction than those in the control group, which is good news for anyone suffering from an inflammatory condition exacerbated by stress, such as psoriasis, lupus, fibromyalgia, asthma, or inflammatory bowel disease.[7]

The results of a different study that were just released also demonstrate the stress- and inflammation-reducing benefits of long-term mindfulness meditation. This study compared meditators with an average of roughly 9,000 lifetime hours of meditation with age- and sex-matched controls. Again, using the Trier Social Stress Test and the topical application of capsaicin, researchers found that the experienced meditators had lower levels of the stress hormone cortisol and lower perceived stress than the control group, as well as a lower inflammatory response. Moreover, experienced meditators reported higher levels of psychological factors associated with well-being and resilience. The study authors concluded that a long-term meditation practice could reduce stress activity and provide therapeutic benefit in chronic inflammatory conditions.[8]

In another study comparing expert meditators with a control group with no meditation experience, researchers found that after undergoing the Trier Social Stress Test, the meditators experienced reduced expression of proinflammatory genes and histone deacetylase genes, which regulate inflammatory pathways, compared with controls. Translation? The experienced meditators exhibited an anti-inflammatory effect that the control group did not. Moreover, the experienced meditators showed a faster recovery from stress.[9]

Social Relations

Research has established a strong connection between social relationships and mortality, and we know that many of the leading causes of death are inflammatory conditions. Social isolation is strongly associated with heart disease, depression, memory loss, decreased overall health and well-being in older adults, overall mortality, and a heightened risk of suicide.[10] We are wired for social connection and interaction, and without it, it's not an exaggeration to say that we begin to deteriorate.

A recent study of 725 adults found that daily social interactions were significantly associated with the proinflammatory cytokine IL-6. A greater proportion of daily positive interactions with close friends or family members predicted lower levels of IL-6, even after adjusting for variables such as age, sex, BMI, smoking status, and alcohol intake.[11] Likewise, a study based on 969 adults ages 35 to 86 found that the frequency of daily positive events was associated with lower IL-6 and CRP in men and women and lower fibrinogen among women. Interestingly, nonpersonal positive events—those that occurred in isolation—did not affect inflammatory biomarkers, underscoring the power of social interactions on inflammation.[12]

A study based on data from 6,729 respondents, which included 2,774 total deaths over 18 years of follow-up, found that a lack of social ties increases the risk of mortality by increasing chronic inflammation. Not to put too fine a point on it, the study authors concluded that "the inflammatory process at work in socially isolated individuals greatly intensifies the likelihood of their dying." The link between chronic inflammation and death is even more pronounced in men, especially strong in older men for all-cause and circulatory disease mortality and in middle-aged men for death from cancer.[13]

One of the times we need the most support in life—when we've lost a loved one—is also associated with inflammation. Researchers studied 260 adults who'd lost one or more loved ones within the past 5 to 63 months and

(continued on page 360)

Chad Neff

AGE: 64

- Reduced total cholesterol by 33 points
- Reduced triglycerides by 108 points
- WEIGHT LOST: 18 pounds
- INCHES LOST: 18

Pat Neff

AGE: 65

- Memory problems and mood swings eliminated
- Regular joint and neck pain relieved
- Daily cough gone
- Elevated glucose dropped 9 points to almost normal
- WEIGHT LOST: 23 pounds
- INCHES LOST: 15

Husband and wife Chad and Pat Neff completed the Whole Body Cure Plan together. They also practice qigong and tai chi together, continue to follow many of the principles of healthy eating they learned together, and were even interviewed together in tag-team style! They also experienced great results together: Pat lost 23 pounds and Chad lost 18, and both report that they kept the weight off and feel better all around. But don't take our word for it—here are Pat and Chad, in their own words.

PAT: I thought the first 2 weeks of only fruits and vegetables was going to be difficult, but I felt much better and more energetic afterward. I had mild arthritis in a few of my fingers, and that improved. I was also surprised that I didn't feel uncomfortably hungry at any point. You could always snack on raw vegetables or a little bit of fruit if you needed something.

(continued)

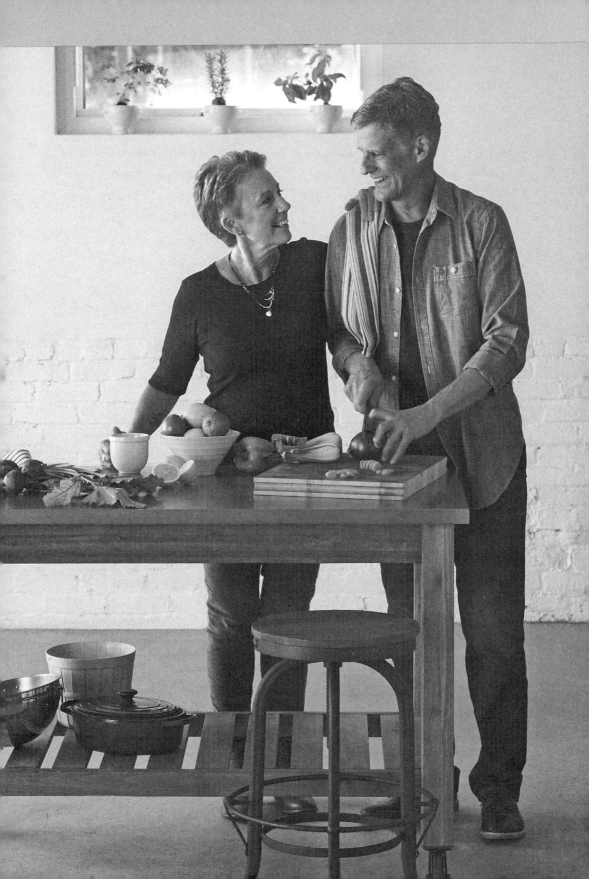

CHAD: It's a big change right away because you're eliminating so many things at once, especially with all the proteins. The protein shakes helped. I also had a bit of mild arthritis to begin with—in my lower back and neck—and that's been much better.

PAT: Chad did all the cooking, and his dishes were all creative and delicious. For example, he made wonderful turkey burgers, and he made chili without the beans—I found out I prefer chili that way.

CHAD: For the turkey burgers, I minced peppers, onions, celery, and garlic in a food processor, lightly sautéed them, and after they cooled a bit, put them in with the turkey. So basically I used vegetables instead of bread crumbs, and the result was that the burgers stayed moist. For the chili, I use lots of peppers of different colors, plus onions, garlic, and tomatoes. You can make it with turkey or with beef, or do a vegetarian version. Another thing we did, which we'd learned from doing a detox diet once before, was to make soups with no cream. Acorn squash soup, for example, usually calls for cream, but you can make it without, and it's still hearty and filling.

PAT: We weren't huge carbohydrate eaters before—we'd have pasta or potatoes on occasion—but we cut carbs entirely. We also cut sugar. As hard as that sounds, I was happy about the no-sugar rule because it cut out my nighttime snacking. Ice cream is my weakness, and I was used to having it at night, but that was out of the question. But guess what happened? The day we finished the program, I wanted a dish of ice cream, and it tasted *terrible*! Dr. Kirshner said that could happen—your taste changes. I just don't want ice cream in the house anymore.

CHAD: We've added in just a few things we used to eat, because neither of us wants to regain the weight we lost. We use just a little dairy now—it's nice to have cream in your coffee.

PAT: Yes! That was my biggest "oh no" moment—not being able to have cream in my coffee. But I will add this: After the plan was over, I followed up on a recommendation from Dr. Kirshner about beet juice, and I found that I really love it. I'm hooked on it.

CHAD: The drinks were one of the toughest things for me. We drank only water, black coffee, and green tea on the plan. But I've learned to add a tiny bit of local raw honey to tea or to warm water. It improves the flavor, and it's good for your immune system. Another thing we added back in and eat occasionally is yogurt. We buy plain 2 percent yogurt and add our own fruit if we want it. You want to avoid that added sugar more than you want to worry about the fat. ■

Pat's and Chad's Tips

PAT: Some people may be worried about the elimination part of the plan, but it's not terrible and it's doable. The 2 weeks of detox was the best kick-off to the whole program, so keep that in mind and stick with it.

CHAD: If you want to be healthy, then you've got to take some time and invest in your health. So many problems come from the gut and from inflammation. It makes sense to eliminate certain foods for a time and see if you experience an improvement—and then, try them one at a time and see if they cause any problems. You'll also see a lot of health benefits simply by cutting out all the sugar and carbohydrates. I didn't need to lose weight, but it was nice to lose it, and I feel better all around.

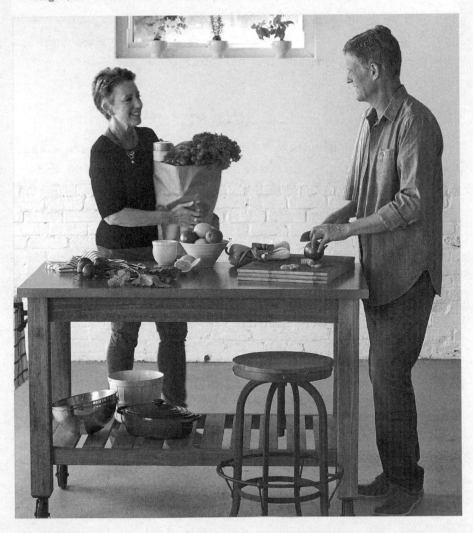

compared them to 269 nonbereaved participants. They found that bereaved participants had higher levels of proinflammatory biomarkers IL-6 and sE-selectin. Further, the number of deaths was associated with progressively higher levels of IL-6, especially among bereaved people with a higher BMI and chronic health problems.[14]

A study of 164 breast cancer survivors found that women with lower social support before cancer treatment experienced higher levels of pain and depressive symptoms than those with strong social support. Moreover, they had higher levels of IL-6, which predicted larger increases in depression. The links between social support, IL-6, pain, and depression held even after accounting for potential variables, including BMI, age, education level, additional illnesses, cancer stage, time since treatment, relationships status, statin use, tamoxifen/aromatase-inhibitor use, and antidepressant use.[15]

Laughter

We know that our emotions affect the body. To cite a familiar example, anger raises our blood pressure, increases our heart and respiratory rates, and can cause sweating and temporary gastrointestinal issues. But research has shown that anger triggers an uptick in IL-6 and CRP, as well. In fact, even the

AN AWE-INSPIRING ANTI-INFLAMMATORY TIP

Researchers studied the effect of positive emotions such as amusement, awe, compassion, contentment, joy, love, and pride on more than 200 volunteers' levels of the proinflammatory cytokine IL-6. They found that while positive emotions were associated with lower levels of IL-6, awe was far and away the best predictor of lower IL-6, even after adjusting for personality and health variables. Examples of volunteers' awe-inspiring experiences included taking nature walks, beholding art, and getting swept away in music.[16] To naturally lower your inflammatory profile, seek out and engage in activities that inspire wonder!

memory of an anger-inciting event has been shown to trigger the production of proinflammatory cytokines IL-6 and TNF-α. Similar physiological effects come from experiences of stress and anxiety.[17]

But just as negative emotions can have negative health consequences, positive emotions have health-promoting effects. One of the most widely studied positive emotional experiences is laughter, and researchers have found that it has a surprisingly potent effect on the immune system and the inflammatory response. Mirthful laughter—the kind of laughter that arises from humor, as opposed to anxiety or embarrassment—has been shown to suppress blood glucose levels after eating in those with type 2 diabetes through natural killer cell activity,[18] to reduce inflammation in blood vessels and increase bloodflow,[19] and in patients with rheumatoid arthritis, to reduce the level of the proinflammatory cytokine IL-6 and increase the level of the anti-inflammatory cytokine IL-4.[20]

In one study on high-risk diabetic patients with high blood pressure and high cholesterol, researchers divided volunteers into a control group and a laughter group and followed them for 12 months. Both groups received therapies for diabetes, high blood pressure, and high cholesterol, but the laughter group also viewed half an hour of comedy per day. After just 2 months, the laughter group had higher HDL ("good") cholesterol levels compared to the control group, and after 4 months, they had significantly lower levels of TNF-α, IFN-γ (interferon gamma), IL-6, and hs-CRP, indicating lower levels of inflammation. By the end of the study, HDL cholesterol had risen by 26 percent in the laughter group and by only 3 percent in the control group. Meanwhile, CRP decreased by 66 percent in the laughter group and by only 26 percent in the control group.[21]

The positive effects of laughter can last up to 12 hours, and it stands to reason that the more laughter in your life, the greater the positive effect.[22] So seek out LOLs whenever you can. The research subjects in the studies cited here got their giggles by watching funny movies and television shows. Other readily available options are comic novels and live comedy shows, or humor is just a click away on the Internet. Or perhaps best of all, spend time with your funniest friends or try laughter yoga, as you'll get the anti-inflammatory benefits of laughter as well as social interaction. While there are no studies that specifically analyzed laughter yoga's effect on inflammatory biomarkers, the practice has been studied extensively, and its documented benefits include improvements in mood, stress, depressive symptoms, pain, heart rate variability, cognitive function, and blood pressure. For more information on laughter yoga, including locations where it's offered and plenty of instructional videos, check out Laughter Yoga University at laughteryoga.org.

Grounding

Grounding, also known as earthing, refers to direct skin contact with the surface of the Earth. Most often, it's done by standing or walking barefoot outdoors, but any contact with the Earth, including sitting or lying down on the ground, qualifies as grounding. The theory behind it is that the Earth, which is electrically conductive, transfers free electrons to us when we make direct contact with the ground. Proponents say that grounding neutralizes the free radicals that build up in the body and accelerate aging, increase inflammation, and cause disease, and they say that grounding results in health benefits such as less stress, better sleep, a more robust immune system, and less pain. It's possible to achieve the effects of grounding through conductive sheets and special shoes that increase the number of free electrons transferred to the body or through simulated methods such as electrode patches affixed to the skin, but all that's truly required for grounding is time set aside and the willingness for your skin to touch "the skin of the Earth." This may be the ultimate in a free and easy way to improve health and well-being.

Recent reviews of the research on grounding published in peer-reviewed journals found that grounding reduces pain, stress, blood thickness, and inflammation; improves sleep; improves mood; increases heart rate variability; and speeds wound healing. (The studies were conducted using a variety of grounding methods, including natural and simulated grounding.) Researchers speculated that the literal disconnection from the Earth that is the result of modern life—exacerbated by rubber-soled shoes that do not conduct electricity, high-rise buildings, elevated beds, and generally spending far less time outdoors—may very well contribute to general physical deterioration as well as the rise in chronic inflammatory diseases. A recent survey of studies on the health effects of grounding concluded that grounding offers a "simple, natural, and accessible health strategy against chronic inflammation."[23]

Studies have also found that simply being in nature can have positive health effects. A recent study found, for example, that people who spent a half-hour or more per week in parks had lower rates of depression and blood pressure—both inflammatory conditions. Those who visited parks more frequently also experienced greater social cohesion. A dose-response analysis suggested that visits to outdoor green spaces of 30 minutes or more per week could reduce the prevalence of depression by up to 7 percent and high blood pressure by up to 9 percent.[24]

Gratitude

A study of 70 patients with asymptomatic heart failure randomized half to 8 weeks of gratitude journaling while half continued with standard treatment. Those who spent 8 weeks focusing on and appreciating the positive aspects of their lives emerged with improved outcomes: They had lower inflammatory scores, higher gratitude scores, and improved heart rate variability during the gratitude journaling sessions.[25]

Another study on patients with asymptomatic heart failure looked at the association between different parameters of health and wellness, including gratitude, spiritual well-being, sleep, mood, fatigue, ability to maintain cardiac function without help, and inflammation. Based on data from 186 patients, researchers found that, overall, gratitude was related to better mood and sleep, more self-efficacy in cardiac function, and lower fatigue and inflammation. They also noted that positive perceptions of daily life seem to be "uniquely associated with inflammation" and that a gratitude practice may reduce inflammatory biomarkers "through changes in affective perceptions of daily life." In other words, focusing on the things for which they were grateful altered patients' perceptions, which in turn lowered their biomarkers of inflammation.[26] Mind over matter at its best!

Even a short gratitude practice can have big effects. A study of 65 women ages 18 to 46 assigned one-third to a mindfulness practice and one-third to gratitude journaling combined with reflection on the things they appreciate; the final third served as controls. By the end of the study, the women in both intervention groups experienced less stress and depression—two of the primary drivers of inflammation—and increased happiness.[27]

Put Your Mind at Ease

If you're nervous about trying a new "mind over matter" technique, let us help you put that fear to rest. There's such a wide array of possibilities out there that with just a little investigation, you're sure to find something that suits you. Meditation, prayer, walks in nature, journaling, breathing exercises, qigong, yoga, and even sitting quietly for a few moments or treating yourself to a power nap are all ways to give yourself an all-natural stress-buster that will have positive effects on body and mind. Finding a practice that works for you—your tastes, your schedule, your ideology, your interests—is one of the keys to cultivating a long-term practice.

Let us also add that it's important to remember that any amount of time you set aside to devote to your chosen practice is fantastic—and well worth it. You need not meditate for hours a day or become a yogi master to experience the benefits of a mindfulness-based practice. Even a few moments a day promotes reduced stress, lower blood pressure, greater peace of mind, improved mood, and, as we've seen, lower inflammation. That's whole-body health at its best.

Appendix

SELF-ASSESSMENT PAGE

DIGESTIVE TRACT	RARELY	WEEKLY	DAILY
Nausea			
Diarrhea			
Constipation			
Bloating after meals			
Bloating not related to meals			
Heartburn			
Less than one bowel movement a day			
Stomach pain			
MUSCULOSKELETAL SYSTEM			
Single joint pain			
Multiple joint pain			
Redness in joints			
Muscle soreness			
Cramping of muscles			
Neck pain			
SKIN			
Acne			
Hives, rashes			
Itchy skin			
Eczema, psoriasis			
Body odor			
MOUTH/THROAT			
Cough			
Sore throat			
Gagging on food			
Gagging on supplements or medications			
Swollen lymph glands			
EYES			
Bags under eyes			
Swollen or red eyelids			
Blurred vision			
HEAD			
Headaches			
Dizziness			
Insomnia			
Faintness			
Mental fatigue			
Balance problems			
Fatigue when reading			
Memory problems			
Mood swings			
Irritability			
WEIGHT			
Overweight			
Sense of puffiness			

Breakfast

1 serving shake: _____

1 serving fat: _____

1 serving vegetable (optional): _____

1 serving fruit (optional): _____

Supplements

1 dose CoCurcumin ☐   **1 dose GI-Revive** ☐

Lunch

2 to 4 servings vegetables (include half as raw): _____

_____

1 serving fat: _____

1 serving fruit: _____

Snack (Optional: Depending on the time difference between lunch and dinner; you may want to have this in the evening.)

½ serving shake _____

Supplements

1 dose CoCurcumin ☐   **1 dose GI-Revive** ☐

Dinner

2 to 4 servings vegetables (include half as raw): _____

_____

_____

1 serving fat: _____

1 serving fruit: _____

_____

Breakfast

1 serving shake: *2 scoops vanilla protein powder*

1 serving fat: *¼ avocado*

1 serving vegetable (optional): *handful spinach*

1 serving fruit (optional): *1½ cups strawberries*

Supplements

1 dose CoCurcumin ☒   1 dose GI-Revive ☒

Lunch

2 to 4 servings vegetables (include half as raw): *large salad with lettuce, tomato, cucumber, radishes*

1 serving fat: *2 tablespoons vinaigrette*

1 serving fruit: *1 apple*

Snack (Optional: Depending on the time difference between lunch and dinner; you may want to have this in the evening.)

½ serving shake *1 scoop chocolate protein powder*

Supplements

1 dose CoCurcumin ☒   1 dose GI-Revive ☒

Dinner

2 to 4 servings vegetables (include half as raw): *sautéed onion, mushrooms, red bell pepper, spinach with 1 cup mashed cauliflower and ½ sweet potato*

1 serving fat: *2 tablespoons olive oil for sautéing*

1 serving fruit: *½ cup pineapple with ¼ cup raspberries and sprinkle of grated gingerroot*

Resources

Protein Powders

Dairy-Based

Solutions4—Vanilla, chocolate, orange, or strawberry
https://www.solutions4.com/solutions4-nutritional-shakes/

Tera's Whey—Vanilla, chocolate, or unflavored
http://simplyteras.com/our-products/

TRUProtiens—Unflavored
https://truproteins.com/clean-whey-unflavored-unsweetened-bulk/

Naked Whey—Unflavored
https://nkdnutrition.com/products/grass-fed-whey-protein-powder

Reserveage—Vanilla, chocolate, or unflavored
http://reserveage.com/product/vanilla-grass-fed-whey-protein/

Plant-Based (Pea Protein)

Orgain—Organic Protein Plant-Based Powder Sweet Vanilla Bean
http://orgain.com/products/organic-protein-powder/#sweet-vanilla-bean

Garden of Life—Raw Protein—Real Vanilla or Real Chocolate
http://www.vitacost.com/garden-of-life-raw-organic-protein-plant
    -formula-vanilla

Swanson Organic—100% Certified Organic Pea Protein Powder Non-GMO
http://www.swansonvitamins.com/swanson-organic-certified-organic
    -pea-protein-powder-non-gmo-1-1-lb-503-grams-pwdr

Plant-Based (Hemp)

Manitoba Harvest—HempPro 70
https://manitobaharvest.com/products/hemp-pro-70/

Grass-Fed Beef-Based (doesn't taste like beef)

Paleo Protein—Vanilla or chocolate
https://paleopro.com/product/paleo-protein-powder-2/

CoCurcumin/Turmeric

Ayush Herbs—CoCurcumin (1 teaspoon)
https://www.ayush.com/store/joint-and-muscle-support/cocurcumin
-52-oz150-g-musculoskeletal-support-52-oz150-g-drink-mix

1MD—Turmeric Curcumin Platinum
https://1md.org/product/turmeric

Healthwise—Turmeric Curcumin Advanced Restore
https://healthwise.life/product/tcar

Digestion

Designs for Health—GI-Revive
http://catalog.designsforhealth.com/GI-Revive-Powder

Kirshner Health Solutions

www.drkirshner.com

Endnotes

Introduction

1   George M. Slavich, "Understanding Inflammation, Its Regulation, and Relevance for Health: A Top Scientific and Public Priority," *Brain, Behavior, and Immunity* 45 (March 2015): 13–14; Donna L. Hoyert and Jiaquan Xu, "Deaths: Preliminary Data for 2011," *National Vital Statistics Reports* 61, no. 6 (October 10, 2012): 1–51, cdc .gov/nchs/data/nvsr/nvsr61/nvsr61_06.pdf.

Chapter 1

1   Nathalie Esser et al., "Inflammation as a Link between Obesity, Metabolic Syndrome, and Type 2 Diabetes," *Diabetes Research and Clinical Practice* 105, no. 2 (2014): 141–50.

2   Ian Graham et al., "Plasma Homocysteine as a Risk Factor for Vascular Disease: The European Concerted Action Project," *JAMA* 277, no. 22 (1997): 1775–81.

3   James T. Wu, "Circulating Homocysteine Is an Inflammation Marker and a Risk Factor of Life-Threatening Inflammatory Diseases," *Journal of Biomedical and Laboratory Sciences* 19, no. 4 (2007): 107–11.

Chapter 2

1   https://ndb.nal.usda.gov/ndb/foods/show/2693?manu=&fgcd=&ds

2   "Beef," George Mateljan Foundation, accessed November 18, 2016, whfoods.com /genpage.php?tname=nutrientprofile&dbid=141.

3   "Bacon, Processed Meats a Cause of Cancer—Your FAQs," American Institute for Cancer Research, October 28, 2015, aicr.org/cancer-research-update/2015/10_28 /cru_Bacon-Processed-Meats-a-Cause-of-Cancer-Your-FAQs.html; Véronique Bouvard et al., "Carcinogenicity of Consumption of Red and Processed Meat," *Lancet Oncology* 16, no. 16 (December 2015): 1599–1600.

4   Ibid.

5   A. Vojdani and C. Vojdani, "Immune Reactivity to Food Coloring," supplement 1, *Alternative Therapies in Health and Medicine* 21 (2015): 52–62.

6   Jaime Uribarri et al., "Advanced Glycation End Products in Foods and a Practical Guide to Their Reduction in the Diet," *Journal of the American Dietetic Association* 110, no. 6 (2010): 911–16.

7   Benoit Chassaing et al., "Dietary Emulsifiers Impact the Mouse Gut Microbiota Promoting Colitis and Metabolic Syndrome," *Nature* 519, no. 7541 (2015): 92–96.

8   A. P. Simopoulos, "The Importance of the Omega-6/Omega-3 Fatty Acid Ratio in Cardiovascular Disease and Other Chronic Diseases," *Experimental Biology and Medicine* 233, no. 6 (2008): 674–88.

9   Xiaofa Qin, "Etiology of Inflammatory Bowel Disease: A Unified Hypothesis," *World Journal of Gastroenterology* 18, no. 15 (2012): 1708–22.

10   A. Noorafshan et al., "Sodium Benzoate, a Food Preservative, Induces Anxiety and Motor Impairment in Rats," *Neurosciences* (Riyadh) 19, no. 1 (2014): 24–28.

11   N. Zengin et al., "The Evaluation of the Genotoxicity of Two Food Preservatives: Sodium Benzoate and Potassium Benzoate," *Food and Chemical Toxicology* 49, no. 4 (2011): 763–69.

12   Alan Chait and Francis Kim, "Saturated Fatty Acids and Inflammation: Who Pays the Toll?," *Arteriosclerosis, Thrombosis, and Vascular Biology* 30, no. 4 (2010): 692–93.

13   Esther Lopez-Garcia et al., "Consumption of *Trans* Fatty Acids Is Related to Plasma Biomarkers of Inflammation and Endothelial Dysfunction," *Journal of Nutrition* 135, no. 3 (March 1, 2005): 562–66.

14   "Shining the Spotlight on Trans Fats," The Nutrition Source, accessed November 20, 2016, hsph.harvard.edu/nutritionsource/transfats/#7.

15   Katherine Esposito et al., "Inflammatory Cytokine Concentrations Are Acutely Increased by Hyperglycemia in Humans," *Circulation* 106, no. 16 (2002): 2067–72.

16   Marian L. Neuhouser et al., "A Low-Glycemic Load Diet Reduces Serum C-Reactive Protein and Modestly Increases Adiponectin in Overweight and Obese Adults," *Journal of Nutrition* 142, no. 2 (2012): 369–74; Patricia Feliciano Pereira et al., "Glycemic Index Role on Visceral Obesity, Subclinical Inflammation and Associated Chronic Diseases," *Nutricion Hospitalaria* 30, no. 2 (2014): 237–43.

17   H. Joe Wang et al., "Alcohol, Inflammation, and Gut-Liver-Brain Interactions in Tissue Damage and Disease Development," *World Journal of Gastroenterology* 16, no. 11 (2010): 1304–13; "Nutrition and Healthy Eating: When to Avoid Alcohol Use," Mayo Clinic, August 30, 2016, mayoclinic.org/healthy-lifestyle/nutrition-and -healthy-eating/in-depth/alcohol/art-20044551?pg=2.

18   Rosa Casas et al., "The Immune Protective Effect of the Mediterranean Diet against Chronic Low-Grade Inflammatory Diseases," *Endocrine, Metabolic & Immune Disorders Drug Targets* 14, no. 4 (2014): 245–54.

19   Karin De Punder and Leo Pruimboom, "The Dietary Intake of Wheat and Other Cereal Grains and Their Role in Inflammation," *Nutrients* 5, no. 3 (2013): 771–87.

20   Ibid.

21   Stephan C. Bischoff et al., "Intestinal Permeability—A New Target for Disease Prevention and Therapy," *BMC Gastroenterology* 14 (November 18, 2014): 189.

22   Biola M. Javierre et al., "Environmental Triggers and Epigenetic Deregulation in Autoimmune Disease," *Discovery Medicine* 12, no. 67 (2011): 535–45.

23   Anselm Mak and Sen Hee Tay, "Environmental Factors, Toxicants and Systemic Lupus Erythematosus," *International Journal of Molecular Sciences* 15, no. 9 (2014): 16043–56.

24   Johanna Bodin et al., "Can Exposure to Environmental Chemicals Increase the Risk of Diabetes Type 1 Development?," *BioMedical Research International* (2015): 208947, doi: 10.1155/2015/208947.

25 Meredith Shiels et al., "Cigarette Smoking and Variations in Systemic Immune and Inflammation Markers," *JNCI: Journal of the National Cancer Institute* 106, no. 11 (2014): dju294, doi: 10.1093/jnci/dju294.

26 Adae O. Amoako and George Guntur A. Pujalte, "Osteoarthritis in Young, Active, and Athletic Individuals," *Clinical Medicine Insights: Arthritis and Musculoskeletal Disorders* 7 (May 22, 2014): 27–32.

27 Luke Spence et al., "Incidence, Etiology and Symptomatology of Upper Respiratory Illness in Elite Athletes," *Medicine and Science in Sports and Exercise* 39, no. 4 (2007): 577–86.

28 Neha Mathur and Bente Klarlund Pedersen, "Exercise as a Mean to Control Low-Grade Systemic Inflammation," *Mediators of Inflammation* (2008): 109502, doi: 10.1155/2008/109502.

29 G. F. Hamilton and J. S. Rhodes, "Exercise Regulation of Cognitive Function and Neuroplasticity in the Healthy and Diseased Brain," *Progress in Molecular Biology and Translational Science* 135 (2015): 381–406.

30 Felice N. Jacka, "Western Diet Is Associated with a Smaller Hippocampus: A Longitudinal Investigation," *BMC Medicine* 13 (2015): 215.

31 C. Y. Hsu et al., "The Association between Insomnia and Increased Future Cardiovascular Events: A Nationwide Population-Based Study," *Psychosomatic Medicine* 7, no. 77 (2015): 743–51; Yun Li et al., "Sleep and Hypertension," *Hypertension* 65 (2015): 644–50; Michael R. Irwin et al., "Sleep Disturbance, Sleep Duration, and Inflammation: A Systematic Review and Meta-Analysis of Cohort Studies and Experimental Sleep Deprivation," *Biological Psychiatry* 80, no. 1 (2016): 40–52.

32 Aric Prather et al., "Sleep Duration, Insomnia, and Markers of Systemic Inflammation: Results from the Netherlands Study of Depression and Anxiety (NESDA)," *Journal of Psychiatric Research* 60 (2015): 95–102.

33 Damien Léger et al., "The Risks of Sleeping 'Too Much.' Survey of a National Representative Sample of 24,671 Adults (INPES Health Barometer)," *PLoS ONE* 9, no. 9 (2014): e106950, doi: 10.1371/journal.pone.0106950.

34 Vilma Aho et al., "Prolonged Sleep Restriction Induces Changes in Pathways Involved in Cholesterol Metabolism and Inflammatory Responses," *Scientific Reports* 6 (April 22, 2016): 24828, doi: 10.1038/srep24828.

35 Michael Berk et al., "So Depression is an Inflammatory Disease, but Where Does the Inflammation Come From?," *BMC Medicine* 11 (2013): 200, doi: 10.1186/1741-7015-11-200.

36 Aho et al., "Prolonged Sleep Restriction Induces Changes," 24828.

37 "How Much Sleep Do We Really Need?," National Sleep Foundation, accessed November 20, 2016, sleepfoundation.org/how-sleep-works/how-much-sleep-do-we-really-need/page/0/2.

38 Johnny Nijm and Lena Jonassan, "Inflammation and Cortisol Response in Coronary Artery Disease," *Annals of Medicine* 41, no. 3 (2009): 224–33.

39 Nicole Powell et al., "Social Stress Up-Regulates Inflammatory Gene Expression in the Leukocyte Transcriptome via B-Adrenergic Induction of Myelopoiesis,"

Proceedings of the National Academy of Sciences of the United States of America 110, no. 41 (2013): 16574–79.

40   "Stress Effects," American Institute of Stress, accessed November 20, 2016, stress .org/stress-effects/.

41   Sandi L. Navarro et al., "Factors Associated with Multiple Biomarkers of Systemic Inflammation," *Cancer Epidemiology, Biomarkers and Prevention* 25, no. 3 (March 2016): 521–31; J. A. Woods et al., "Exercise, Inflammation and Aging," *Aging and Disease* 3, no. 1 (2012): 130–40.

Chapter 3

1   "Life Expectancy at Birth (Years), 2000–2015: Both Sexes: 2015," World Health Organization, accessed November 20, 2016, gamapserver.who.int/gho/interactive _charts/mbd/life_expectancy/atlas.html.

2   National Institute on Aging, National Institutes of Health, and World Health Organization, *Global Health and Aging*, October 2011, nia.nih.gov/research /publication/global-health-and-aging/living-longer.

3   Andrea Metti et al., "Change in Inflammatory Markers and Cognitive Status among Oldest Old Women from the Study of Osteoporotic Fractures," *Journal of the American Geriatrics Society* 62, no. 4 (2014): 662–66.

4   Patricia Griffin et al., "Integration of Immunity with Physical and Cognitive Function in Definitions of Successful Aging," *Aging and Disease* 3, no. 1 (2012): 34–50.

5   "Life Expectancy at Birth (Years), 2000–2015," gamapserver.who.int/gho/interactive _charts/mbd/life_expectancy/atlas.html.

6   "Older Persons' Health," Centers for Disease Control and Prevention, last modified October 6, 2016, cdc.gov/nchs/fastats/older-american-health.htm.

7   Tasnime Akbaraly et al., "Chronic Inflammation as a Determinant of Future Aging Phenotypes," *CMAJ* 185, no. 16 (2013): E763–E770, doi: 10.1503/cmaj.122072.

8   Monika Puzianowska-Kuźnicka et al., "Interleukin-6 and C-Reactive Protein, Successful Aging, and Mortality: the PolSenior Study," *Immunity & Ageing* 13 (2016): 21.

9   Ravi Varadhan et al., "Simple Biologically Informed Inflammatory Index of Two Serum Cytokines Predicts 10 Year All-Cause Mortality in Older Adults," *Journals of Gerontology Series A: Biological Sciences and Medical Sciences* 69, no. 2 (2014): 165–73; Akbaraly et al., "Chronic Inflammation as a Determinant," E763–E770; Ying Chen and John Lyga, "Brain-Skin Connection: Stress, Inflammation and Skin Aging," *Inflammation & Allergy Drug Targets* 13, no. 3 (2014): 177–90.

10   Sean X. Leng et al., "Inflammation and Frailty in Older Women," *Journal of the American Geriatrics Society* 55, no. 6 (2007): 864–71.

11   Caroline Buffière et al., "Slight Chronic Elevation of C-Reactive Protein Is Associated with Lower Aerobic Fitness but Does Not Impair Meal-Induced Stimulation of Muscle Protein Metabolism in Healthy Old Men," *Journal of Physiology* 593, no. 5 (2015): 1259–72.

12   Francesco Prattichizzo et al., "'Inflammaging' as a Druggable Target: A Senescence-Associated Secretory Phenotype—Centered View of Type 2 Diabetes," *Oxidative Medicine and Cellular Longevity* 2016 (2016): 1810327, dx.doi.org/10.1155/2016/1810327.

13   Varadhan et al., "Simple Biologically Informed Inflammatory Index," 165–73.

14   Alicja Puchta et al., "TNF Drives Monocyte Dysfunction with Age and Results in Impaired Anti-Pneumococcal Immunity," *PLoS Pathogens* 12, no. 1 (2016): e1005368, dx.doi.org/10.1371/journal.ppat.1005368.

15   Ibid.

16   Karl-Heinz Wagner et al., "Biomarkers of Aging: From Function to Molecular Biology," *Nutrients* 8, no. 6 (2016): E338, doi: 10.3390/nu8060338.

17   Francis Rodier and Judith Campisi, "Four Faces of Cellular Senescence," *Journal of Cell Biology* 192, no. 4 (2011): 547–56.

18   Jean-Phillipe Coppé et al., "The Senescence-Associated Secretory Phenotype: The Dark Side of Tumor Suppression," *Annual Review of Pathology* 5 (2010): 99–118; Rodier and Campisi, "Four Faces of Cellular Senescence," 547–56; Adam Freund et al., "Inflammatory Networks during Cellular Senescence: Causes and Consequences," *Trends in Molecular Medicine* 16, no. 5 (2010): 238–46.

19   Masood A. Shammas, "Telomeres, Lifestyle, Cancer, and Aging," *Current Opinion in Clinical Nutrition and Metabolic Care* 14, no. 1 (2011): 28–34; Alexandra Bernadotte et al., "Markers of Cellular Senescence. Telomere Shortening as a Marker of Cellular Senescence," *Aging* 8, no. 1 (2016): 3–11.

20   Georgios Nikolakis et al., "Skin Mirrors Human Aging," *Hormone Molecular Biology and Clinical Investigation* 16, no. 1 (2013): 13–28.

21   Chen and Lyga, "Brain-Skin Connection," 177–90.

22   Harrison P. Nguyen and Rajani Katta, "Sugar Sag: Glycation and the Role of Diet in Aging Skin," *Skin Therapy Letter* 20, no. 6 (2015): 1–5.

23   Ibid.

24   "Stopping Skin Cancer Epidemic Starts with Children," Skin Cancer Foundation, July 21, 2008, skincancer.org/media-and-press/Press-Release-2008/stopping-skin-cancer-epidemic-starts-with-children.

25   "Sunscreen FAQs," American Academy of Dermatology, accessed November 20, 2016, aad.org/media/stats/prevention-and-care/sunscreen-faqs.

26   H. C. Okada et al., "Facial Changes Caused by Smoking: A Comparison Between Smoking and Nonsmoking Identical Twins," *Plastic and Reconstructive Surgery* 132, no. 5 (2013): 1085–92.

27   Andrea Vierkotter et al., "Airborne Particle Exposure and Extrinsic Skin Aging," *Journal of Investigative Dermatology* 130, no. 12 (2010): 2719–26; Kyung Eun Kim et al., "Air Pollution and Skin Diseases: Adverse Effects of Airborne Particulate Matter on Various Skin Diseases," *Life Sciences* 152 (May 2016): 126–34.

28   Michelle Garay et al., "Pollution Doubles Skin Damage from Solar Ultraviolet Radiation," supplement 1, *Journal of the American Academy of Dermatology* 64, no. 2 (2011): AB23.

29   J. Krutmann et al., "Pollution and Skin: From Epidemiological and Mechanistic

Studies to Clinical Implications," *Journal of Dermatological Science* 76, no. 33 (2014): 163–68.

30 Yasumichi Arai et al., "Inflammation, but Not Telomere Length, Predicts Successful Ageing at Extreme Old Age: A Longitudinal Study of Semi-Supercentenarians," *EBioMedicine* 2, no. 10 (2015): 1549–58.

31 Nguyen and Katta, "Sugar Sag," 1–5; Ricki J. Colman et al., "Caloric Restriction Reduces Age-Related and All-Cause Mortality in Rhesus Monkeys," *Nature Communications* 5 (2014): 3557, doi:10.1038/ncomms4557.

32 Valter D. Longo et al., "Interventions to Slow Aging in Humans: Are We Ready?," *Aging Cell* 14, no. 4 (2015): 497–510.

33 S. N. Meydani et al., "Long-Term Moderate Calorie Restriction Inhibits Inflammation without Impairing Cell-Mediated Immunity: A Randomized Controlled Trial in Non-Obese Humans," *Aging* 8, no. 7 (2016): 1416–31.

34 Valter D. Longo and Mark P. Mattson, "Fasting: Molecular Mechanisms and Clinical Applications," *Cell Metabolism* 19, no. 2 (2014): 181–92.

35 Shibu M. Poulouse et al., "Improving Brain Signaling in Aging: Could Berries Be the Answer?," *Expert Review of Neurotherapeutics* 12, no. 8 (2012): 887–89.

36 Elizabeth E. Devore et al., "Dietary Intake of Berries and Flavonoids in Relation to Cognitive Decline," *Annals of Neurology* 72, no. 1 (2012): 135–43.

37 Amy Jennings et al., "Intakes of Anthocyanins and Flavones Are Associated with Biomarkers of Insulin Resistance and Inflammation in Women," *Journal of Nutrition* 144, no. 2 (2014): 202–8.

38 Martha Clare Morris et al., "MIND Diet Slows Cognitive Decline with Aging," *Alzheimer's & Dementia: Journal of the Alzheimer's Association* 11, no. 9 (2015): 1015–22. Martin Root et al., "Flavonol Intake and Cognitive Decline in Middle-Aged Adults," *Journal of Medicinal Food* 18, no. 12 (2015): 1327–32.

39 "Flavonoids," Linus Pauling Institute Micronutrient Information Center, accessed November 20, 2016, lpi.oregonstate.edu/mic/dietary-factors/phytochemicals /flavonoids.

40 Christopher T. Ford et al., "Identification of (Poly)phenol Treatments That Modulate the Release of Proinflammatory Cytokines by Human Lymphocytes," *British Journal of Nutrition*, 115, no. 10 (2016): 1699–1710.

41 Eunmiri Roh et al., "Molecular Mechanisms of Green Tea Polyphenols with Protective Effects against Skin Photoaging," *Critical Reviews in Food Science and Nutrition* (June 26, 2015): Epub ahead of print.

42 Giuseppe Derosa et al., "Effect of Curcumin on Circulating Interleukin-6 Concentrations: A Systematic Review and Meta-Analysis of Randomized Controlled Trials," *Pharmacological Research* 111 (September 2016): 394–404.

43 Y. Liu et al., "Inhibitory Effects of Black Pepper (*Piper Nigrum*) Extracts and Compounds on Human Tumor Cell Proliferation, Cyclooxygenase Enzymes, Lipid Peroxidation and Nuclear Transcription Factor-Kappa-B," *Natural Products Communication* 5, no. 8 (2010): 1253–57.

44 Guido Shoba et al., "Influence of Piperine on the Pharmacokinetics of Curcumin in Animals and Human Volunteers," *Planta Medica* 64, no. 4 (1998): 353–56.

45 Brad J. Douglass and Dallas L. Clouatre, "Beyond Yellow Curry: Assessing

Commercial Curcumin Absorption Technologies," *Journal of the American College of Nutrition* 34, no. 4 (2015): 347–58.

46   Nguyen and Katta, "Sugar Sag," 1–5.

47   Lisa Parkinson and Russell Keast, "Oleocanthal, a Phenolic Derived from Virgin Olive Oil: A Review of the Beneficial Effects on Inflammatory Disease," *International Journal of Molecular Sciences* 15, no. 7 (2014): 12323–34.

48   Mitra Rozati et al., "Cardio-Metabolic and Immunological Impacts of Extra Virgin Olive Oil Consumption in Overweight and Obese Older Adults: A Randomized Controlled Trial," *Nutrition & Metabolism* 12 (August 7, 2015): 28.

49   Andrea Ticinesi et al., "Nutrition and Inflammation in Older Individuals: Focus on Vitamin D, *n*-3 Polyunsaturated Fatty Acids and Whey Proteins," *Nutrients* 8, no. 4 (2016): 186.

50   T. M. Freitas-Simoes et al., "Nutrients, Foods, Dietary Patterns and Telomere Length: Update of Epidemiological Studies and Randomized Trials," *Metabolism: Clinical and Experimental* 65, no. 4 (2016): 406–15.

51   Cindy W. Leung et al., "Soda and Cell Aging: Associations Between Sugar-Sweetened Beverage Consumption and Leukocyte Telomere Length in Healthy Adults from the National Health and Nutrition Examination Surveys," *American Journal of Public Health* 104, no. 12 (2014): 2425–31.

52   Rajani Katta and Samir P. Desai, "Diet and Dermatology: The Role of Dietary Intervention in Skin Disease," *Journal of Clinical and Aesthetic Dermatology* 7, no. 7 (2014): 46–51.

53   P. O. Duarte et al., "Cardiovascular Risk Factors and Inflammatory Activity among Centenarians with and without Dementia," *Aging Clinical and Experimental Research* (July 2016): Epub ahead of print, doi: 10.1007/s40520-016-0603-9.

54   Yang Claire Yang et al., "Social Support, Social Strain and Inflammation: Evidence from a National Longitudinal Study of U.S. Adults." *Social Science & Medicine* 107 (April 2014): 124–35.

55   S. L. van Ockenburg et al., "Stressful Life Events and Leukocyte Telomere Attrition in Adulthood: A Prospective Population-Based Cohort Study," *Psychological Medicine* 45, no. 14 (2015): 2975–84; Maya B. Mathur et al., "Perceived Stress and Telomere Length: A Systematic Review, Meta-Analysis, and Methodologic Considerations for Advancing the Field," *Brain, Behavior, and Immunity* 54 (May 2016): 158–69.

56   J. D. Creswell et al., "Alterations in Resting-State Functional Connectivity Link Mindfulness Meditation with Reduced Interleukin-6: A Randomized Controlled Trial," *Biological Psychiatry* 80, no. 1 (2016): 53–61.

57   David S. Black and George M. Slavich, "Mindfulness Meditation and the Immune System: A Systematic Review of Randomized Controlled Trials," *Annals of the New York Academy of Sciences* 1373, no. 1 (2016): 13–24.

Chapter 4

1   Emma Young, "Gut Instincts: The Secrets of Your Second Brain," New Scientist, December 12, 2012, newscientist.com/article/mg21628951.900-gut-instincts-the

-secrets-of-your-second-brain; Behtash Ghazi Nezami and Shanthi Srinivasan, "Enteric Nervous System in the Small Intestine: Pathophysiology and Clinical Implications," *Current Gastroenterology Reports* 12, no. 5 (2010): 358–65.

2   Nezami and Srinivasan, "Enteric Nervous System in the Small Intestine," 358–65.

3   Staffan Holmqvist et al., "Direct Evidence of Parkinson Pathology Spread from the Gastrointestinal Tract to the Brain in Rats," *Acta Neuropathologica* 128, no. 6 (2014): 805–20.

4   Kirsty Brown et al., "Diet-Induced Dysbiosis of the Intestinal Microbiota and the Effects on Immunity and Disease," *Nutrients* 4, no. 8 (2012): 1095–1119.

5   Amy Langdon et al., "The Effects of Antibiotics on the Microbiome throughout Development and Alternative Approaches for Therapeutic Modulation," *Genome Medicine* 8, no. 1 (2016): 39, doi: 10.1186/s13073-016-0294-z.

6   T. G. Dinan et al., "Collective Unconscious: How Gut Microbes Shape Human Behavior," *Journal of Psychiatric Research* 63 (April 2015): 1–9.

7   Lawrence A. David et al., "Diet Rapidly and Reproducibly Alters the Human Gut Microbiome," *Nature* 505, no. 7484 (2014): 559–63.

8   Annick Hartstra et al., "Insights into the Role of the Microbiome in Obesity and Type 2 Diabetes," *Diabetes Care* 38, no. 1 (2015): 159–65.

9   Brown et al., "Diet-Induced Dysbiosis," 1095–1119.

10   John R. Kelly et al., "Transferring the Blues: Depression-Associated Gut Microbiota Induces Neurobehavioural Changes in the Rat," *Journal of Psychiatric Research* 82 (November 2016): 109–18.

11   Ruth Ann Luna and Jane A. Foster, "Gut Brain Axis: Diet Microbiota Interactions and Implications for Modulation of Anxiety and Depression," *Current Opinion in Biotechnology* 32 (April 2015): 35–41.

12   Sophie Dutheil et al., "High-Fat Diet Induced Anxiety and Anhedonia: Impact on Brain Homeostasis and Inflammation," *Neuropsychopharmacology* 41, no. 7 (2016): 1874–87.

13   Luna and Foster, "Gut Brain Axis," 35–41.

14   Noboyuki Sudo et al., "Postnatal Microbial Colonization Programs the Hypothalamic-Pituitary-Adrenal System for Stress Response in Mice," *Journal of Physiology* 558 (July 1, 2004): 263–75.

15   Charlotte D'Mello et al., "Probiotics Improve Inflammation-Associated Sickness Behavior by Altering Communication between the Peripheral Immune System and the Brain," *Journal of Neuroscience* 35, no. 30 (2015): 10821–30.

16   Theodor Bokic et al., "Potential Causes and Present Pharmacotherapy of Irritable Bowel Syndrome (IBS): An Overview," *Pharmacology* 96, no. 1–2 (2015): 76–85.

17   T. G. Dinan et al., "Psychobiotics: A Novel Class of Psychotropic," *Biological Psychiatry* 74, no. 10 (2013): 720–26.

18   Kirsten Tillisch et al., "Consumption of Fermented Milk Product with Probiotic Modulates Brain Activity," *Gastroenterology* 144, no. 7 (2013): 1394–1401.

19   Laura Steenbergen et al., "A Randomized Controlled Trial to Test the Effect of Multispecies Probiotics on Cognitive Reactivity to Sad Mood," *Brain, Behavior, and Immunity* 48 (August 2015): 258–64.

20   Michael Messaoudi et al., "Assessment of Psychotropic-Like Properties of a Probiotic Formulation (*Lactobacillus Helveticus* R0052 and *Bifidobacterium Longum* R0175) in Rats and Human Subjects," *British Journal of Nutrition* 105, no. 5 (2011): 755–64.

21   Matthew Hilimire et al., "Fermented Foods, Neuroticism, and Social Anxiety: An Interaction Model," *Psychiatry Research* 228, no. 2 (2015): 203–8.

22   Ibid.

23   Lynnette R. Ferguson. "Nutritional Modulation of Gene Expression: Might This Be of Benefit to Individuals with Crohn's Disease?," *Frontiers in Immunology* 6 (September 11, 2015): 467.

24   Franziska Durchschein et al., "Diet Therapy for Inflammatory Bowel Diseases: The Established and the New," *World Journal of Gastroenterology* 22, no. 7 (2016): 2179–94.

25   Moftah Alhagamhmad et al., "An Overview of the Bacterial Contribution to Crohn Disease Pathogenesis," *Journal of Medical Microbiology* 65 (October 2016): 1049–59.

26   Viran Gunaskeera et al., "Treatment of Crohn's Disease with an IgG4-Guided Exclusion Diet: A Randomized Controlled Trial," *Digestive Diseases and Sciences* 61, no. 4 (2016): 1148–57.

27   Ibid.

28   A. Tjonneland et al., "Linoleic Acid, a Dietary N-6 Polyunsaturated Fatty Acid, and the Aetiology of Ulcerative Colitis: A Nested Case-Control Study within a European Prospective Cohort Study," *Gut* 58, no. 12 (2009): 1606–11.

29   Durchschein et al., "Diet Therapy for Inflammatory Bowel Diseases," 2179–94.

30   Danuta Owczarek et al., "Diet and Nutritional Factors in Inflammatory Bowel Diseases," *World Journal of Gastroenterology* 22, no. 3 (2016): 895–905.

31   Durchschein et al., "Diet Therapy for Inflammatory Bowel Diseases," 2179–94.

32   Brown et al., "Diet-Induced Dysbiosis," 1095–119.

33   Bokic et al., "Potential Causes and Present Pharmacotherapy," 76–85.

34   Ruth E. Ley et al., "Microbial Ecology: Human Gut Microbes Associated with Obesity," *Nature* 444 (December 21, 2006): 1022–23.

35   Peter J. Turnbaugh et al., "An Obesity-Associated Gut Microbiome with Increased Capacity for Energy Harvest," *Nature* 444 (December 21, 2006): 1027–31.

36   Peter J. Turnbaugh et al., "A Core Gut Microbiome in Obese and Lean Twins," *Nature* 457 (January 22, 2009): 480–84.

37   Vanessa K. Ridaura et al., "Cultured Gut Microbiota from Twins Discordant for Obesity Modulate Adiposity and Metabolic Phenotypes in Mice," *Science* 341, no. 6150 (2013): doi: 10.1126/science.1241214.

38   Ibid.

39   Young, "Gut Instincts," newscientist.com/article/mg21628951.900-gut-instincts-the-secrets-of-your-second-brain.

40   Leandro Lobo et al., "The Interplay between Microbiota and Inflammation: Lessons from Peritonitis and Sepsis," *Clinical & Translational Immunology* 5, no. 7 (2016): E90, doi: 10.1038/cti.2016.32.

41   Kristin Schmidt et al., "Prebiotic Intake Reduces the Waking Cortisol Response and Alters Emotional Bias in Healthy Volunteers." *Psychopharmacology* 232, no. 10 (2015): 1793–1801.

Chapter 5

1   "How Are Overweight and Obesity Diagnosed?," National Heart, Lung, and Blood Institute, last modified July 13, 2012, https://www.nhlbi.nih.gov/health/health-topics/topics/obe/diagnosis.

2   http://apps.who.int/iris/bitstream/10665/148114/1/9789241564854_eng.pdf?ua=1

3   "Overweight and Obesity Statistics," National Institute of Diabetes and Digestive and Kidney Diseases, October 2012, niddk.nih.gov/health-information/health-statistics/Pages/overweight-obesity-statistics.aspx.

4   "Obesity Rates & Trends: Obesity among WIC Participants," The State of Obesity, November, 2016, stateofobesity.org/rates/.

5   "Leading Causes of Death," Centers for Disease Control and Prevention, last modified October, 7, 2016, cdc.gov/nchs/fastats/leading-causes-of-death.htm.

6   Amy R. Johnson et al., "The Inflammation Highway: Metabolism Accelerates Inflammatory Traffic in Obesity," *Immunological Reviews* 249, no. 1 (2012): 218–38.

7   Peter Mancuso, "The Role of Adipokines in Chronic Inflammation," *ImmunoTargets and Therapy* 5 (May 23, 2016): 47–56.

8   Johnson et al., "The Inflammation Highway," 218–38; Mancuso, "The Role of Adipokines," 47–56.

9   Ibid.

10   Eleni Karfopoulou et al., "Dietary Patterns in Weight Loss Maintenance: Results from the MedWeight Study," *European Journal of Nutrition* (2016): Epub ahead of print, doi:10.1007/s00394-015-1147-z.

11   Mark Lemstra et al., "Weight Loss Intervention Adherence and Factors Promoting Adherence: A Meta-Analysis," *Patient Preference and Adherence* 10 (August 12, 2016): 1547–59.

12   Jean-Philippe Chaput and Angelo Tremblay, "Adequate Sleep to Improve the Treatment of Obesity," *CMAJ* 184, no. 18 (2012): 1975–76.

13   Ines Santos et al., "Weight Control Behaviors of Highly Successful Weight Loss Maintainers: The Portuguese Weight Control Registry," *Journal of Behavioral Medicine* (2016): Epub ahead of print, doi:10.1007/s10865-016-9786-y.

14   Martinus Evans et al., "The Weight Loss Blogosphere: An Online Survey of Weight Loss Bloggers," *Translational Behavioral Medicine* 6, no. 3 (2016): 403–9.

15   Flavia M. Silva et al., "Effect of Diet on Adiponectin Levels in Blood," *Nutrition Reviews* 69, no. 10 (2011): 599–612.

16   Frank B. Hu et al., "Diet, Lifestyle, and the Risk of Type 2 Diabetes Mellitus in Women," *New England Journal of Medicine* 345 (September 13, 2001): 790–97.

17   "Diabetes," World Health Organization, November 2016, who.int/mediacentre/factsheets/fs312/en/.

18   "Simple Steps to Preventing Diabetes," The Nutrition Source, accessed November 22, 2016, hsph.harvard.edu/nutritionsource/preventing-diabetes-full -story/#ref53.

19   Nisa M. Maruther et al., "Early Response to Preventive Strategies in the Diabetes Prevention Program," *Journal of Internal General Medicine* 28, no. 12 (2013): 1629–36.

20   Vicki Conn et al., "Insulin Sensitivity following Exercise Interventions: Systematic Review and Meta-Analysis of Outcomes among Healthy Adults," *Journal of Primary Care & Community Health* 5, no. 3 (2014): 211–22; Kimberley L. Way et al., "The Effect of Regular Exercise on Insulin Sensitivity in Type 2 Diabetes Mellitus: A Systematic Review and Meta-Analysis," *Diabetes & Metabolism Journal* 40, no. 4 (2016): 253–71.

21   Justina Godos et al., "Adherence to the Mediterranean Diet Is Inversely Associated with Metabolic Syndrome Occurrence: A Meta-Analysis of Observational Studies," *International Journal of Food Sciences and Nutrition* (August 25, 2016): 1–11.

22   Hiba Bawadi et al., "Energy Balance and Macronutrient Distribution in Relation to C-Reactive Protein and HbA1c Levels among Patients with Type 2 Diabetes," *Food & Nutrition Research* 60 (May 27, 2016): 29904, doi: 10.3402/fnr.v60.29904.

23   Reza Meshkani and Sanaz Vakili, "Tissue Resident Macrophages: Key Players in the Pathogenesis of Type 2 Diabetes and Its Complications," *Clinica Chimica Acta* (2016): Epub ahead of print, doi: 10.1016/j.cca.2016.08.015.

24   Lara R. Dugas et al., "The Obese Gut Microbiome across the Epidemiologic Transition," *Emerging Themes in Epidemiology* 13 (January 11, 2016): 2, doi: 10.1186/s12982-015-0044-5.

25   R. Jumpertz et al., "Energy-Balance Studies Reveal Associations Between Gut Microbes, Caloric Load, and Nutrient Absorption in Humans," *American Journal of Clinical Nutrition* 94, no. 1 (2011): 58–65.

26   R. S. Kootte et al., "The Therapeutic Potential of Manipulating Gut Microbiota in Obesity and Type 2 Diabetes Mellitus," *Diabetes, Obesity and Metabolism* 14, no. 2 (2012): 112–20.

27   Gabriel A. Al-Ghalith et al., "The Guts of Obesity: Progress and Challenges in Linking Gut Microbes to Obesity," *Discovery Medicine* 19, no. 103 (2015): 81–88; Ana P. B. Moreira et al., "Influence of a High-Fat Diet on Gut Microbiota, Intestinal Permeability and Metabolic Endotoxaemia," *British Journal of Nutrition* 108, no. 5 (2012): 801–9.

28   Kootte et al., "The Therapeutic Potential of Manipulating Gut Microbiota," 112–20.

29   Davide Festi et al., "Gut Microbiota and Metabolic Syndrome," *World Journal of Gastroenterology* 20, no. 43 (2014): 16079–94.

30   Yukio Kadooka et al., "Regulation of Abdominal Adiposity by Probiotics (*Lactobacillus Gasseri* SBT2055) in Adults with Obese Tendencies in a Randomized Controlled Trial," *European Journal of Clinical Nutrition* 64, no. 6 (2010): 636–43.

31   Yukio Kadooka et al., "Effect of *Lactobacillus Gasseri* SBT2055 in Fermented Milk on Abdominal Adiposity in Adults in a Randomised Controlled Trial," *British Journal of Nutrition* 110, no. 9 (2013): 1696–1703.

32   Kootte et al., "The Therapeutic Potential of Manipulating Gut Microbiota," 112–20.

33   Fanny B. Morel et al., "α-Galacto-oligosaccharides Dose-Dependently Reduce Appetite and Decrease Inflammation in Overweight Adults," *Journal of Nutrition* 145, no. 9 (2015): 2052–59.

34   Elizabeth Selvin et al., "The Effect of Weight Loss on C-Reactive Protein: A Systematic Review," *Archives of Internal Medicine* 167, no. 1 (2007): 31–39.

35   Faidon Magkos et al., "Effects of Moderate and Subsequent Progressive Weight Loss on Metabolic Function and Adipose Tissue Biology in Humans with Obesity," 23, no. 4 (2016): 591–601.

36   Uma Mudaliar et al., "Cardiometabolic Risk Factor Changes Observed in Diabetes Prevention Programs in US Settings: A Systematic Review and Meta-Analysis," *PLoS Medicine* 13, no. 7 (2016): e1002095, doi: 10.1371/journal.pmed.1002095.

37   Joshua D. Brown et al., "Effects on Cardiovascular Risk Factors of Weight Losses Limited to 5–10," *Translational Behavioral Medicine* 6, no. 3 (2016): 339–46.

38   Kathryn M. Ross et al., "Successful Weight Loss Maintenance Associated with Morning Chronotype and Better Sleep Quality," *Journal of Behavioral Medicine* 39, no. 3 (2016): 465–71.

39   Emily Jane Gallagher and Derek LeRoith, "Obesity and Diabetes: The Increased Risk of Cancer and Cancer-Related Mortality," *Physiological Reviews* 95, no. 3 (2015): 727–48; Melina Arnold et al., "Duration of Adulthood Overweight, Obesity, and Cancer Risk in the Women's Health Initiative: A Longitudinal Study from the United States," *PLoS Medicine* 13, no. 8 (2016): e1002081, doi: 10.1371/journal .pmed.1002081.

40   Nidia Celest Horie et al., "Cognitive Effects of Intentional Weight Loss in Elderly Obese Individuals with Mild Cognitive Impairment," *Journal of Clinical Endocrinology & Metabolism* 101, no. 3 (2016): 1104–12.

41   Y. F. Chuang et al., "Midlife Adiposity Predicts Earlier Onset of Alzheimer's Dementia, Neuropathology and Presymptomatic Cerebral Amyloid Accumulation," *Molecular Psychiatry* 21, no. 7 (2015): 910–15.

42   Charles Swencionis et al., "Weight Change, Psychological Well-Being, and Vitality in Adults Participating in a Cognitive-Behavioral Weight Loss Program," *Health Psychology* 32, no. 4 (2013): 439–46.

43   Dario Giugliano et al., "The Effects of Diet on Inflammation: Emphasis on the Metabolic Syndrome," *Journal of the American College of Cardiology* 48, no. 4 (2006): 677–85.

44   Lisa Te Morenga et al., "Dietary Sugars and Body Weight: Systematic Review and Meta-Analyses of Randomised Controlled Trials and Cohort Studies," *BMJ* 346 (2013): e7492, doi: http://dx.doi.org/10.1136/bmj.e7492.

45   Wenpeng You and Maciej Henneberg, "Meat in Modern Diet, Just as Bad as Sugar, Correlates to Worldwide Obesity: An Ecological Analysis," *Journal of Nutrition & Food Sciences* 6, no. 4 (2016): doi: 10.4172/2155-9600.1000517.

46   "Bacon, Processed Meats a Cause of Cancer—Your FAQs," American Institute for Cancer Research, October 28, 2015, aicr.org/cancer-research-update/2015/10_28 /cru_Bacon-Processed-Meats-a-Cause-of-Cancer-Your-FAQs.html.

47   Rachel C. Masters et al., "Whole and Refined Grain Intakes are Related to Inflammatory Protein Concentrations in Human Plasma," *Journal of Nutrition* 140, no. 3 (2010): 587–94.

48   Xiaona Zhao et al., "Trans-Fatty Acids Aggravate Obesity, Insulin Resistance and Hepatic Steatosis in C57BL/6 Mice, Possibly by Suppressing the IRS1 Dependent Pathway," *Molecules* 21, no. 6 (2016): 705.

49   E. Patterson et al., "Health Implications of High Dietary Omega-6 Polyunsaturated Fatty Acids," *Journal of Nutrition and Metabolism* (2012): 539426, http://dx.doi .org/10.1155/2012/539426.

50   Silvia Lorente-Cebrián et al., "Role of Omega-3 Fatty Acids in Obesity, Metabolic Syndrome, and Cardiovascular Diseases: A Review of the Evidence," *Journal of Physiology and Biochemistry* 69, no. 3 (2013): 633–51.

51   Marta Guasch-Ferre et al., "Olive Oil Consumption and Risk of Type 2 Diabetes in US Women," *American Journal of Clinical Nutrition* 102, no. 2 (2015): 479–86.

52   C. Santangelo et al., "Consumption of Extra-Virgin Olive Oil Rich in Phenolic Compounds Improves Metabolic Control in Patients with Type 2 Diabetes Mellitus: A Possible Involvement of Reduced Levels of Circulating Visfatin," *Journal of Endocrinological Investigation* (2016): Epub ahead of print, doi:10.1007 /s40618-016-0506-9.

53   Rachel C. Brown et al., "Association of Nut Consumption with Cardiometabolic Risk Factors in the 2008/2009 New Zealand Adult Nutrition Survey," *Nutrients* 7, no. 9 (2015): 7523–42.

54   Mahmoud Parham et al., "Effects of Pistachio Nut Supplementation on Blood Glucose in Patients with Type 2 Diabetes: A Randomized Crossover Trial," *Review of Diabetic Studies* 11, no. 2 (2014): 190–96.

55   Pablo Hernández-Alonso et al., "Beneficial Effect of Pistachio Consumption on Glucose Metabolism, Insulin Resistance, Inflammation, and Related Metabolic Risk Markers: A Randomized Clinical Trial," *Diabetes Care* 37, no. 11 (2014): 3098–3105.

56   Kerry S. Kuehl, "Cherry Juice Targets Antioxidant Potential and Pain Relief," *Medicine and Sport Science* 59 (2012): 86–93.

57   M. Trinder et al., "Probiotic Lactobacilli: A Potential Prophylactic Treatment for Reducing Pesticide Absorption in Humans and Wildlife," *Beneficial Microbes* 6, no. 6 (2015): 841–47.

58   Jaako Mursu et al., "Intake of Fruit, Berries, and Vegetables and Risk of Type 2 Diabetes in Finnish Men: The Kuopio Ischaemic Heart Disease Risk Factor Study," *American Journal of Clinical Nutrition* 99, no. 2 (2014) 328–33.

59   Tamara Y. Forbes-Hernandez, "The Healthy Effects of Strawberry Polyphenols: Which Strategy behind Antioxidant Capacity?," supplement 1, *Critical Reviews in Food Science and Nutrition* 56 (July 29, 2016): S46–S59.

60   Sandi L. Navarro et al., "Cruciferous Vegetables Have Variable Effects on Biomarkers of Systemic Inflammation in a Randomized Controlled Trial in Healthy Young Adults," *Journal of Nutrition* 144, no. 11 (2014): 1850–57; Yu Jiang et al., "Cruciferous Vegetable Intake Is Inversely Correlated with Circulating Levels of Proinflammatory

Markers in Women," *Journal of the Academy of Nutrition and Dietetics* 114, no. 5 (2014): 700–708.

61   Wan-Shui Yang et al., "Tea Consumption and Risk of Type 2 Diabetes: A Dose-Response Meta-Analysis of Cohort Studies," *British Journal of Nutrition* 111, no. 8 (2014): 1329–39.

62   P. L. Janssens, "Nutraceuticals for Body-Weight Management: The Role of Green Tea Catechins," *Physiology & Behavior* 162 (August 1, 2016): 83–87.

63   Ana F. Vinha et al., "Pre-Meal Tomato (*Lycopersicon Esculentum*) Intake Can Have Anti-Obesity Effects in Young Women?" *International Journal of Food Sciences and Nutrition* 65, no. 8 (2014): 1019–26.

64   Britt Burton-Freeman et al., "Protective Activity of Processed Tomato Products on Postprandial Oxidation and Inflammation: A Clinical Trial in Healthy Weight Men and Women," *Molecular Nutrition and Food Research* 56, no. 4 (2012): 622–31.

65   H. P. Vasantha Rupasinghe et al., "Phytochemicals in Regulating Fatty Acid β-Oxidation: Potential Underlying Mechanisms and Their Involvement in Obesity and Weight Loss," *Pharmacology & Therapeutics* 165 (September 2016): 153–63.

Chapter 6

1   Darrel J. Gaskin and Patrick Richard, "The Economic Costs of Pain in the United States," *Journal of Pain* 13, no. 8 (2012): 715–24.

2   Albert Dahan et al., "Comorbidities and the Complexities of Chronic Pain," *Anesthesiology* 10, no. 121 (2014): 675–77.

3   María Dueñas et al., "A Review of Chronic Pain Impact on Patients, Their Social Environment and the Health Care System," *Journal of Pain Research* 9 (June 2016): 457–67.

4   Naomi Eisenberger et al., "In Sickness and in Health: The Co-Regulation of Inflammation and Social Behavior," *Neuropsychopharmacology* (2016): Epub ahead of print, doi: 10.1038/npp.2016.141.

5   Keiko Yamada et al., "Influence of Work-Related Psychosocial Factors on the Prevalence of Chronic Pain and Quality of Life in Patients with Chronic Pain." *BMJ* 6, no. 4 (2016): e010356, doi: 10.1136/bmjopen-2015-010356; Rannveig Fanavoll et al., "Psychosocial Work Stress, Leisure Time Physical Exercise and the Risk of Chronic Pain in the Neck/Shoulders: Longitudinal Data from the Norwegian HUNT Study," *International Journal of Occupational Medicine and Environmental Health* 29, no. 4 (2016): 585–95.

6   Jan Jaracz et al., "Unexplained Painful Physical Symptoms in Patients with Major Depressive Disorder: Prevalence, Pathophysiology and Management," *CNS Drugs* 30, no. 4 (2016): 293–304.

7   Diane Smith et al., "Chronic Pain and Mortality: A Systematic Review," *PLoS One* 9, no. 6 (2014): e99048, doi: 10.1371/journal.pone.0099048.

8   A. L. Hassett et al., "The Risk of Suicide Mortality in Chronic Pain Patients," *Current Pain and Headache Reports* 18, no. 8 (2014): 436; J. M. Hooley et al., "Chronic Pain and Suicide: Understanding the Association," *Current Pain and Headache Reports* 18, no. 8 (2014): 435.

9   Nicola Torrance et al., "Severe Chronic Pain Is Associated with Increased 10 Year Mortality. A Cohort Record Linkage Study," *European Journal of Pain* 14, no. 4 (2010): 380–86.

10   Milind M. Muley et al., "Preclinical Assessment of Inflammatory Pain," *CNS Neuroscience & Therapeutics* 22, no. 2 (2016): 88–101.

11   Ibid.

12   Jennifer M. Hootman et al., "Updated Projected Prevalence of Self-Reported Doctor-Diagnosed Arthritis and Arthritis-Attributable Activity Limitation Among US Adults, 2015-2040," *Arthritis & Rheumatology* 68, no. 7 (2016): 1582–87.

13   Kunal Kulkarni et al., "Obesity and Osteoarthritis," *Maturitas* 89 (July 2016): 22–28.

14   W. J. Carman et al., "Obesity as a Risk Factor for Osteoarthritis of the Hand and Wrist: A Prospective Study," *American Journal of Epidemiology* 139, no. 2 (1994): 119–29.

15   Siew-Li Goh et al., "Relative Efficacy of Different Types of Exercise for Treatment of Knee and Hip Osteoarthritis: Protocol for Network Meta-Analysis of Randomised Controlled Trials," *Systematic Reviews* 5, no. 1 (2016): 147.

16   Kok Yong Chin, "The Spice for Joint Inflammation: Anti-Inflammatory Role of Curcumin in Treating Osteoarthritis," *Drug Design, Development and Therapy* 10 (September 20, 2016): 3029–42.

17   Guido Shoba et al, "Influence of Piperine on the Pharmacokinetics of Curcumin in Animals and Human Volunteers," *Planta Medica* 64:4 (1998): 353–56.

18   Brad J. Douglass and Dallas L. Clouatre, "Beyond Yellow Curry: Assessing Commercial Curcumin Absorption Technologies," *Journal of the American College of Nutrition* 34:4 (2015): 347–58.

19   Krishnapura Srinivasan, "Biological Activities of Red Pepper (*Capsicum annuum*) and Its Pungent Principle Capsaicin: A Review," *Critical Reviews in Food Science and Nutrition* 56, no. 9 (2016): 1488–1500.

20   Salahuddin Ahmed, "Green Tea Polyphenol Epigallocatechin 3-Gallate in Arthritis: Progress and Promise," *Arthritis Research & Therapy* 12, no. 2 (2010): 208.

21   "Prevalence," National Fibromyalgia Association, accessed November 23, 2016, fmaware.org/about-fibromyalgia/prevalence/.

22   Kathleen A. Sluka and Daniel J. Clauw, "Neurobiology of Fibromyalgia and Chronic Widespread Pain," *Neuroscience* (2016): Epub ahead of print, doi: 10.1016 /j.neuroscience.2016.06.006.

23   Ibid.

24   A. Rossi et al., "Fibromyalgia and Nutrition: What News?," supplement 1, *Clinical and Experimental Rheumatology* 33, no. 88 (2015): S117–25.

25   C. E. Gota et al., "Fibromyalgia and Obesity: The Association between Body Mass Index and Disability, Depression, History of Abuse, Medications, and Comorbidities," *Journal of Clinical Rheumatology* 21, no. 6 (2015): 289–95.

26   Kenji Sanada et al., "Effects of Non-Pharmacological Interventions on Inflammatory Biomarker Expression in Patients with Fibromyalgia: A Systematic Review," *Arthritis Research & Therapy* 17 (September 26, 2015): 272, doi: 10.1186 /s13075-015-0789-9.

27   Kathleen Holton, "The Role of Diet in the Treatment of Fibromyalgia," *Pain Management* 6, no. 4 (2016): 317–20.

28   Kathleen Holton et al., "The Effect of Dietary Glutamate on Fibromyalgia and Irritable Bowel Symptoms," supplement 6, *Clinical and Experimental Rheumatology* 30, no. 74 (2012): 10–17.

29   Holton, "The Role of Diet in the Treatment of Fibromyalgia," 317–20.

30   Tyng-Guey Wang et al., "Is Serum Hypovitaminosis D Associated with Chronic Widespread Pain Including Fibromyalgia? A Meta-Analysis of Observational Studies," *Pain Physician* 18, no. 5 (2015): 877–87.

31   J. McBeth et al., "Extended Report: Musculoskeletal Pain Is Associated with Very Low Levels of Vitamin D in Men: Results from the European Male Ageing Study," *Annals of the Rheumatic Diseases* 69, no. 8 (2010): 1448–52.

32   Roland von Känel et al., "Vitamin D and Central Sensitivity in Patients with Chronic Pain," *Pain Medicine* 15, no. 9 (2014): 1609–18.

33   M. Okumus et al., "Fibromyalgia Syndrome: Is It Related to Vitamin D Deficiency in Premenopausal Female Patients?," *Pain Management Nursing* 14, no. 4 (2013): E156–63.

34   F. Wepner et al., "Effects of Vitamin D on Patients with Fibromyalgia Syndrome: A Randomized Placebo-Controlled Trial," *Pain* 155, no. 2 (2014): 261–68.

35   D. J. Armstrong et al., "Vitamin D Deficiency Is Associated with Anxiety and Depression in Fibromyalgia," *Clinical Rheumatology* 26, no. 4 (2007): 551–54.

36   http://nutritiondata.self.com/foods-000102000000000000000.html

37   M. Haugen et al., "Diet and Disease Symptoms in Rheumatic Diseases—Results of a Questionnaire Based Survey," *Clinical Rheumatology* 10, no. 4 (1991): 401–7.

38   F. Puccio et al., "Food Allergy Is an Important Diseases Associated to Fibromyalgia," supplement 3, *Clinical and Translational Allergy* 3 (July 25, 2013): P120, doi: 10.1186/2045-7022-3-S3-P120.

39   Ellen Gold et al., "The Association of Inflammation with Premenstrual Symptoms," *Journal of Women's Health* (2016): Epub ahead of print, doi: 10.1089/jwh.2015.5529.

40   Parvaneh Mirabi et al., "Effect of Medicinal Herbs on Primary Dysmenorrhoea—A Systematic Review," *Iranian Journal of Pharmaceutical Research* 13, no. 3 (2014): 757–67.

41   Seyedeh Zahra Masoumi et al., "Evaluation of Mint Efficacy Regarding Dysmenorrhea in Comparison with Mefenamic Acid: A Double Blinded Randomized Crossover Study," *Iranian Journal of Nursing and Midwifery Research* 21, no. 4 (2016): 363–67.

42   Molouk Jaafarpour et al., "Comparative Effect of Cinnamon and Ibuprofen for Treatment of Primary Dysmenorrhea: A Randomized Double-Blind Clinical Trial," *Journal of Clinical and Diagnostic Research* 9, no. 4 (2015): QC04–7.

43   Nahid Rahbar, "Effect of Omega-3 Fatty Acids on Intensity of Primary Dysmenorrhea," *International Journal of Gynecology and Obstetrics* 117, no. 1 (2012): 45–47.

44   Jaracz et al., "Unexplained Painful Physical Symptoms," 293–304.

45   Dahan et al., "Comorbidities and the Complexities," 675–77.

46   Jun-Ming Zhang and Jianxiong An. "Cytokines, Inflammation and Pain." *International Anesthesiology Clinics* 45.2 (2007): 27–37.

47   N. Eijkelkamp et al., "IL4-10 Fusion Protein Is a Novel Drug to Treat Persistent Inflammatory Pain," *Journal of Neuroscience* 36, no. 28 (2016): 7353–63.

48   Veronica I. Shubayev et al., "Chapter 8: Cytokines in Pain," in *Translational Pain Research: From Mouse to Man*, eds. L. Kruger and A. R. Light (Boca Raton, FL: CRC Press/Taylor & Francis, 2010), ncbi.nlm.nih.gov/books/NBK57275/.

49   Ibid.

50   Dahan et al., "Comorbidities and the Complexities," 675–77.

51   Rebecca Gordon and Saul Bloxham, "A Systematic Review of the Effects of Exercise and Physical Activity on Non-Specific Chronic Low Back Pain," *Healthcare* 4, no. 2 (2016): 22.

52   Andrew J. Vickers et al., "Acupuncture for Chronic Pain: Individual Patient Data Meta-Analysis," *Archives of Internal Medicine* 172, no. 19 (2012): 1444–53.

53   Robert Sielski et al., "Efficacy of Biofeedback for Chronic Back Pain: A Meta-Analysis," *International Journal of Behavioral Medicine* (2016): Epub ahead of print, doi: 10.1007/s12529-016-9572-9.

54   Lawrence Leung, "Pain Catastrophizing: An Updated Review," *Indian Journal of Psychological Medicine* 34, no. 3 (2012): 204–17.

55   J. Lasselin et al., "Low-Grade Inflammation May Moderate the Effect of Behavioral Treatment for Chronic Pain in Adults," *Journal of Behavioral Medicine* (2016): Epub ahead of print, doi: 10.1007/s10865-016-9769-z.

56   Whitney Scott et al., "A Comprehensive Examination of Changes in Psychological Flexibility Following Acceptance and Commitment Therapy for Chronic Pain," *Journal of Contemporary Psychotherapy* 46, no. 3 (2016): 139–48; L. S. Hughes et al., "Acceptance and Commitment Therapy (ACT) for Chronic Pain: A Systematic Review and Meta Analyses," *Clinical Journal of Pain* (2016): Epub ahead of print, doi: 10.1097/AJP.0000000000000425.

57   Fadel Zeidan et al., "The Effects of Brief Mindfulness Meditation Training on Experimentally Induced Pain," *Journal of Pain* 11, no. 3 (2010): 199–209.

Chapter 7

1   J. Sokolove et al., "Increased Inflammation and Disease Activity among Current Cigarette Smokers with Rheumatoid Arthritis: A Cross-Sectional Analysis of US Veterans," *Rheumatology* (2016): Epub ahead of print, doi: 10.1093/rheumatology/kew285.

2   Serena Schippa and Maria Pia Conte, "Dysbiotic Events in Gut Microbiota: Impact on Human Health," *Nutrients* 6, no. 12 (2014): 5786–805.

3   Elizabeth C. Rosser and Claudia Mauri, "A Clinical Update on the Significance of the Gut Microbiota in Systemic Autoimmunity," *Journal of Autoimmunity* (2016): Epub ahead of print, doi: 10.1016/j.jaut.2016.06.009; Kirsty Brown et al., "Diet-Induced Dysbiosis of the Intestinal Microbiota and the Effects on Immunity and Disease," *Nutrients* 4, no. 8 (2012): 1095–119.

4   Aaron Lerner et al., "The World Incidence and Prevalence of Autoimmune Diseases Is Increasing," *International Journal of Celiac Disease* 3, no. 4 (2015): 151–55.

5   Aaron Lerner and Torsten Matthias, "Changes in Intestinal Tight Junction Permeability Associated with Industrial Food Additives Explain the Rising Incidence of Autoimmune Disease," *Autoimmunity Reviews* 14, no. 6 (2015): 479–89.

6   Pietro E. Lazzerini et al., "Systemic Inflammation and Arrhythmic Risk: Lessons from Rheumatoid Arthritis," *European Heart Journal* (2016): Epub ahead of print, doi: http://dx.doi.org/10.1093/eurheartj/ehw208; Pietro E. Lazzerini et al., "Association between High Sensitivity C-Reactive Protein, Heart Rate Variability and Corrected QT Interval in Patients with Chronic Inflammatory Arthritis," *European Journal of Internal Medicine* 24, no. 4 (2013): 368–74.

7   Pietro E. Lazzerini et al., "Antiarrhythmic Potential of Anticytokine Therapy in Rheumatoid Arthritis: Tocilizumab Reduces Corrected QT Interval by Controlling Systemic Inflammation," *Arthritis Care & Research* 67, no. 3 (2015): 332–39.

8   Ibid.

9   K. R. Feingold and C. Grunfield, "Effect of Inflammation on HDL Structure and Function," *Current Opinion in Lipidology* (2016): Epub ahead of print, doi: 10.1097/MOL.0000000000000333.

10   R. Casas et al., "Long-Term Immunomodulatory Effects of a Mediterranean Diet in Adults at High Risk of Cardiovascular Disease in the PREvención con DIeta MEDiterránea Randomized Controlled Trial," *Journal of Nutrition* (2016): Epub ahead of print, doi: 10.3945/jn.115.229476.

11   Andrea Picchianti Diamanti et al., "Microbiota and Chronic Inflammatory Arthritis: An Interwoven Link," *Journal of Translational Medicine* 14, no. 1 (2016): 233.

12   Ibid.

13   Karin Klack et al., "Diet and Nutritional Aspects in Systemic Lupus Erythematosus," *Revista Brasileira de Reumatologia* 52, no. 3 (2012): 384–408.

14   Mariane Curado Borges et al., "Polyunsaturated Omega-3 Acids and Systemic Lupus Erythematosus: What Do We Know?," *Revista Brasileira de Reumatologia* 54, no. 6 (2014): 459–66.

15   Cristina Arriens et al., "Placebo-Controlled Randomized Clinical Trial of Fish Oil's Impact on Fatigue, Quality of Life, and Disease Activity in Systemic Lupus Erythematosus," *Nutrition Journal* 14 (August 18, 2015): 82.

16   Carol M. Greco et al., "Updated Review of Complementary and Alternative Medicine Treatments for Systemic Lupus Erythematosus," *Current Rheumatology Reports* 15, no. 11 (2013): 378.

17   Anna Abou-Raya et al., "The Effect of Vitamin D Supplementation on Inflammatory and Hemostatic Markers and Disease Activity in Patients with Systemic Lupus Erythematosus: A Randomized Placebo-Controlled Trial," *Journal of Rheumatology* 40, no. 3 (2013): 265–72.

18   Ibid.

19   Parvi Khajehdehi, "Oral Supplementation of Turmeric Decreases Proteinuria, Hematuria, and Systolic Blood Pressure in Patients Suffering from Relapsing or

Refractory Lupus Nephritis: A Randomized and Placebo-Controlled Study," *Journal of Renal Nutrition* 22, no. 1 (2012): 50–57.

20 J. J. Bright, "Curcumin and Autoimmune Disease," *Advances in Experimental Medicine and Biology* 595 (2007): 425–51.

21 S. van Beugen et al., "Predictors of Perceived Stigmatization in Patients with Psoriasis," *British Journal of Dermatology* (July 20, 2016): Epub ahead of print, doi: 10.1111/bjd.14875.

22 R. C. Lamb et al., "Screening for Anxiety and Depression in People with Psoriasis: A Cross Sectional Study in a Tertiary Referral Setting," *British Journal of Dermatology* (July 20, 2016): Epub ahead of print, doi: 10.1111/bjd.14833.

23 Krzystof Owczarek and Mariusz Jaworski, "Quality of Life and Severity of Skin Changes in the Dynamics of Psoriasis," *Advances in Dermatology and Allergology/ Postępy Dermatologii i Alergologii* 33, no. 2 (2016): 102–8.

24 Bhavnit K. Bhatia et al., "Diet and Psoriasis: Part 2. Celiac Disease and Role of a Gluten-Free Diet," *Journal of the American Academy of Dermatology* 71, no. 2 (2014): 350–58.

25 J. F. Ludvigsson et al., "Psoriasis in a Nationwide Cohort Study of Patients with Celiac Disease," *Journal of Investigative Dermatology* 131, no. 10 (2011): 2010–16.

26 B. Correia et al., "Obesity: A Key Component of Psoriasis," *Acto Bio-Medica* 86, no. 2 (2015): 121–29.

27 Peter Jensen et al., "Effect of Weight Loss on the Severity of Psoriasis," *JAMA Dermatology* 149, no. 7 (2013): 795–801.

28 Peter Jensen et al., "Long-Term Effects of Weight Reduction on the Severity of Psoriasis in a Cohort Derived from a Randomized Trial: A Prospective Observational Follow-Up Study," *American Journal of Clinical Nutrition* 104, no. 2 (2016): 259–65.

29 Andreas Daiber et al., "Targeting Vascular (Endothelial) Dysfunction," *British Journal of Pharmacology* (2016): Epub ahead of print, doi: 10.1111/bph.13517.

30 Kerstin Wolk and Robert Sabat, "Adipokines in Psoriasis: An Important Link Between Skin Inflammation and Metabolic Alterations," *Reviews in Endocrine & Metabolic Disorders* (2016): Epub ahead of print, doi: 10.1007/s11154-016-9381-0.

31 H. B. Naik et al., "Severity of Psoriasis Associates with Aortic Vascular Inflammation Detected by FDG PET/CT and Neutrophil Activation in a Prospective Observational Study," *Arteriosclerosis, Thrombosis, and Vascular Biology* 35, no. 12 (2015): 2667–76.

32 "Anti-Inflammatory Diet," National Psoriasis Foundation, accessed November 25, 2016, psoriasis.org/treating-psoriasis/complementary-and-alternative/diet-and -nutrition/anti-inflammatory-diet.

33 "What Is Celiac Disease?," Celiac Disease Foundation, accessed November 25, 2016, celiac.org/celiac-disease/what-is-celiac-disease/.

34 R. Pillon et al., "Prevalence of Celiac Disease in Patients with Severe Food Allergy," *Allergy* 70, no. 10 (2015): 2346–49.

35 Aya M. Westbrook et al., "Mouse Models of Intestinal Inflammation and Cancer," *Archives of Toxicology* 90, no. 9 (2016): 2109–30.

36   Irene Marafini et al., "Celiac Disease-Related Inflammation Is Marked by Reduction of Nkp44/Nkp46-Double Positive Natural Killer Cells," *PLoS ONE* 11, no. 5 (2016): e0155103, doi: 10.1371/journal.pone.0155103.

37   M. W. Schaart and M. L. Mearin, "Early Nutrition: Prevention of Celiac Disease?," supplement 1, *Journal of Pediatric Gastroenterology and Nutrition* 59 (July 2014): S18–S20.

38   M. L. Mearin, "Celiac Disease: Prevention in Children," *Digestive Diseases* 33, no. 2 (2015): 162–66.

39   M. L. Mearin, "The Prevention of Celiac Disease," *Best Practices & Research: Clinical Gastroenterology* 29, no. 3 (2015): 493–501.

40   Giovanni Marasco et al., "Gut Microbiota and Celiac Disease," *Digestive Diseases and Sciences* 61, no. 6 (2016): 1461–72.

41   Ruby Pawankar, "Allergic Diseases and Asthma: A Global Public Health Concern and a Call to Action," *World Allergy Organization Journal* 7, no. 1 (2014): 12.

42   Ruby Pawankar et al., eds., *World Allergy Organization (WAO) White Book on Allergy: Update 2013*, worldallergy.org/UserFiles/file/WhiteBook2-2013-v8.pdf.

43   Sally F. Bloomfield et al., "Time to Abandon the Hygiene Hypothesis: New Perspectives on Allergic Disease, the Human Microbiome, Infectious Disease Prevention and the Role of Targeted Hygiene," *Perspectives in Public Health* 136, no. 4 (2016): 213–24.

44   Ibid.

45   Richard R. Rosenkranz et al., "Dietary Factors Associated with Lifetime Asthma or Hayfever Diagnosis in Australian Middle-Aged and Older Adults: A Cross-Sectional Study," *Nutrition Journal* 11 (2012): 84.

46   Pawankar, "Allergic Diseases and Asthma," 12.

47   Brown et al., "Diet-Induced Dysbiosis of the Intestinal Microbiota," 1095–119.

48   Pawankar et al., eds., *World Allergy Organization (WAO) White Book on Allergy*, worldallergy.org/UserFiles/file/WhiteBook2-2013-v8.pdf.

49   Ekaterina Maslova et al., "Consumption of Artificially-Sweetened Soft Drinks in Pregnancy and Risk of Child Asthma and Allergic Rhinitis," *PLoS ONE* 8, no. 2 (2013): e57261, http://dx.doi.org/10.1371/journal.pone.0057261.

50   George du Toit et al., "Randomized Trial of Peanut Consumption in Infants at Risk for Peanut Allergy," *New England Journal of Medicine* 372 (2015): 803–13.

51   David M. Fleischer et al., "Consensus Communication on Early Peanut Introduction and the Prevention of Peanut Allergy in High-Risk Infants," *Pediatrics* 136, no. 3 (2015): 600–604.

52   M. Kuitunen, "Probiotics and Prebiotics in Preventing Food Allergy & Eczema," *Current Opinion in Preventing Food Allergy and Eczema* 13, no. 3 (2013): 280–86.

53   Yannick Perrin et al., "Comparison of Two Oral Probiotic Preparations in a Randomized Crossover Trial Highlights a Potentially Beneficial Effect of *Lactobacillus Paracasei* NCC2461 in Patients with Allergic Rhinitis," *Clinical and Translational Allergy* 4, no. 1 (2014): 1.

54   A. Singh et al., "Immune-Modulatory Effect of Probiotic *Bifidobacterium Lactis* NCC2818 in Individuals Suffering from Seasonal Allergic Rhinitis to Grass Pollen:

An Exploratory, Randomized, Placebo-Controlled Clinical Trial," *European Journal of Clinical Nutrition* 67, no. 2 (2013): 161–67.

Chapter 8

1 Aoife O'Donovan et al., "Altered Inflammatory Activity Associated with Reduced Hippocampal Volume and More Severe Posttraumatic Stress Symptoms in Gulf War Veterans," *Psychoneuroendocrinology* 51 (January 2015): 557–66.

2 Brianne M. Bettcher et al., "C-Reactive Protein Is Related to Memory and Medial Temporal Brain Volume in Older Adults," *Brain, Behavior, and Immunity* 26, no. 1 (2012): 103–8.

3 Theoharis Theoharides et al., "Brain 'Fog,' Inflammation and Obesity: Key Aspects of Neuropsychiatric Disorders Improved by Luteolin," *Frontiers in Neuroscience* 9 (July 3, 2015): 225.

4 D. B. McKim et al., "Neuroinflammatory Dynamics Underlie Memory Impairments after Repeated Social Defeat," *Journal of Neuroscience* 36, no. 9 (2016): 2590–2604.

5 Emmanuelle Kesse-Guyot et al., "Total and Specific Polyphenol Intakes in Midlife Are Associated with Cognitive Function Measured 13 Years Later," *Journal of Nutrition* 142, no. 1 (2012): 76–83.

6 Belkacemi Abdenour and Ramassamy Charles, "Innovative Anthocyanin Formulation Protects Neuronal-Like Cells against Oxidative Stress-Induced Damage: Pharmacotherapeutic Application for Alzheimer's Disease," supplement 1, *Free Radical Biology & Medicine* 75, no. 1 (2014): S1–S45.

7 Shibu M. Poulose et al., "Effects of Pterostilbene and Resveratrol on Brain and Behavior," *Neurochemistry International* 89 (October 2015): 227–33.

8 "World Alzheimer Report 2015: The Global Impact of Dementia: An Analysis of Prevalence, Incidence, Cost and Trends: Summary Sheet," Alzheimer's Disease International, accessed November 25, 2016, alz.co.uk/research/World AlzheimerReport2015-sheet.pdf.

9 "Alzheimer's & Dementia," Alzheimer's Association, accessed November 25, 2016, alz.org/dementia/types-of-dementia.asp.

10 Alain Koyama et al., "The Role of Peripheral Inflammatory Markers in Dementia and Alzheimer's Disease: A Meta-Analysis," *Journals of Gerontology: Series A Biological Sciences and Medical Sciences* 68, no. 4 (2013): 433–40.

11 Guochao Zhong et al., "Smoking Is Associated with an Increased Risk of Dementia: A Meta-Analysis of Prospective Cohort Studies with Investigation of Potential Effect Modifiers," *PLoS ONE* 10, no. 3 (2015): e0118333, doi: 10.1371/journal .pone.0118333.

12 Maximilian Wiesmann et al., "Vascular Aspects of Cognitive Impairment and Dementia," *Journal of Cerebral Blood Flow & Metabolism* 33, no. 11 (2013): 1696–1706.

13 Behnaz Shakersain et al., "Prudent Diet May Attenuate the Adverse Effects of Western Diet on Cognitive Decline," *Alzheimer's & Dementia* 12, no. 2 (2016): 100–109.

14   Sophie Dutheil et al., "High-Fat Diet Induced Anxiety and Anhedonia: Impact on Brain Homeostasis and Inflammation," *Neuropsychopharmacology* 41, no. 7 (2016): 1874–87.

15   Deepak Kumar et al., "Amyloid-β Peptide Protects Against Microbial Infection in Mouse and Worm Models of Alzheimer's Disease," *Science Translational Medicine* 8, no. 340 (2016): 340–72.

16   "Human Amyloid-Beta Acts as Natural Antibiotic in the Brain: Alzheimer's-Associated Amyloid Plaques May Trap Microbes," ScienceDaily, May 25, 2016, sciencedaily.com/releases/2016/05/160525161351.htm.

17   Ibid.

18   Ruth Itzhaki et al., "Microbes and Alzheimer's Disease," *Journal of Alzheimer's Disease* 51, no. 4 (2016): 979–84.

19   Breno S. Diniz et al., "Higher Serum sTNFR1 Level Predicts Conversion from Mild Cognitive Impairment to Alzheimer's Disease," *Journal of Alzheimer's Disease* 22, no. 4 (2010): 1305–11.

20   X. Cheng et al., "Targeting TNF: A Therapeutic Strategy for Alzheimer's Disease," *Drug Discovery Today* 19, no. 11 (2014): 1822–27.

21   Mark E. McCaulley and Kira A. Grush, "Alzheimer's Disease: Exploring the Role of Inflammation and Implications for Treatment," *International Journal of Alzheimer's Disease* (2015): http://dx.doi.org/10.1155/2015/515248.

22   John C. Breitner et al., "Extended Results of the Alzheimer Disease Anti-Inflammatory Prevention Trial (ADAPT)," *Alzheimer's & Dementia* 7, no. 4 (2011): 402–11.

23   Tony Wyss-Coray and Joseph Rogers, "Inflammation in Alzheimer Disease—A Brief Review of the Basic Science and Clinical Literature," *Cold Spring Harbor Perspectives in Medicine* 2, no. 1 (2012): doi: 10.1101/cshperspect.a006346.

24   Hui Chen et al., "Folic Acid Supplementation Mitigates Alzheimer's Disease by Reducing Inflammation: A Randomized Controlled Trial," *Mediators of Inflammation* (2016): http://dx.doi.org/10.1155/2016/5912146.

25   Abraham Reichenberg et al., "Cytokine-Associated Emotional and Cognitive Disturbances in Humans," *JAMA Psychiatry* 58, no. 5 (2001): 445–52.

26   Ellen Gold et al., "The Association of Inflammation with Premenstrual Symptoms," *Journal of Women's Health* (May 2016): Epub ahead of print, doi:10.1089/jwh.2015.5529.

27   J. L. Gordon et al., "Cardiovascular, Hemodynamic, Neuroendocrine, and Inflammatory Markers in Women with and without Vasomotor Symptoms," *Menopause* (2016): Epub ahead of print, doi: 10.1097/GME.0000000000000689.

28   Marie-Claude Audet et al., "Cytokine Variations and Mood Disorders: Influence of Social Stressors and Social Support," *Frontiers in Neuroscience* 8 (2014): 416.

29   Charles L. Raison et al., "A Randomized Controlled Trial of the Tumor Necrosis Factor-Alpha Antagonist Infliximab in Treatment Resistant Depression: Role of Baseline Inflammatory Biomarkers," *JAMA Psychiatry* 70, no. 1 (2013): 31–41.

30   Juan Joseph Young et al., "Is There Progress? An Overview of Selecting Biomarker Candidates for Major Depressive Disorder," *Frontiers in Psychiatry* 7 (2016): 72.

31   M. Soledad Cepeda et al., "Depression Is Associated with High Levels of C-Reactive Protein and Low Levels of Fractional Exhaled Nitric Oxide," *Journal of Clinical Psychiatry* (2016): Epub ahead of print, doi: 10.4088/JCP.15m10267.

32   Aoife O'Donovan et al., "Suicidal Ideation Is Associated with Elevated Inflammation in Patients with Major Depressive Disorder," *Depression and Anxiety* 30, no. 4 (2013): 307–14.

33   Maria Almond, "Depression and Inflammation: Examining the Link," *Current Psychiatry* 12, no. 6 (2013): 24–32.

34   Charles L. Raison et al., "Neuropsychiatric Adverse Effects of Interferon-A: Recognition and Management," *CNS Drugs* 19, no. 2 (2005): 105–23.

35   Robert Dantzer et al., "From Inflammation to Sickness and Depression: When the Immune System Subjugates the Brain," *Nature Reviews Neuroscience* 9, no. 1 (2008): 46–56.

36   J. Krogh et al., "The Association Between Depressive Symptoms, Cognitive Function, and Inflammation in Major Depression," *Brain, Behavior, and Immunity* 35 (January 2014): 70–76.

37   Judith H. Lichtman et al., "Depression and Coronary Heart Disease," *Circulation* 118, no. 17 (2008): 1768–75.

38   Brenda Pennix, "Depression and Cardiovascular Disease: Epidemiological Evidence on Their Linking Mechanisms," *Neuroscience & Biobehavioral Reviews* (2016): Epub ahead of print, doi:10.1016/j.neubiorev.2016.07.003.

39   Ole Kohler et al., "Effect of Anti-inflammatory Treatment on Depression, Depressive Symptoms, and Adverse Effects," *JAMA Psychiatry* 71, no. 12 (2014): 1381–91.

40   Felger, "The Role of Dopamine in Inflammation-Associated Depression," doi: 10.1007/7854_2016_13.

41   Maria Almond, "Depression and Inflammation: Examining the Link," *Current Psychiatry* 12, no. 6 (2013): 24–32.

42   F. N. Kaufmann et al., "Curcumin in Depressive Disorders: An Overview of Potential Mechanisms, Preclinical and Clinical Findings," *European Journal of Pharmacology* 5, no. 784 (2016): 192–98.

43   Cecile Grudet et al., "Suicidal Patients Are Deficient in Vitamin D, Associated with a Pro-Inflammatory Status in the Blood," *Psychoneuroendocrinology* 50 (December 2014): 210–19.

44   Giuseppe Grosso et al., "Role of Omega-3 Fatty Acids in the Treatment of Depressive Disorders: A Comprehensive Meta-Analysis of Randomized Clinical Trials," *PLoS ONE* 9, no. 5 (2014): e96905, doi: 10.1371/journal.pone.0096905.

45   D. Révész et al., "Depressive and Anxiety Disorders and Short Leukocyte Telomere Length: Mediating Effects of Metabolic Stress and Lifestyle Factors," *Psychological Medicine* 46, no. 11 (2016): 2337–49.

46   Josine E. Verhoeven et al., "Anxiety Disorders and Accelerated Cellular Ageing," *British Journal of Psychiatry* 206, no. 5 (2015): 371–78.

47   Martin Root et al., "Flavonol Intake and Cognitive Decline in Middle-Aged Adults," *Journal of Medicinal Food* 18, no. 12 (2015): 1327–32.

48   Theoharides et al., "Brain 'Fog,' Inflammation and Obesity," 225.

Chapter 9

1   "Heart Disease and Stroke Statistics—At-a-Glance," American Heart Association, accessed November 25, 2016, heart.org/idc/groups/ahamahpublic/@wcm/@sop/@smd/documents/downloadable/ucm_470704.pdf.

2   J. Lee et al., "Cigarette Smoking and Inflammation: Cellular and Molecular Mechanisms," *Journal of Dental Research* 91, no. 2 (2012): 142–49.

3   Andreas Daiber et al., "Targeting Vascular (Endothelial) Dysfunction," *British Journal of Pharmacology* (2016): Epub ahead of print, doi: 10.1111/bph.13517.

4   H. B. Naik et al., "Severity of Psoriasis Associates with Aortic Vascular Inflammation Detected by FDG PET/CT and Neutrophil Activation in a Prospective Observational Study," *Arteriosclerosis, Thrombosis, and Vascular Biology* 35, no. 12 (2015): 2667–76.

5   J. I. Silverberg and P. Greenland, "Eczema and Cardiovascular Risk Factors in 2 Adult U.S. Populations," *Journal of Allergy and Clinical Immunology* 135, no. 3 (2015): 721–28.

6   Lee et al., "Cigarette Smoking and Inflammation," 142–49.

7   Ibid.

8   Arif Yurdagul et al., "The Arterial Microenvironment: The Where and Why of Atherosclerosis," *Biochemical Journal* 473, no. 10 (2016): 1281–95.

9   "Who Is at Risk for Atherosclerosis?," National Heart, Lung, and Blood Institute, last modified June 22, 2016, www.nhlbi.nih.gov/health/health-topics/topics/atherosclerosis/atrisk.

10   Frederik Strang and Heribert Schunkert, "C-Reactive Protein and Coronary Heart Disease: All Said—Is Not It?," *Mediators of Inflammation* (2014): http://dx.doi.org/10.1155/2014/757123; Oliver Zimmermann et al., "C-Reactive Protein in Human Atherogenesis: Facts and Fiction," *Mediators of Inflammation* (2014): http://dx.doi.org/10.1155/2014/561428.

11   Yurdagul et al., "The Arterial Microenvironment," 1281–95.

12   Carmen P. Wong et al., "Induction of Regulatory T Cells by Green Tea Polyphenol EGCG," *Immunology Letters* 139, no. 1–2 (2011): 7–13.

13   S. Gao et al., "Curcumin Induces M2 Macrophage Polarization by Secretion IL-4 and/or IL-13," *Journal of Molecular and Cellular Cardiology* 85 (August 2015): 131–39.

14   Saleta Sierra et al., "Intestinal and Immunological Effects of Daily Oral Administration of *Lactobacillus Salivarius* CECT5713 to Healthy Adults," *Anaerobe* 10, no. 3 (2010): 195–200.

15   James E. McLaren et al., "Cytokines, Macrophage Lipid Metabolism and Foam Cells: Implications for Cardiovascular Disease Therapy," *Progress in Lipid Research* 50, no. 4 (2011): 331–47.

16   Alan R. Tall and Laurent Yvan-Charvet, "Cholesterol, Inflammation, and Innate Immunity," *Nature Reviews Immunology* 15, no. 2 (2015): 104–16.

17   Paul M. Ridker, "Clinical Application of C-Reactive Protein for Cardiovascular Disease Detection and Prevention," *Circulation* 107, no. 3 (2003): 363–69.

18   Strang and Schunkert, "C-Reactive Protein and Coronary Heart Disease," http://dx.doi.org/10.1155/2014/757123.

19   Francisco A. H. Fonseca and Maria Cristina de Oliveira Izar, "High-Sensitivity C-Reactive Protein and Cardiovascular Disease across Countries and Ethnicities," *Clinics* 71, no. 4 (2016): 235–42.

20   Diederik F. van Wijk et al., "C-Reactive Protein Identifies Low-Risk Metabolically Healthy Obese Persons: The European Prospective Investigation of Cancer–Norfolk Prospective Population Study," *Journal of the American Heart Association* 5, no. 6 (2016): doi: 10.1161/JAHA.115.002823.

21   James E. Brown et al., "Intermittent Fasting: A Dietary Intervention for Prevention of Diabetes and Cardiovascular Disease?," *British Journal of Diabetes and Vascular Disease* 13, no. 2 (2013): 68–72.

22   Mabrouka E. L. Oudi et al., "Homocysteine and Markers of Inflammation in Acute Coronary Syndrome," *Experimental & Clinical Cardiology* 15, no. 2 (2010): E25–28.

23   Paul Ganguly and Sreyoshi Fatima Alam, "Role of Homocysteine in the Development of Cardiovascular Disease," *Nutrition Journal* 14 (2015): 6.

24   Ibid.

25   Michelle A. Albert et al., "Effect of Statin Therapy on C-Reactive Protein Levels: The Pravastatin Inflammation/CRP Evaluation (PRINCE): A Randomized Trial and Cohort Study," *JAMA* 286, no. 1 (2001): 64–70.

26   Paul M. Ridker, "A Test in Context: High-Sensitivity C-Reactive Protein," *Journal of the American College of Cardiology* 67, no. 6 (2016): 712–23.

27   O. L. Bokeriya, "Meta-Analysis of Clinical Studies on the Use of Statins for Prevention of Atrial Fibrillation Soon After Coronary Bypass Surgery," *Klinicheskia Meditsina* 94, no. 2 (2016): 85–92.

28   Minxiong Li et al., "The Prevention of Statins against AKI and Mortality Following Cardiac Surgery: A Meta-Analysis," *International Journal of Cardiology* 222 (November 1, 2016): 260–66.

39   Zhennan Li, "Effects of Statin Therapy on Progression of Mild Noncalcified Coronary Plaque Assessed by Serial Coronary Computed Tomography Angiography: A Multicenter Prospective Study," *American Heart Journal* 180 (2016): 29–38.

30   Ryan Ungaro et al., "Statins Associated with Decreased Risk of New Onset Inflammatory Bowel Disease," *American Journal of Gastroenterology* (2016): Epub ahead of print, doi: 10.1038/ajg.2016.233.

31   Lynnette J. Riddell et al., "Dietary Strategies for Lowering Homocysteine Concentrations," *American Journal of Clinical Nutrition* 71, no. 6 (2000): 1448–54.

32   Rory Collins et al., "Interpretation of the Evidence for the Efficacy and Safety of Statin Therapy," *Lancet* (2016): Epub ahead of print, doi: 10.1016/S0140 -6736(16)31357-5.

33   A.J. Rahal et al., "Do Statins Really Cause Diabetes? A Meta-Analysis of Major Randomized Controlled Clinical Trials," *Saudi Medical Journal* 37, no. 10 (2016): 1051–60.

34   "Heart Disease and Aspirin Therapy," American Heart Association, January 23, 2015, news.heart.org/heart-disease-aspirin-therapy/.

35   "How Does Smoking Affect the Heart and Blood Vessels?," National Heart, Lung, and Blood Institute, last modified June 22, 2016, www.nhlbi.nih.gov/health /health-topics/topics/smo.

36   Andrew S. Greenberg and Martin S. Obin, "Obesity and the Role of Adipose Tissue in Inflammation and Metabolism," *American Journal of Clinical Nutrition* 83, no. 2 (2006): S461S–65.

37   Harman S. Mattu and Harpal S. Randeva, "Role of Adipokines in Cardiovascular Disease," *Journal of Endocrinology* 216, no. 1 (2013): T17–36.

38   Robert Soufer et al., "Body Mass Index and Risk for Mental Stress Induced Ischemia in Coronary Artery Disease," *Molecular Medicine* 22 (2016): Epub ahead of print, doi: 10.2119/molmed.2016.00128.

39   B. J. Howard et al., "Associations of Overall Sitting Time and TV Viewing Time with Fibrinogen and C Reactive Protein: The AusDiab Study," *British Journal of Sports Medicine* 49, no. 4 (2015): 255–58.

40   F. B. Benatti and M. Reid-Larsen, "The Effects of Breaking up Prolonged Sitting Time: A Review of Experimental Studies," *Medicine and Science in Sports and Exercise* 47, no. 10 (2015): 2053–61.

41   Michael Gleeson et al., "The Anti-Inflammatory Effects of Exercise: Mechanisms and Implications for the Prevention and Treatment of Disease," *Nature Reviews: Immunology* 11, no. 9 (2011): 607–15.

42   Tracy L. Hammonds et al., "Effects of Exercise on C-Reactive Protein in Healthy Patients and in Patients with Heart Disease: A Meta-Analysis," *Heart & Lung* 45, no. 3 (2016): 273–82.

Chapter 10

1   Angus G. Dalgleish et al., "Randomised, Open-Label, Phase II Study of Gemcitabine with and without IMM-101 for Advanced Pancreatic Cancer," *British Journal of Cancer* (2016): Epub ahead of print, doi: 10.1038/bjc.2016.271.

2   Haitian Lu et al., "Inflammation, a Key Event in Cancer Development," *Molecular Cancer Research* 4, no. 4 (2006): 221–33; Seth Rakoff-Nahoum, "Why Cancer and Inflammation?," *Yale Journal of Biology and Medicine* 79, no. 3–4 (2006): 123–130; Rudi Beyaert et al., "Cancer Risk in Immune-Mediated Inflammatory Diseases (IMID)," *Molecular Cancer* 12 (2013): 98.

3   Ibid.

4   Madhuri Koti et al., "A Distinct Pre-Existing Inflammatory Tumour Microenvironment Is Associated with Chemotherapy Resistance in High-Grade Serous Epithelial Ovarian Cancer," *British Journal of Cancer* 112 (2015): 1215–22.

5   Orsolya Kiraly et al., "Inflammation-Induced Cell Proliferation Potentiates DNA Damage-Induced Mutations *In Vivo*," *PLoS Genetics* 11, no. 2 (2015): e1004901, http://dx.doi.org/10.1371/journal.pgen.1004901.

6   Kristine H. Allin et al., "Inflammatory Biomarkers and Risk of Cancer in 84,000 Individuals from the General Population," *International Journal of Cancer* 139, no. 7 (2016): 1493–1500.

7   "Harms of Cigarette Smoking and Health Benefits of Quitting," National Cancer Institute, December 3, 2014, cancer.gov/about-cancer/causes-prevention/risk /tobacco/cessation-fact-sheet.

8   "Cancer," World Health Organization, last modified February 2015, who.int /mediacentre/factsheets/fs297/en/.

9   "Bacon, Processed Meats a Cause of Cancer—Your FAQs," American Institute for Cancer Research, October 28, 2015, aicr.org/cancer-research-update/2015/10_28 /cru_Bacon-Processed-Meats-a-Cause-of-Cancer-Your-FAQs.html.

10   Rebecca L. Siegel et al., "Cancer Statistics, 2017," *CA: A Cancer Journal for Clinicians* 67, no. 1 (2017): 7–30.

11   Ibid.

12   Ibid.

13   Ibid.

14   Ibid.

15   Ibid.

16   "Colorectal Cancer Risk Factors," American Cancer Society, last modified January 20, 2016, cancer.org/cancer/colonandrectumcancer/detailedguide/colorectal -cancer-risk-factors.

17   Sara Wirén et al., "Pooled Cohort Study on Height and Risk of Cancer and Cancer Death," *Cancer Causes & Control* 25, no. 2 (2014): 151–59.

18   "Can Infections Cause Cancer?," American Cancer Society, last modified July 11, 2016, cancer.org/cancer/cancercauses/othercarcinogens/infectiousagents /infectiousagentsandcancer/infectious-agents-and-cancer-intro.

19   Matthew P. Thompson and Razelle Kurzrock, "Epstein-Barr Virus and Cancer," *Clinical Cancer Research* 10, no. 3 (2004): 803–21.

20   Taslima Lina et al., "Immune Evasion Strategies Used by *Helicobacter Pylori*," *World Journal of Gastroenterology* 20, no. 36 (2014): 12753–66.

21   Ibid.

22   "HPV and Cancer," National Cancer Institute, February 19, 2015, cancer.gov /about-cancer/causes-prevention/risk/infectious-agents/hpv-fact-sheet.

23   Lauri E. Markowitz et al., "Prevalence of HPV after Introduction of the Vaccination Program in the United States," *Pediatrics* 137, no. 3 (2016): e20151968, doi: 10.1542 /peds.2015-1968.

24   Frederik Hvid-Jensen et al., "Incidence of Adenocarcinoma among Patients with Barrett's Esophagus," *New England Journal of Medicine* 365, no. 15 (2011): 1375–83.

25   Elizabeth R. Rayburn et al., "Anti-Inflammatory Agents for Cancer Therapy," *Molecular and Cellular Pharmacology* 1, no. 1 (2009): 29–43.

26   Xin-Zu Chen et al. "Association of *Helicobacter Pylori* Infection and Chronic Atrophic Gastritis with Risk of Colonic, Pancreatic and Gastric Cancer: A Ten-Year Follow-up of the ESTHER Cohort Study," *Oncotarget* 7, no. 13 (2016): 17182–93.

27   Eun Ran Kim and Dong Kyung Chang, "Colorectal Cancer in Inflammatory Bowel Disease: The Risk, Pathogenesis, Prevention and Diagnosis," *World Journal of Gastroenterology* 20, no. 29 (2014): 9872–81.

28   Yin Cao et al., "Regular Aspirin Use Associates with Lower Risk of Colorectal Cancers with Low Numbers of Tumor-Infiltrating Lymphocytes," *Gastroenterology* (July 27, 2016): doi: 10.1053/j.gastro.2016.07.030.

29   "Lung Cancer Fact Sheet," American Lung Association, last modified November 3, 2016, www.lung.org/lung-health-and-diseases/lung-disease-lookup/lung-cancer /learn-about-lung-cancer/lung-cancer-fact-sheet.html.

30   Amy R. Johnson et al., "The Inflammation Highway: Metabolism Accelerates Inflammatory Traffic in Obesity," *Immunological Reviews* 249, no. 1 (2012): 218–38.

31   Elizabeth D. Kantor et al., "Adolescent Body Mass Index and Erythrocyte Sedimentation Rate in Relation to Colorectal Cancer Risk," *Gut* 65, no. 8 (2016): 1289–95.

32   Melina Arnold et al., "Duration of Adulthood Overweight, Obesity, and Cancer Risk in the Women's Health Initiative: A Longitudinal Study from the United States," *PLoS Medicine* 13, no. 8 (2016): e1002081, http://dx.doi.org/10.1371/journal .pmed.1002081.

33   Catherine Duggan et al., "Dietary Weight Loss and Exercise Effects on Serum Biomarkers of Angiogenesis in Overweight Postmenopausal Women: A Randomized Controlled Trial," *Cancer Research* 76, no. 14 (2016): 4226–35.

34   Véronique Bouvard et al., "Carcinogenicity of Consumption of Red and Processed Meat," *Lancet Oncology* 16, no. 16 (2015): 1599–1600.

35   Mingyang Song et al., "Nutrients, Foods, and Colorectal Cancer Prevention," *Gastroenterology* 148, no. 6 (2015): 1244–60.

36   Ibid.

37   Yue Zhou et al., "Natural Polyphenols for Prevention and Treatment of Cancer," *Nutrients* 8, no. 8 (2016): 515.

38   Marta Sancho and Nuria Mach, "Effects of Wine Polyphenols on Cancer Prevention," *Nutricion Hospitalaria* 31, no. 2 (2015): 535–51; Elizabeth Mostofsky et al., "Key Findings on Alcohol Consumption and a Variety of Health Outcomes from the Nurses' Health Study," *American Journal of Public Health* 106, no. 9 (2016): 1586–91.

39   Jennie Connor, "Alcohol Consumption as a Cause of Cancer," *Addiction* (July 21, 2016): Epub ahead of print, doi: 10.1111/add.13477.

40   Helmut K. Seitz and Peter Becker, "Alcohol Metabolism and Cancer Risk," *Alcohol Research and Health* 30, no. 1 (2007): 38–47.

41   Yin Cao et al., "Light to Moderate Intake of Alcohol, Drinking Patterns, and Risk of Cancer: Results from Two Prospective US Cohort Studies," *BMJ* 351 (August 18, 2015): doi: http://dx.doi.org/10.1136/bmj.h4238.

42   S. Bell et al., "Ten-Year Alcohol Consumption Typologies and Trajectories of C-Reactive Protein, Interleukin-6 and Interleukin-1 Receptor Antagonist over the Following 12 Years: A Prospective Cohort Study," *Journal of Internal Medicine* (2016): Epub ahead of print, doi: 10.1111/joim.12544.

43   Imke Janssen et al., "Moderate Wine Consumption Is Associated with Lower Hemostatic and Inflammatory Risk Factors over 8 Years: The Study of Women's Health across the Nation (SWAN)," *Nutrition and Aging* 2, no. 2–3 (2014): 91–99.

44   Fangyi Gu et al., "Sleep Duration and Cancer in the NIH-AARP Diet and Health Study Cohort," *PLoS ONE* 11, no. 9 (2016): e0161561, http://dx.doi.org/10.1371/journal.pone.0161561.

45   Jenny Theorell-Haglow et al., "Both Habitual Short Sleepers and Long Sleepers Are at Greater Risk of Obesity: A Population-Based 10-Year Follow-Up in Women," *Sleep Medicine* 15, no. 10 (2014): 1204–11.

46   "How Much Sleep Do We Really Need?," National Sleep Foundation, accessed November 25, 2016, sleepfoundation.org/how-sleep-works/how-much-sleep-do-we-really-need/page/0/2.

47   Andrea Detter, "Dramatic Remissions Seen in Immunotherapy Trial of Blood Cancer Patients," Fred Hutchinson Cancer Research Center, February, 16, 2016, fredhutch.org/en/news/center-news/2016/02/immunotherapy-remission-blood-cancer-AAAS-riddell.html.

48   Dalgleish et al., "Randomised, Open-Label, Phase II Study," doi: 10.1038/bjc.2016.271.

Chapter 11

1   Miles McEvoy, "Organic 101: What the USDA Organic Label Means," *USDA Blog*, March 22, 2012, blogs.usda.gov/2012/03/22/organic-101-what-the-usda-organic-label-means/.

2   Marcin Barański et al., "Higher Antioxidant and Lower Cadmium Concentrations and Lower Incidence of Pesticide Residues in Organically Grown Crops: A Systematic Literature Review and Meta-Analyses," *British Journal of Nutrition* 112, no. 5 (2014): 794–811.

3   Dominika Srednicka-Tober et al., "Composition Differences between Organic and Conventional Meat: A Systematic Literature Review and Meta-Analysis," *British Journal of Nutrition* 115, no. 6 (2016): 994–1011.

4   Brad J. Douglass and Dallas L. Clouatre, "Beyond Yellow Curry: Assessing Commercial Curcumin Absorption Technologies," *Journal of the American College of Nutrition* 34:4 (2015): 347–58.

5   Chandra L. Jackson and Frank B. Hu, "Long-Term Associations of Nut Consumption with Body Weight and Obesity," supplement 1, *American Journal of Clinical Nutrition* 100 (July 2014): S408–S11.

Chapter 12

1   Luke Spence et al., "Incidence, Etiology and Symptomatology of Upper Respiratory Illness in Elite Athletes," *Medicine and Science in Sports and Exercise* 39, no. 4 (2007): 577–86.

2   Adae O. Amoako and George Guntur A. Pujalte, "Osteoarthritis in Young, Active, and Athletic Individuals," *Clinical Medicine Insights: Arthritis and Musculoskeletal Disorders* 7 (May 22, 2014): 27–32.

3   Jeffrey B. Kreher and Jennifer B. Schwartz, "Overtraining Syndrome: A Practical Guide," *Sports Health* 4, no. 2 (2012): 128–38.

4   T. L. Yost and A. G. Taylor, "Qigong as a Novel Intervention for Service Members with Mild Traumatic Brain Injury," *Explore: The Journal of Science and Healing* 9, no. 3 (2013): 142–49.

5   S. C. Kuan et al., "Effectiveness of Qigong in Promoting the Health of Wheelchair-Bound Older Adults in Long-Term Care Facilities," *Biological Research in Nursing* 14, no. 2 (2012): 139–46.

6   Byeongsang Oh et al., "A Critical Review of the Effects of Medical Qigong on Quality of Life, Immune Function, and Survival in Cancer Patients," *Integrated Cancer Therapies* 11, no. 2 (2012): 101–10; Roger Jahnke et al., "A Comprehensive Review of Health Benefits of Qigong and Tai Chi," *American Journal of Health Promotion* 24, no. 6 (2010): E1–E25; Ryan Abbott and Helen Lavretsky, "Tai Chi and Qigong for the Treatment and Prevention of Mental Disorders," *Psychiatric Clinics of North America* 36, no. 1 (2013): 109–19; A. W. K. Chan et al., "Tai Chi Qigong Improves Lung Functions and Activity Tolerance in COPD Clients: A Single Blind, Randomized Controlled Trial," *Complementary Therapies in Medicine*, 19, no. 1 (2013): 3–11.

7   Chong-Wen Wang et al., "Managing Stress and Anxiety through Qigong Exercise in Healthy Adults: A Systematic Review and Meta-Analysis of Randomized Controlled Trials," *BMC Complementary and Alternative Medicine* 14 (January 9, 2014): 8.

8   Ryan Abbott and Helen Lavretsky, "Tai Chi and Qigong for the Treatment and Prevention of Mental Disorders," *Psychiatric Clinics of North America* 36, no. 1 (2013): 109–19.

9   Liu X. et al., "A Systematic Review and Meta-Analysis of the Effects of Qigong and Tai Chi for Depressive Symptoms," *Complementary Therapies in Medicine* 23, no. 4 (2015): 516–34.

10   Ming-Chien Chyu et al., "Complementary and Alternative Exercises for Management of Osteoarthritis," *Arthritis* 2011 (2011): http://dx.doi.org/10.1155/2011/364319.

11   Ibid.

12   L. Skoglund et al., "Qigong Training and Effects on Stress, Neck-Shoulder Pain and Life Quality in a Computerised Office Environment," *Complementary Therapies in Clinical Practice* 17, no. 1 (2011): 54–57.

13   L. Skoglund et al., "Qigong Reduces Stress in Computer Operators," *Complementary Therapies in Clinical Practice* 13, no. 2 (2007): 78–84.

14   Jana Sawynok and Mary Lynch, "Qigong and Fibromyalgia: Randomized Controlled Trials and Beyond," *Evidence-Based Complementary and Alternative Medicine* 2014 (2014): http://dx.doi.org/10.1155/2014/379715.

15   Rainbow T. H. Ho et al., "A Randomized Controlled Trial of Qigong Exercise on Fatigue Symptoms, Functioning, and Telomerase Activity in Persons with Chronic Fatigue or Chronic Fatigue Syndrome," *Annals of Behavioral Medicine* 44, no. 2 (2012): 160–70.

16   Guan-Cheng Sun et al., "Effects of Qigong on Glucose Control in Type 2 Diabetes," *Diabetes Care* 33, no. 1 (2010): E8.

17   Ran Li et al., "The Effect of Baduanjin on Promoting the Physical Fitness and Health of Adults," *Evidence-Based Complementary and Alternative Medicine* 2014 (2014): http://dx.doi.org/10.1155/2014/784059.

18   Xingjiang Xiong et al., "Qigong for Hypertension: A Systematic Review," *Medicine* 94, no. 1 (2015): E352.

19   Shane R. Freeman et al., "Sit, Breathe, Smile: Effects of Single and Weekly Seated Qigong on Blood Pressure and Quality of Life in Long-Term Care," *Complementary Therapies in Clinical Practice* 20, no. 1 (2014): 48–53.

20   B. M. Y. Cheung et al., "Randomised Controlled Trial of Qigong in the Treatment of Mild Essential Hypertension," *Journal of Human Hypertension* 19, no. 9 (2005): 697–704.

21   P. J. Klein et al., "Qigong in Cancer Care: A Systematic Review and Construct Analysis of Effective Qigong Therapy," *Support Care in Cancer* 24, no. 7 (2016): 3209–22.

22   Byeongsang Oh et al., "Impact of Medical Qigong on Quality of Life, Fatigue, Mood and Inflammation in Cancer Patients: A Randomized Controlled Trial," *Annals of Oncology* 21, no. 3 (2010): 608–14.

23   Hsing-Hsia Chen et al., "The Effects of Baduanjin Qigong in the Prevention of Bone Loss for Middle-Aged Women," *American Journal of Chinese Medicine* 34, no. 5 (2006): 741–47.

24   Eu Suen Chan et al., "Biochemical and Psychometric Evaluation of Self-Healing Qigong as a Stress Reduction Tool among First Year Nursing and Midwifery Students," *Complementary Therapies in Clinical Practice* 19, no. 4 (2013): 179–83.

Chapter 13

1   T. L. Ngo, "Review of the Effects of Mindfulness Meditation on Mental and Physical Health and Its Mechanisms of Action," *Santé Mentale au Québec* 38, no. 2 (2013): 19–34; Melissa A. Rosenkranz et al., "A Comparison of Mindfulness-Based Stress Reduction and an Active Control in Modulation of Neurogenic Inflammation," *Brain, Behavior, and Immunity* 27, no. 1 (2013): 174–84.

2   David S. Black and George M. Slavich, "Mindfulness Meditation and the Immune System: A Systematic Review of Randomized Controlled Trials," *Annals of the New York Academy of Sciences* 1373, no. 1 (2016): 13–24.

3   E. Walsh et al., "Brief Mindfulness Training Reduces Salivary IL-6 and TNF-α in Young Women with Depressive Symptomatology," *Journal of Consulting and Clinical Psychology* (2016): Epub ahead of print, doi: 10.1037/ccp0000122.

4   David S. Black et al., "Mindfulness Meditation and Improvement in Sleep Quality and Daytime Impairment among Older Adults with Sleep Disturbances: A Randomized Clinical Trial," *JAMA Internal Medicine* 175, no. 4 (2015): 494–501.

5   Autumn M. Gallegos et al., "Mindfulness-Based Stress Reduction to Enhance Psychological Functioning and Improve Inflammatory Biomarkers in Trauma-Exposed Women: A Pilot Study," *Psychological Trauma: Theory, Research, Practice, and Policy* 7, no. 6 (2015): 525–32.

6   J. David Creswell et al., "Mindfulness-Based Stress Reduction Training Reduces Loneliness and Proinflammatory Gene Expression in Older Adults: A Small Randomized Controlled Trial," *Brain, Behavior, and Immunity* 26, no. 7 (2012): 1095–101.

7   Rosenkranz et al., "A Comparison of Mindfulness-Based Stress Reduction," 174–84.

8   Melissa A. Rosenkranz et al., "Reduced Stress and Inflammatory Responsiveness in Experienced Meditators Compared to a Matched Healthy Control Group," *Brain, Behavior, and Immunity* 68 (June 2016): 117–25.

9   Perla Kaliman et al., "Rapid Changes in Histone Deacetylases and Inflammatory Gene Expression in Expert Meditators," *Psychoneuroendocrinology* 40 (February 2014): 96–107.

10   Yang Claire Yang et al., "Social Isolation and Adult Mortality: The Role of Chronic Inflammation and Sex Differences," *Journal of Health and Social Behavior* 54, no. 2 (2013): 183–203.

11   Amoha Bajaj et al., "Daily Social Interactions, Close Relationships, and Systemic Inflammation in Two Samples: Healthy Middle-Aged and Older Adults," *Brain, Behavior, and Immunity* 58 (November 2016): 152–64.

12   Nancy L. Sin et al., "Daily Positive Events and Inflammation: Findings from the National Study of Daily Experiences," *Brain, Behavior, and Immunity* 43 (January 2015): 130–38.

13   Ibid.

14   M. Cohen et al., "The Association between Bereavement and Biomarkers of Inflammation," *Behavioral Medicine* 41, no. 2 (2015): 49–59.

15   Spenser Hughes et al., "Social Support Predicts Inflammation, Pain, and Depressive Symptoms: Longitudinal Relationships among Breast Cancer Survivors," *Psychoneuroendocrinology* 42 (April 2014): 38–44.

16   Jennifer E. Stellar et al., "Positive Affect and Markers of Inflammation: Discrete Positive Emotions Predict Lower Levels of Inflammatory Cytokines," *Emotion* 15, no. 2 (2015) 129–33.

17   Samuel Brod et al., "'As Above, so Below' Examining the Interplay between Emotion and the Immune System," *Immunology* 143, no. 3 (2014): 311–18.

18   T. Hayashi and K. Murakami, "The Effects of Laughter on Postprandial Glucose Levels and Gene Expression in Type 2 Diabetic Patients," *Life Sciences* 85, no. 5–6 (2009): 185–87.

19   Michael Miller and William F. Fry, "The Effect of Mirthful Laughter on the Human Cardiovascular System," *Medical Hypotheses* 73, no. 5 (2009): 636.

20   T. Matsuzaki et al., "Mirthful Laughter Differentially Affects Serum Pro- and Anti-Inflammatory Cytokine Levels Depending on the Level of Disease Activity in Patients with Rheumatoid Arthritis," *Rheumatology* 45, no. 2 (2006): 182–86.

21   Lee S. Berk and Stanley Tan, "Mirthful Laughter, as Adjunct Therapy in Diabetic Care, Increases HDL Cholesterol and Attenuates Inflammatory Cytokines and C-RP and Possible CVD Risk," supplement 990, *FASEB Journal* 23, no. 1 (April 2009).

22   Brod et al., "'As Above, so Below,'" 311–18.

23   Gaétan Chevalier et al., "Earthing: Health Implications of Reconnecting the Human Body to the Earth's Surface Electrons," *Journal of Environmental and Public Health* (2012): doi: 10.1155/2012/291541; Gaétan Chevalier, "The Effect of Grounding the Human Body on Mood," *Psychological Reports* 116, no. 2 (2015): 534–42; James L. Oschman et al., "The Effects of Grounding (Earthing) on Inflammation, the

Immune Response, Wound Healing, and Prevention and Treatment of Chronic Inflammatory and Autoimmune Diseases," *Journal of Inflammation Research* 8 (2015): 83–96.

24   Danielle F. Shanahan et al., "Health Benefits from Nature Experiences Depend on Dose," *Scientific Reports* 6 (2016): doi: 10.1038/srep28551.

25   L. S. Redwine et al., "Pilot Randomized Study of a Gratitude Journaling Intervention on Heart Rate Variability and Inflammatory Biomarkers in Patients with Stage B Heart Failure," *Psychosomatic Medicine* 78, no. 6 (2016): 667–76.

26   Paul J. Mills et al., "The Role of Gratitude in Spiritual Well-Being in Asymptomatic Heart Failure Patients," *Spirituality in Clinical Practice* 2, no. 1 (2015): 5–17.

27   Karen O'Leary and Dockray Samantha, "The Effects of Two Novel Gratitude and Mindfulness Interventions on Well-Being," *Journal of Alternative and Complementary Medicine* 21, no. 4 (2015): 243–45.

Index

Underscored page references indicate boxed text.

L

Lactobacillus, 93, 102–3
Lactobacillus acidophilus, 154
Lactobacillus gasseri, 93
Lamb recipes
    Grilled Lamb Chops with Orange
        Relish, 289
    Lamb Burgers with Tomato, 288
    Lamb Kabobs with Mushrooms and
        Tomatoes, 287
Laughter, 360–62
Laughter yoga, 361–62
Leaky gut, 23, 27, 92, 134
Learning Early about Peanut Allergy
        (LEAP) study, 151, 154
Legumes, 235
Leptin, 85–86
Lewy bodies, 60
Linoleic acid, 71. *See also* Omega-6
Lipopolysaccharides (LPSs), 92, 93
Lipp, Terry, 74–76
Logs, 218, 367, 368
Longevity, inflammation and, 48
Long-term inflammation, 6–7. *See also*
        chronic inflammation
LPSs, 92, 93
Lunch
    reset phase, 217
    during rest of plan, 222
    testing phase, 221
Lung cancer, 194
Lupus, 28, 138–40
Luteolin, 173

M

Macrophages, 84–85, 90–91, 178
Major depressive disorder (MDD), 168,
        169, 170, 171
Mallard, Donna, 182–83
Manipulation and mobilization
        techniques, 125
MBSR, 127, 351–54
MCI, 158–59
MDD. *See* major depressive disorder
Meat
    aging and, 53–54

beef recipes
    Beef and Vegetable Roast, 267
    Burgers with Caramelized Onion,
        268
    Grilled Beef and Arugula Salad,
        270
    Grilled Steak with Avocado, 265
    Mediterranean Beef Stew, 266
    Thai Beef Lettuce Wraps, 269
lamb recipes
    Grilled Lamb Chops with Orange
        Relish, 289
    Lamb Burgers with Tomato, 288
    Lamb Kabobs with Mushrooms
        and Tomatoes, 287
processed, 17–18, 206
red
    cancer and, 206
    chronic inflammation from, 17–18
    irritable bowel syndrome and, 72
    weight gain from, 99–100
    weight gain from, 99–100
    in Whole Body Cure Eating Plan,
        230–31
Medications. *See also specific types*
    for allergies, 149
    for chronic pain, 120, 122–24
    for heart disease risk, 184–86
    for rheumatoid arthritis, 136
    statins, 184–86
Meditation, mindfulness
    chronic pain treatment, 127
    combating stress with, 55–56
    general discussion, 351–55
Mediterranean diet, 52, 86, 137
Memory loss, 158–61, 172–73
Mental health, 163–66. *See also*
        depression
Metabolic arthritis, 112
Metabolic conditions
    fat cells, 84–88
    insulin resistance, 88–93, 97
    overweight and obesity, 81–84
    qigong, relieving with, 300–301
    type 2 diabetes, 88–93, 97
    weight gain, 99–101
    weight loss, 97–98, 101–4
Metabolic endotoxemia, 92, 93
Metabolic syndrome, 89, 142, 170

Michael, Ann, 118–19
Microbiome, gut
  diet, effect of, 63–65
  general discussion, 61–63
  obesity and, 91–93
  psychological conditions and, 65–66
  rheumatoid arthritis and, 137
Mild cognitive impairment (MCI), 158–59
Mind-body connection, 350
Mindfulness, 351
Mindfulness-based stress reduction
    (MBSR), 127, 351–54
Mindfulness meditation
  chronic pain treatment, 127
  combating stress with, 55–56
  general discussion, 351–55
Minerals, 117
Mint, 121
Monosodium glutamate (MSG), 116,
    238
Mood. *See also* depression
  early warning sign of inflammation, 12
  general discussion, 166–67
  stabilizing with phytonutrients,
    172–73
  weight loss, improving with, 98
MSG, 116, 238
Muscle relaxants, 124
My Transformation participants
  Ann Michael, 118–19
  Chad and Pat Neff, 256–59
  Donna Mallard, 182–83
  Haunani Kekuna, 94–96
  Joanne Nadovich, 204–5
  Tammy Pfeiffer, 24–25
  Terry Bortz, 152–53
  Terry Lipp, 74–75

N

Nadovich, Joanne, 204–5
National Psoriasis Foundation, 142–43
National Sleep Foundation, 32
National Weight Control Registry
    (NWCR), 98
Nature, spending time in, 363
Neff, Chad, 356–59

Neff, Pat, 356–59
Neuroinflammation
  dementia, 161–66
  general discussion, 156–58
  memory loss, 158–61
  mood, 166–72
Neurotransmitters, 59
NF-κB, 192
Nondairy fermented foods, 68
Nonsteroidal anti-inflammatory drugs
    (NSAIDs)
  for chronic pain, 120, 122
  for dementia, 165
  for depression, 170
  for heart disease risk, 186
  for rheumatoid arthritis, 136
Nuclear factor kappa B (NF-κB), 192
Nutrition. *See* diet
Nuts, 102, 231–32, 290
NWCR, 98

O

Obesity
  chronic inflammation and, 7
  conditions related to, 83
  fat cells, 84–88
  gut health and, 73, 77–79, 91–93
  meaning of term, 81–84
  risk factor for
    cancer, 202–3
    fibromyalgia, 115–16
    heart disease, 180, 188
    insulin resistance and type 2
        diabetes, 88–93, 97
    osteoarthritis, 112
    psoriasis, 141–42
  stress and, 78
  weight gain, foods related to, 99–101
  weight loss
    benefits of, 97–98
    foods that promote, 101–4
    tips for, 86–87
Oils, 52–53, 101–2, 228
Oleocanthal, 52
Oligofructose, 93
Olive oil, 52–53, 101–2

lupus and, 139–40
rheumatoid arthritis and, 137–38
Vitamins
  for fibromyalgia, 117
  homocysteine levels, lowering with,
    185
  in pill form, 22

W

Waist circumference, 9, 20, 90, 93, 301
Water filtration system, 29
Weight
  conditions linked to, 83
    cancer, 202–3
    fibromyalgia, 115–16
    heart disease, 188
    insulin resistance and Type 2
      Diabetes, 88–93, 97
    psoriasis, 141–42
  fat cells, 84–88
  gut health and, 73, 77–79
  obesity, meaning of term, 81–84
  weight gain, foods related to, 99–101
  weight loss
    benefits of, 97–98
    foods that promote, 101–4
    tips for, 86–87
Weight-bearing exercise, 31
Western diet
  autoimmune disorders and, 133–34
  chronic pain and, 126
  dementia and, 162–63
  inflammatory bowel disease and, 69
Wheat, 22
White blood cell count, 193
Whole Body Cure Eating Plan
  alcohol, 236
  beans and legumes, 235
  beverages, 232
  chemical additives, 238

dairy, 234, 235
eating out, 233
fats, 228
food sensitivities, eliminating
  eating after testing phase, 222–23
  order for introducing foods into
    diet, 221–22
  reset phase, 216–18
  testing phase, 218–21
foods to avoid, 235–38
fruits, 226–27
grains and flours, 236–37
meat, poultry, fish, and eggs,
  230–31
nuts and seeds, 231–32
organic foods, 216
overview, 214
processed foods, 237–38
protein shakes, 228–29
real foods, 214–15
reincorporating foods, 233–35
sea salt, 233
soy, 234
sugar and sugar substitutes, 237
supplements, 229
vegetables, 224–26
Whole-body pain relief, 128–29
Whole foods vs. supplements, 22
Whole grains, 22
Wine, 207, 235, 236
Winter, eating vegetables during,
  227
World Health Organization's
  International Agency for
  Research, 17

Y

Yeast infection, antibiotic-induced, 62
Yoga, 296, 361–62
Yogurt, 68, 72